Pathogenesis, Treatment and Prevention of Leishmaniasis

Pathogenesis, Treatment and Prevention of Leishmaniasis

Edited by

Mukesh Samant
Cell and Molecular Biology Laboratory, Department of Zoology,
Kumaun University, SSJ Campus, Almora, Uttarakhand, India

Satish Chandra Pandey
Cell and Molecular Biology Laboratory, Department of Zoology,
Kumaun University, SSJ Campus, Almora, Uttarakhand, India

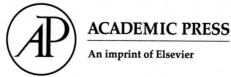

ACADEMIC PRESS

An imprint of Elsevier

Academic Press is an imprint of Elsevier
125 London Wall, London EC2Y 5AS, United Kingdom
525 B Street, Suite 1650, San Diego, CA 92101, United States
50 Hampshire Street, 5th Floor, Cambridge, MA 02139, United States
The Boulevard, Langford Lane, Kidlington, Oxford OX5 1GB, United Kingdom

British Library Cataloguing-in-Publication Data
A catalogue record for this book is available from the British Library

Library of Congress Cataloging-in-Publication Data
A catalog record for this book is available from the Library of Congress

ISBN: 978-0-12-822800-5

For Information on all Academic Press publications
visit our website at https://www.elsevier.com/books-and-journals

Publisher: Stacy Masucci
Acquisitions Editor: Kattie Washington
Editorial Project Manager: Sara Pianavilla
Production Project Manager: Maria Bernard
Cover Designer: Greg Harris

Typeset by MPS Limited, Chennai, India

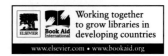

Working together
to grow libraries in
developing countries

www.elsevier.com • www.bookaid.org

Contents

5. DNA microarray analysis of *Leishmania* parasite: strengths and limitations   85

Satish Chandra Pandey, Saurabh Gangola, Saurabh Kumar, Prasenjit Debborma, Deep Chandra Suyal, Arjita Punetha, Tushar Joshi, Pankaj Bhatt and Mukesh Samant

6. Drug resistance and repurposing of existing drugs in Leishmaniasis   103

Ashutosh Paliwal, Rekha Gahtori, Amrita Kumari and Pooja Pandey

List of contributors

Pankaj Bhatt Integrative Microbiology Research Centre, South China Agricultural University, Guangzhou, China

Deepa Bisht Department of Biotechnology, Kumaun University, Sir J C Bose Technical Campus, Bhimtal, India

Subhash Chandra Department of Botany, Kumaun University, SSJ Campus, Almora, India

Khushboo Dasauni Department of Biotechnology, Kumaun University, Sir J C Bose Technical Campus, Bhimtal, India

Prasenjit Debborma School of Agriculture, Graphic Era Hill University, Dehradun, India

Rekha Gahtori Department of Biotechnology, Kumaun University, Sir J C Bose Technical Campus, Bhimtal, India

Saurabh Gangola School of Agriculture, Graphic Era Hill University, Bhimtal, India

Vinita Gouri Cell and Molecular Biology Laboratory, Department of Zoology, Kumaun University, SSJ Campus, Almora, India

Diksha Joshi Cell and Molecular Biology Laboratory, Department of Zoology, Kumaun University, SSJ Campus, Almora, India

Tanuja Joshi Department of Botany, Kumaun University, SSJ Campus, Almora, India

Tushar Joshi Department of Botany, Kumaun University, SSJ Campus, Almora, India; Department of Biotechnology, Kumaun University, Sir J C Bose Technical Campus, Bhimtal, India

Keerti Molecular Biology and Genetics Unit, Jawaharlal Nehru Centre for Advanced Scientific Research, Bengaluru, India

Prashant Khare Department of Microbiology, All India Institute of Medical Sciences, Bhopal, India

Awanish Kumar Department of Biotechnology, National Institute of Technology, Raipur, India

Saurabh Kumar Division of Crop Research, ICAR-Research Complex for Eastern Region, Patna, India

Vivek Kumar Department of Botany, Government Post Graduate College, Champawat, India

Amrita Kumari Department of Biotechnology, Kumaun University, Sir J C Bose Technical Campus, Bhimtal, India

Shalini Mathpal Department of Biotechnology, Kumaun University, Sir J C Bose Technical Campus, Bhimtal, India; Department of Botany, Kumaun University, SSJ Campus, Almora, India

Tapan Kumar Nailwal Department of Biotechnology, Kumaun University, Sir J C Bose Technical Campus, Bhimtal, India

Ashutosh Paliwal Department of Biotechnology, Kumaun University, Sir J C Bose Technical Campus, Bhimtal, India

Veni Pande Cell and Molecular Biology Laboratory, Department of Zoology, Kumaun University, SSJ Campus, Almora, India

Anupam Pandey Department of Biotechnology, Kumaun University, Sir J C Bose Technical Campus, Bhimtal, India; ICAR-Directorate of Coldwater Fisheries Research, Nainital, India

Pooja Pandey Department of Biotechnology, Kumaun University, Sir J C Bose Technical Campus, Bhimtal, India

Satish Chandra Pandey Cell and Molecular Biology Laboratory, Department of Zoology, Kumaun University, SSJ Campus, Almora, India

Arjita Punetha Department of Environmental Science, GBPUAT, Pantnagar, India

Utkarsha Sahu Department of Microbiology, All India Institute of Medical Sciences, Bhopal, India

Mukesh Samant Cell and Molecular Biology Laboratory, Department of Zoology, Kumaun University, SSJ Campus, Almora, India

Priyanka Sharma Department of Botany, Kumaun University, DSB Campus, Nainital, India

Deep Chandra Suyal Department of Microbiology, Akal College of Basic Sciences, Eternal University, Baru Sahib, Sirmaur, India

Ankita H. Tripathi Department of Biotechnology, Kumaun University, Sir J C Bose Technical Campus, Bhimtal, India

Lokesh Kumar Tripathi Department of Biotechnology, Kumaun University, Sir J C Bose Technical Campus, Bhimtal, India

Priyanka H. Tripathi Department of Biotechnology, Kumaun University, Sir J C Bose Technical Campus, Bhimtal, India; ICAR-Directorate of Coldwater Fisheries Research, Nainital, India

Shobha Upreti Cell and Molecular Biology Laboratory, Department of Zoology, Kumaun University, SSJ Campus, Almora, India

Preface

This book presents a comprehensive overview of leishmaniasis, caused by the protozoan parasite *Leishmania*, which affects people worldwide. The disease is spread between mammalian hosts by Phlebotomine sand flies and caused by at least 20 members of the genus *Leishmania*. Leishmaniasis is amongst the most severe infectious diseases, with a wide range of clinical manifestations ranging from cutaneous, mucocutaneous, to fatal visceral infections. About 350 million individuals are at risk of developing *Leishmania*, with at least 500,000 new cases of VL and 1.5 million new cases of CL with substantial morbidity being reported per year. The book starts with an overview of leishmaniasis, presenting historical and prospective viewpoints and goes on to cover the clinical symptoms, mechanisms of infection, immunology, invasion, diagnostics, drugs, resistance, vaccines, and experimental models of *Leishmania*. Moreover, the book focuses on recent advances and challenges in the discovery of promising drug targets, biomarker identification, and innovative leishmaniasis vaccine strategies. This book is useful for parasitologists, academicians, as well as students at the undergraduate, graduate, and doctoral levels, to understand the fundamental biology of *Leishmania*, its mode of action, and how it is treated around the world. We are grateful to our contributing authors for their willingness to collaborate with us in the preparation of this book. Finally, we are thankful to the Almighty, the Great, for providing us the power and wisdom to accomplish this task.

Editors
Mukesh Samant and
Satish Chandra Pandey

Chapter 1

Leishmaniasis: an overview of evolution, classification, distribution, and historical aspects of parasite and its vector

Lokesh Kumar Tripathi and Tapan Kumar Nailwal
Department of Biotechnology, Kumaun University, Sir J C Bose Technical Campus, Bhimtal, India

1.1 Introduction

Neglected diseases pose great health problems that induce significant socio-economic impact globally. Treatments of neglected diseases still remain uncertain as their control and preventive strategies and proper management have varied little for decades due to minimal interests of policy makers, researchers, scientists, and funding agencies. Leishmaniasis is one such neglected, tropical, parasitic disease that afflicts the poverty-stricken and marginalized populations. With nearly two million active cases adding in over 90 countries where this disease is endemic, nearly 80% of the affected populations are estimated to earn, on an average, less than $2 per day and suffer death loss, around 59,000 lives. Furthermore, less than half a billion people existing in rampant areas are currently at risk of acquiring this disease or another form of it (Alvar et al., 2012). On the basis of morbidity, out of 16 categories belonging to neglected tropical diseases reported between the years (2005−2013), apart from malaria, leishmaniasis is ranked as the second vilest disease and also ranks second, with dengue being first, with an increment in frequency of 5.7−5.9 million disability adjusted life years (DALYs) (Murray, Berman, Davies, & Saravia, 2005). This disease typically becomes an epidemic in areas where disasters, famine, drought, floods, and civil wars are apparent (Bern, Maguire, & Alvar, 2008). Leishmaniasis rife is in all continents except for Antarctica and is more prevalent in Southern and in Central America, and is considered as new world and prevalent in south Europe, Africa, the Middle East, as well as Central Asian, and the

Pathogenesis, Treatment and Prevention of Leishmaniasis. DOI: https://doi.org/10.1016/B978-0-12-822800-5.00004-4

subcontinent of India, which here, is regarded as old world. It epitomizes a multifaceted disease with extensive clinical manifestations and is epidemiologically diverse. It is a non-transmissible, vector-harbored disease caused by kinetoplastid parasites in various leishmanial species (Oryan, 2015; Shirian, Oryan, Hatam, Panahi, & Daneshbod, 2014). These obligatory parasites reside intracellularly and are transmitted to mammalian species when bitten by sand-flies (females) which belong to genera of *Lutzomyia* and *Phlebotomus* via anthroponotic or zoonotic modes (Caldart et al., 2017; Tsakmakidis et al., 2017). Approximately, 70 species of mammals including humans are recognized as potent hosts for distinct *Leishmania* species in various terrestrial regions of world, however, few serve as parasite reservoirs. Even though, natural infection is apparent in rodents (De Araujo, Boite, Cupolillo, Jansen, & Roque, 2013; Roque & Jansen, 2014) and canines (Montoya et al., 2016), these parasites are also capable of inducing infection in Xenarthrans (de Castro Ferreira et al., 2017), Hyraxes, Marsupials (De Rezende et al., 2017), Chiropterans (Maroli et al., 2007), Procyonids, felids (Dahroug et al., 2011; Soares et al., 2013), Perissodactyla (Malta et al., 2010), and primates (Lewis, 1971), thus determining potentiality of cyclic spread. Various species (> 30), that belong to *Leishmania* genus have been identified on the basis of their genetic as well as biochemical characterization (Kamhawi, 2006). However, only two species cause a lethal form of this disease. In accordance with topographical regions and quantifiable medical symptoms existing in affected individuals, leishmanial parasites occur as either amastigotes or promastigotes. Furthermore, promastigotes forms have been classified into five types:procyclic, haptomonad, necto-monad, lepto-monadm and metacyclic promastigotes (Kloehn et al., 2015). Metacyclic promastigotes are considered as an infective stage which is highly adaptable for effective transmission within a human host (Kloehn et al., 2015). Microscopically, promastigotes represent lengthy cells that contain a nucleus, however within amastigotes the nucleus went into a semi-quiescent physiological state and had a truncated replication frequency of less than two weeks during in vivo infection (Handman & Bullen, 2002). Transmission mode of parasites requires a host (human) for blood-fed female sand flies. Two genera, *Lutzomyia* and *Phlebotomus*, that represent new and old-world species respectively, serve as vectors. However, not all sand-fly species serve as vector reservoirs for parasite transmission and thus portray a digenetic lifecycle (Zink et al., 2006).

1.2 History of leishmaniasis

1.2.1 Ancient and middle ages

Prehistorically, several accounts of lesions had been suggestive of Oriental sores from tablets from 7th century BCE, originating from Assyrian King

Ashurbanipal's library. In a paleo-parasitological analysis, leishmanial mito-chondrial DNA were identified in four out of forty-two specimens of mum-mified fossils from Middle Kingdom tomb in West Thebes which dates back to 2050−1650 BCE. Sequencing analysis of such DNA samples exposed that these mummies had suffered from *Leishmania donovani* infection, causal parasite for visceral leishmaniasis (VL) in ancient Egypt (Maspero, 1896). Ancient Egyptian medical records such as, Ebers Papyrus, which dates back to 1500 BCE, also mentioned leishmaniasis (Frias, Leles, & Araujo, 2013). These records documented reports clinical condition of a skin disease, Nile pimple, that allegedly refersto as a cutaneous form of leishmaniasis. Furthermore, macrophages infected with Leishmania were also determined by immunological analysis in a six-year old Peruvian mummy dated to 800 BCE (Boelaert & Sundar, 2014). Individuals that were healed from the Oriental sores were protected from further infections and also provide evi-dences about knowledge of Arabic societies for the presence of leishmaniasis (Edrissian et al., 2016). This insight was used by the people from Central Asia and the Middle East for acquiring active immunization against the Oriental sore. Persian polymath Rhazes (854−935) of Baghdad, illustrated in his archives, indicated the occurrence of cutaneous sores (Russell, 1756). Avicenna (980−1037), philosopher as well as a physician from Persia, remains to be the first to accurately describe the Oriental sore (Balkh sore)-as a skin dryness disorder that formed lesions caused by *Leishmania tropica*, from northerly regions of Afghanistan.

1.2.2 Leishmaniasis during 16th century up-till 19th century

Numerous incidents were documented during this time period that expressed Oriental sores in the Middle Eastern regions. Most of such information, describes similar conditions hence named after the places where these were acquired and most of them continue to be well known today such as, Aleppo boil, Baghdad boil, Jericho boil, etc. In 1756, Alexander Russell, a Scottish physician, printed a thorough clinical report of dry and wet forms of the Oriental sore while practicing in Aleppo, Syria (Costa, Matheson, Iachetta, Llagostera, & Appenzeller, 2009). Russell's description provided insights about how the natives differentiate among male and female disease types, which relates to wet zoonotic cutaneous leishmaniasis (CL) caused by *Leishmania major* and dry CL forms that were anthroponotic and triggered by *L. tropica*. Furthermore, his records advocated the use of mercurial plaster as themost effective treatment. Soon after colonization of the Americas by Spanish rulers at the beginning of 16th century, there were reports from mis-sionaries related to blemishing facial conditions evocative of mucocutaneous leishmanasis (MCL) (Lainson, 2010). One such description of MCL from a Spanish presenter named Pedro Pizarro, in 1571, described the damage of the nose and lips of cocoa growers that used to work in lower eastern slopes of the Peruvian Andes (Twining, 1827). However, no compelling reports about VL are present before the 19th century. One published book about kala-azar by an army surgeon, Twining (1827); gave details about patients from Bengal, India, where patients had enlarged spleens, acute anemia, and sporadic fever (Gibson, 1983). Later in 1832, Twining in another book, further elaborated kala-azar symptoms that included skin dryness with a scale-like appearance. Outbreak of kala-azar had been previously documented in 1825 from a Mahomedpore village in lower Bengal, India (Gibson, 1983) and soon from there this disease went west and contacted Burdwan, West-Bengal in 1860 (Leishman, 1903). Further, it became an epidemic and spread north in Assam in subsequent years (Kerr, 2000). With a mortality of 30% in the affected areas kala-azar lingered for decades. Kala-azar or back disease indicated shadowy skin discoloration with progression of infection among people with a fair skin tone. The quest for causal mediators for various leishmaniasis forms initiated during late 1800s, in which Piotr Fokich Borovsky, a Russian army doctor, in 1898, first described protozoan present Oriental sore lesions.

1.2.3   Lieshmaniasis in 20th century

It was William Boog Leishman, a pathologist from Scotland, in 1903, who observed ovoid bodies in smears that he had collected from a soldier who had died from splenomegaly. W.B. Leishman served the British Army in India and was stationed at Dum Dum town, not far from Calcutta. He soon observed similar ovoid structures from a disease-ridden experimental rat and printed this finding in 1903 which concluded ovoid structures were disintegrated arrangement of trypanosomes. He termed this illness as dum-dum fever, a type of Trypanosomiasis (Donovan, 1903). Soon another report with similar findings emerged from an Irish doctor Charles Donovan, a professor at Madras Medical College. His publication also suggested similar ovoid bodies in spleen smears from native Indian patients who suffered with remittent fever and had enlarged spleen (Ross, 1903). Donovan also sent one slide of organism to Charles Louis Alphonse Laveran who authorized protozoan parasites at that time in France. Laveran stated this new parasite to be of genus *Piroplasma*. At the meantime, a British doctor Ronald Ross, in 1889, the government of India ordered Ross to examine kala-azar situation in the region, for which he soon published his findings in 1903 that concluded these ovoid bodies discovered by both Leishman and Donovan, were not collapsed form of trypanosomes rather a new protozoan microorganism that resembled the clinical manifestation with that of kala-azar (Ross, 1903). In another publication Ross also proposed a name to these ovoid bodies as *L. donovani*. Soon in 1908, a related VL instigating species *Leishmania infantum*, was reported by bacteriologist from France, Charles Jules Henry Nicolle (1866−1936) in which young ones that suffered with splenic anemia in Tunisia (Nicolle, 1908). In 1903, James Homer Wright (1869−1928), pathologist from America, was credited for his discovery of *Helcosomai tropicum*, from a sore specimen in an American girl. Max Luhe, a German physician in 1906 changed this name to *L. tropica* (Luhe & Barth, 1906). Two Russian physicians, Wassily L. Yakimoff (1870−1940) and Nathan I. Schokhor (1887−1941) in 1914, based on parasite size apparent in skin lesions, suggested division of *L. tropica* into two subspecies namely, *L. tropica* minor with small amastigotes and *L. tropica-* major that had large amastigotes (Yakimoff and Schokhor, 1914) and thus, for next six decades, their classification was considered as standard. However, later it become evident that these two subspecies of *L. tropica* produced two forms of lesions and were distinct with their epidemiology (Schnur, 1987). *L. tropica* minor was associated in producing dry nodule lesions and occurred in townships whereas *L. tropica* major produced drizzly ulcer type lesions that occurred frequently in rustic regions. (Bray, Ashford, & Bray, 1973) classified these subspecies as *L. tropica* and *L. major*, respectively due to the above differentiation. They also reported identification of another species, *Leishmania aethiopica* that caused a varied form of CL in Ethiopia. First description of new world *Leishmania* parasites were, autonomously reported in 1909 by Adolpho C. Lindenberg (1872−1944), of Brazil and Antonio Carini (1872−1950) of Italy, from skin lesions of patients suffering with Bauru ulcers in Sao Paulo, Brazil. Gaspar de Oliveira Vianna (1885−1914), a Brazilian scientist in 1911 (Vianna, 1911), also studied similar leishmanial specimens and came to a conclusion that this parasite was distinct morphologically from *L. tropica* and named this parasite as *Lapsus calami* (daMatta, 1916), but later corrected it to Leishmania *braziliensis*, by Alfredo Augusto da Matta (1870−1954), one of Vianna's colleague, in 1916. VL, was first documented in Latin America in 1930s. Since Aristides Marques da Cunha (1887−1949) and Evandro Serafim Lobo Chagas (1905−1940) (da Cunha and Chagas, 1937), had faced difficulty with laboratory animal infection with Brazilian parasites while there was no ambiguity with *L. donovani* and *L. infantum*, causal parasites of old-world visceral form. Both Cunha and Chagas realized the discovery of the novel species was accountable for the visceral form in the new world and thus named it *Leishmania chagasi* in 1937. Cunha however, after a year, succeeded in infecting laboratory animals with American VL cultures and thus concluded this parasite was identical to *L. infantum*, found in Latin America (Mauricio, Howard, Stothard, & Miles, 1999). Recently, modern molecular analysis techniques have proved indistinguishable differences between *L. chagasi* and *L. infantum* strains, and also supported this notion (Reuss et al., 2012). One recently discovered species *Leishmania martiniquensis*, isolated in 1995, had obtained its taxonomical position in 2002 and was found identical to *Leishmania siamensis*, on the basis of DNA analysis. This parasite is associated with infection in cattle and horses in Europe and in the United States (Leelayoova et al., 2013), and also

VL in humans in Thailand (Adler and Ber, 1941). Finally, transmission mode via sand fly bite was confirmed by a British-Israeli parasitologist, Saul Adler, in 1941. He had effectively infected five volunteers with sandflies contagious with *L. tropica* (Poinar and Poinar, 2004a,b).

1.3 Fossil evidence for origin of *Leishmania* genus

Prehistorically, occurrence of similar species to *Leishmania* was recognized in two fossils that got preserved in millions of years old amber. The first evidence emerged from a wiped-out sand-fly, *Palaeomyia burmitis*, preserved in an approximately, 100 million years old Cretaceous Burmese amber (Poinar and Poinar, 2004a,b). Here, from the blood-crammed alimentary canal, a new fossilized genus of *Paleoleishmania* was identified and subsequently named as *Paleoleishmania proterus* (Poinar and Poinar, 2004a,b). Amastigotes along with promastigotes and paramastigotes were observed from blood that suggests that this sand-fly sucked blood from vertebrates, conclusively from reptiles (Poinar, 2008), and hence acquired this parasite from the blood (Poinar and Poinar, 2004a,b). Existence of amastigotes indicated a digenic life-cycle of *P. proterus*. Second fossil evidence from approximately 20 million years old Dominican amber indicated a related microorganism, *Paleoleishmania neotropicum*, from gut and proboscis of another vanished sand fly, *Lutzomyia adiketis*. Here to muchsurprise, vertebrate blood was absent (Nowak, 1999) and the presence of amastigotes raised query sinceno monogenetic flagellated microorganism were inhabitants of *L. adiketis*, yet again, relating to the digenic lifecycle of *P. neotropicum* with host vertebrate. Such fossils served as the most probable evidence and suggest that Neotropical sandflies served as vectors for *Leishmania*-like parasitic microorganisms from mid-Oligocene to early Miocene time period.

1.4 Evolution of *Leishmania*

1.4.1 Palearctic hypothesis

Palearctic hypothesis is backed by investigations from fossil records that suggest evolution of inherited phlebotomine sand flies and murid rodents during Paleocene (66−56 mya), in Palaerctic region (Lysenko, 1971) that comprise of geographical areas of Europe, Asia (northern Himalayas, north Arabia, and northern Saharan Africa), as suggested by Lysenko in 1971. Murid rodents, most probably served as reservoir mammalian hosts and their burrows provided humidity and protected the vector sand flies from the cold (Kerr, 2000). *Leishmania* together with vector flies and murid hosts, most likely, wentto the Nearctic region (North America that included Greenland, Central Florida and Mexican highlands) during Eocene (56−34 mya) while the Bering land bridge remained an integral part. As the Bering isthmus went astray, new world *Lutzomyia* sand flies, evolved in Nearctic during Oligocene (34–23 mya) (Tuon, Neto, & Amato, 2008), approximately three million years afterwards, with new configuration of Panama land bridge, the Neotropical region, which included South America, Central America, lowlands of south Mexico, islands in the Caribbean and south Florida, in Pliocene (5.33–2.86 mya) (Noyes, 1998). They were colonized by sigmodontine rodents and *Lutzomyia* sandflies. Rise in temperature served as the primary reason for sand flies inhabitation and propagation in the forest canopy that led to conclude that arboreal mammals might have become new hosts for the parasite, thus explaining the diversity expansion of *Leishmania* by sand fly vector in the new world in comparison to that of the old world.

1.4.2 Neotropical hypothesis

The origin of *Leishmania* genus in the Neotropical region was described by Noyes (Croan, Morrison, & Ellis, 1997). It was speculated that new and large diversity of new world *Leishmania* species in comparison to the old world signaled for origin in Neotropical region (Nowak, 1991). However, foundation for newer species does not always ascend at a steady frequency specified for extensive inhabitation time. Alterations in climatic conditions, varied range of hosts, lead to geographical isolation. With above considerations, new world leishmanial speciation may have credited to express fast-tracked progress in Neotropical region. As speculated, sloths must have served as first vertebrate host for the parasite and later got adapted to porcupines during the Eocene. Moreover, the parasite could have introduced in Nearctic region via infected porcupines and further to Palearctic region via unknown mammal during Miocene (Croan et al., 1997). Yet, that hypothesis becomes unsuited with a minimum of two recognized facts. Firstly, fossil records do not specify that porcupines were present up till late Pliocene soon after formation of Isthmus of Panama isthmus (Momen and Cupolillo, 2000), hence around 30–50 million years later as assumed by this hypothesis. The second fact signifies that *Lutzomyia* sand flies were the only vectors present in Neotropical region and thus have evolved only during Oligocene in Nearctic which was about 30 million years, hence, very delayed for a potent insect carrier for parasite.

1.4.3 Hypothesis of multiple origin

This hypothesis discussed severance and ensuing autonomous evolution of two subgenera *Viannia* and *Leishmania*, with the separation of South America from Africa 100 mya (Yurchenko, Lukes, Jirku, Zeledon, & Maslov, 2006). Being only a pompous hypothesis, involves vicariance as a mode for evolution of major clades of *Leishmania*. It too describes ancient departure of *Paraleishmania* from every species of *Leishmania*. Proposed expansion and modification of this hypothesis can be termed as the supercontinent hypothesis, for *Leishmania* genus origination. Here, ancestor of *Leishmania* emerged from some monoxenous parasites on Gondwana (Fernandes, Nelson, & Beverley, 1993). The supercontinent proposal suggested mammalian adaptation might have occurred around 90 mya when mammalian species began to spread out and Africa went into complete isolation. Moreover, tiers of genetic diversity between subgenera of *Viannia* and *Leishmania* have been previously referred to as an expression of vicariance after partition of South America and Africa (Stevens and Rambaut, 2001). The above thoughts are consistent with expected divergence time period presented by two sets of data, first genome-wide and the other based on genes, altogether with distinct calibrated statistics. Single migration event of a lineage in the subgenus (*Leishmania*), back to the new world was essential hypothetically. Migration is reasoned to befallen through Neartic and Beringia during mid Miocene (30 mya), when adequate temperature was present for sand fly survival (Galati, 2003). Moreover, divergent *Leishmania amazonensis* isolates are also acknowledged in west and central China which are unswerving with clade's phylogenetic position of old-world species of *Leishmania*. The worldwide distribution of phlebotomine sand fly genera, entirely oblige as parasite vectors, most likely caused due to fragmentation of Pangaea, following breakage of continents.

1.5 Sand fly classification

More than 800 sand fly species are recognized with approximately 464 of them constituting new world species and 375 representing the oldworld species (Perfil'ev, 1968). Previously, phenotypic approaches were employed to derive overall likeness/relationship between genera and subgenera of sand flies in both old and the new world rather than ancestor−descendant matches. Such approaches allowed proliferation of the taxa, specifically at subgeneric level. It also led to simplify and merge higher taxonomic categories into species. Sand flies are placed in *Nematocera* (sub-order) of *Diptera* (order) that belongs to the (subfamily) of *Phlebotominae* in *Psychodidae* (family). The knowledge of Phlebotomine sand-fly systematics has advanced with introduction of new approaches such as, molecular and phylogenetic analysis, multivariate morphometrics, analysis of isozymes and chromosomes and lately mass spectrometry. Average flight range of sand flies i.e., 1.5 km/day, have also allowed speculating about intra-specific and inter-specific variations within subgenera and populations. Taxonomic history of sand fly can be fragmented into two distinct periods. Phlebotometry, that analyzed morphological external features such as, male genitalia structures, wing venation indices, etc. were used to distinguish taxa, and were prominent during the first period. Whereas the second period focused on internal structures such as, spermathecae and pharynx descriptions (Theodor, 1958). Classification presented by Theodor and Lewis proposed a subdivision of Phlebotomine sand-flies both for old and new world species that included two genera namely, *Phlebotomus* and *Sergentomyia* for old world species and for the new world species, (*Lutzomyia, Brumptomyia* and *Warileya*) genera had been assigned. This classification was later reviewed by Young and Duncan (1994), and remains a choice among most taxonomists. In 2003, Galati recognized 464 species of new world Neotropical Phlebotomine sandflies that classify 23 genera, 20 subgenera, 3 species groups, and 28 series and further reorganized *Phlebotominae* subfamily into two tribes namely, *Hertigiini* and *Phlebotomini* (Galati, 2003). In 2014, Galati proposed a classification in which *Phlebotomini* tribe included 931 species, out of which 916 species were validated and 15 species are of uncertain taxonomic status altogether, classified under six subtribes (*Phlebotomina, Australo-phlebotomina, Brumptomyiina, Sergentomyiina, Lutzomyiina,* and *Psychodopygina*). Tribe *Hertigiini* was also differentiated into two subtribes of *Hertigiina* and *Idiophlebotomina*. At present, *Phlebotominae* is subdivided into six genera on the basis of traditional and practical approach, out of which three genera represent the old world namely, *Phlebotomus* comprised of 13 subgenera, 10 subgenera of *Sergentomyia*, and 4 species from *Chinius* (Table 1.1). The new world includes 3 genera that are, *Lutzomyia* with 26 subgenera,

TABLE 1.1 Genera and subgenera of the old world sandflies.

Genera	Phlebotomus	Sergentomyia	Chinius
Subgenera	Adlerius	Capensomyia	Chinius junlianensis
	Anaphlebotomus	Grassomyia	Chinius barbazani
	Australophlebotomus	Neophlebotomus	Chinius eunicegalatiae
	Euphlebotomus	Parrotomyia	Chinius samarensis
	Idiophlebotomus	Parvidens	
	Kasauliuls	Rondonomyia	
	Larroussius	Sergentomyia	
	Madaphlebotomus	Sintonius	
	Paraphlebotomus	Spelaeomyia	
	Phlebotomus	Vattieromyia	
	Spelaeophlebotomus		
	Synphlebotomus		
	Transphlebotomus		

TABLE 1.2 Genera and subgenera of the new world sandflies.

Genera	*Warileya* (includes 6 species)	*Lutzomyia*	*Brumptomyia* (includes 26 species)
Subgenera	Subgenera of *Lutzomyia*		
		Coromyia	*Pressatia*
		Dampfomyia	*Psathyromyia*
		Evandromyia	*Trichophoromyia*
		Helcocyrtomyia	*Trichopygomyia*
		Micropygomyia	*Viannamyia*
		Nyssomyia	*Psychodopygus*
			Sciopemyia

Brumptomyia that holds 24 species, and *Warileya* with six species widely used for classifying sand flies (Galati, 2014) (Table 1.2).

1.6   Geographical distribution of sandflies

1.6.1   Old world sandflies

Three genera namely, *Phlebotomus, Chinius, and Sergentomyia* constitute old world sand-flies that are prominent in various regions of the world. The Palearctic region that encompasses central Asia (Bailly-Chaumara, Abonnec, & Pastre, 1971), including China, southern Europe, northern Africa, and the MiddleEast (Lewis, 1974, 2010; Rispal and Leger, 1998), being the primary temperate region in old world, have more than 200 species of sand flies viz., *Phlebotomus* subgenera (*Adlerius, Anaphlebotomus, Euphlebotomus, Idiophlebotomus, Larroussius, Paraphlebotomus, Phlebotomus, Synphlebotomus* and *Transphlebotomus*) present. Other genera such as *Chinius* and *Sergentomyia* are also found but *Phlebotomus* genus is the most dominant. In the Afrotropical region, various subgenera of *Anaphlebotomus, Larroussius, Paraphlebotomus, Phlebotomus, Spelaeophlebotomus*, and from *Phlebotomus* genus, along with *Sergentomyia* genus are dispersed. Malagasy region which contains Madagascar and islands in the Indian Ocean, has species that belong to *Phlebotomus* genera namely *Anaphlebotomus* and *Madaphlebotomus* subgenera as well as *Sergentomyia*. However, reports that suggest disease vector sand fly species are not present as such (Leger, Depaquit, & Gay, 2012). The Oriental region includes more than 120 species of *Phlebotomus, Chinius*, and *Sergentomyia* genera. *Phlebotomus argentipes* is one such important vector of kala-azar in the east Indian region and in far east areas such as Vietnam; sand fly bites are quite rare, with only Philippines as an exception (Lewis, 2010; Lewis and Dyce, 1988). Lastly in the

Australian region, Australasian phlebotomine fauna reveal a bipolar origin. *Phlebotomus* genus, eight species of Australo-phlebotomus are present, these originates from south where one species of subgenus *Idiophlebotomus* and 24 species of *Sergentomyia* genus from north are present (Schodde and Calaby, 1972) (Table 1.3). Several species of sand flies also co-occur, for example, *Sundasciurus Hoogstraali, S. vanilla,* co-occur both in Australia as well as in New Guinea, thus chains the hypothesis about concurrent expansion of New Guinea sand fly fauna together with east Australian sand flies as proposed by Schodde and Calaby (Flegontov et al., 2013).

1.6.2   New world sand flies

Three genera are found in Nearctic and Neotropical regions namely, *Lutzomyia, Warileya,* and *Brumptomyia* in the new world. Genus *Lutzomyia* is a large genus that constitutes more than 400 species in various subgenera, *Coromyia, Evandromyia, Helcocyrtomyia, Dampfomyia, Micropygomyia, Nyssomyia, Pressatia, Pintomyia, Psychodopygus, Sciopemyia, Viannamyia,* and *Trichopygomyia* and other ungrouped species. Genus *Lutzomyia* is more diverse when compared to counterparts of the old world. However, in a few subgenera such as *Nyssomyia, Psychodopygus,* and *Lutzomyia* vector species are found. Temperate regions in North America have sandflies with little interest but in tropical America, these are abundant. Genus *Lutzomyia* is the primary and widely dispersed in terms of species diversity and have great medical importance. Species of this genus are distributed in various regions that range from southern areas of Nearctic and throughout Neotropical ecozone. Sandflies are abundant in forest of Central and Southern America. Genus *Warileya* includes six species, primarily found in Neotropical region whereas 24 species of Genus *Brumptomyia* are roughly dispersed in Central and Southern America (Table 1.3). However, no species are reported to bite humans. *Brumptomyia* genus species constitute a sandflies group usually related with armadillo burrows. Identification of species of *Brumptomyia* genus is totally based on male structures (Maslov, Votypka, Yurchenko, & Lukes, 2013; Hamilton et al., 2015). In the Nearctic region only 14 species majorly from *Micropygomyia* subgenus, are present, however five species to this ecozone are restricted. Many species prefer hot and humid environments hence becoming unfavorable for the development of phlebotomine in particular for undeveloped stages. This feature supports the ideas of originating phlebotomine sandflies in the tropics with very few scattered species into temperate regions (Perfil'ev, 1968). Approximately over 450 sandfly species are found in Neotropical regions. Neotropical ecozone, which is the distribution center of Lutzomyia genus now a days, once thought to be forest, covered lowlands present in the eastern great Andes. This situation is certainly a dry periods consequence that isolate specific populations occurred during Pleistocene from which some isolated reproductively and might have

TABLE 1.3 Geographical distribution of *Leishmania* species and respective vector (sandfly genus) and reservoirs.

Region	*Leishmania* species	Sand fly genus	Reservoirs
Indian	*Leishmania donovani* (*Leishmania archibaldi*), *Leishmania tropica*, *Leishmania hemidactyli*, *Leishmania siamensis*	*Sergentomyia*	Carnivora, Dog, Gerbil, Human, Lizard
Australian	*Leishmania australiensis*	*Sergentomyia*	Kangaroo, Macropode
Malagasy	No autochthonous leishmaniasis	*Sergentomyia*	Unknown
Nearctic	*Leishmania infantum* (*Leishmania chagasi*), *L. siamensis*, *Leishmania lindenbergi*, *Leishmania panamensis*, *Leishmania utingensis*, *Leishmania mexicana* (*Leishmania pifanoi*), *Leishmania martiniquensis*,	*Brumptomyia*	Cat, Cattel, Dog, Hare, Horse, Equine, Heteromys, Human, Neotoma, Oryzomys, Peromysus, Sigmodon, Ototylomys
Neotropical	*L. utingensis*, *L. mexicana* (*L. pifanoi*), *L. infantum* (*L. chagasi*), *Leishmania shawi*, *Leishmania peruviana*, *Leishmania naiffi*, *Leishmania deanei*, *Leishmania henrici*, *Leishmania venezuelensis*, *Leishmania herreri*, *L. panamensis*, *Leishmania lainsoni*, *Leishmania hertigi*, *Leishmania forattinii*, *L. lindenbergi*, *Leishmania enrietti*, *Leishmania guyanensis*, *Leishmania equatorensis*,	*Brumptomyia*, *Warileya*	Cat, Carnivora, Dog, Agouti, Akodon, Cingulata, Dasypus, Coendou, Hoplomys, Pilosa, Equine, Primates, Sloth, Marsupialia, Rodentia, Hare, Echimyid, Dasyprocta, Heteromys, Myrmecophaga, Neacomys, Phyllotis, Oryzomys, Tamandua

(*Continued*)

TABLE 1.3 (Continued)

Region	*Leishmania* species	Sand fly genus	Reservoirs
	Leishmania aristidesi, Leishmania colombiensis, Leishmania braziliensis, Leishmania garnhami		
Palearctic	*Leishmania chameleonis, Leishmania adleri, L. donovani (L. archibaldi), Leishmania major (Leishmania killicki), Leishmania tarentolae, Leishmania nicollei, Leishmania zmeevi, L. martiniquensis, Leishmania arabica, Leishmania agamae, Leishmania turanica, Leishmania gulikae, Leishmania ceramodactyli, Leishmania helioscope, Leishmania gymnodactyli, Leishmania promastigotae, Leishmania sofieffi, Leishmania gerbilli, Leishmania phrynocephali*	*Chinius, Sergentomyia*	Cat, Cattel, Dog, Gerbil, Lizard, Human, Horse, Hare, Lizard, Equine, Hyrax,
Afrotropical	*L. adleri, Leishmania aethiopica, Leishmania davidi, L. donovani (L. archibaldi), L. major, L. gymnodactyli, L. tropica, Leishmania hoogstraali, L. platycephala, Leishmania zuckermani, L. tarentolae, Leishmania senegalensis*	*Sergentomyia*	Arvicanthis, Carnivora, Dendrohyrax, Dog, Felis, Genette, Gerbil, Hyrax, Lizard, Procavia, Mastomys, Heterohyrax

colonized in much more humid conditions in areas of northern and western regions of the subcontinent (Leger et al., 2012).

1.7 *Leishmania* classification and distribution

The family *Trypanosomatidae* comprise of three genera (dixenous) namely, *Leishmania, Phytomonas, and Trypanosoma*, eleven genera (monoxenous) and three genera, *Angomonas, Strigomonas, and Kentomonas*, all distinguish with the existence of subfamily *Strigomonadinae*, an endosymbiotic bacterium (Dantas-Torres et al., 2010).

Classification of *Leishmania* is as follows:

Kingdom: *Protista*

Class: *Kinetoplastea* (Slama et al., 2014)

Sub-class: *Meta-kinetoplastina* (Slama et al., 2014)

Order: *Trypanosomatida*

Family: *Trypanosomatidae*

Subfamily: *Leishmaniinae* (Killick-Kendrick, Killick-Kendrick, Tang, & Bastien, 1996)

Genus: *Leishmania*

Species of *Leishmania* genus are heteroxenous, (able to colonize two hosts). These species survive in intestinal tract of Phlebotomine sand flies and in phagocytes of reticulo-endothelial system of mammals (Lainson, 2010). *Leishmania* species that infect mammals are distributed globally from tropical and subtropical areas that include the American continents as well as basin of Mediterranean, southeast European countries, Africa, Asia and more recently in Australia. From Malagasy region, no autochthonous case has been reported, with an exception of canine leishmaniasis case, published (Moreno, Rioux, Lanotte, Pratlong, & Serres, 1986) which presented an overview of leishmaniasis occurrence and causative species found in all affected countries. Semi-arid areas developed by mankind in the old world, typical *Leishmania* transmissions have occurred peri-domestically, while parasites in the new world are usually related with sylvatic habitats. Even though *Leishmania* parasites are mainly gut-dwellers, they were hardly ever detected in sand fly salivary glands. Presence in salivary gland is inferred with high intensity infection of metacyclic promastigotes present in stomodeal valve and the thoracic mid-gut of vector.

On the basis of extrinsic characters, Linnean classifications for *Leishmania* were first proposed from 1916 to 1961. Nicolle (1908) suggested an early classification, which separated *L. infantum* that caused VL in the Mediterranean, from *L. donovani* that was the etiological species for kala-azar in India. Biagi, in 1964, classified various *Leishmania* species of the new world (Thomaz-Soccol et al., 1993). However, the disease may display similar clinical symptoms due to distinct *Leishmania* species, for e.g., VL with cutaneous; Adler, pointed out such difficulties in 1964 (Cupolillo, Grimaldi, & Momen, 1994). In 1987, Lainson and Shaw were presented new classifications that divided

Leishmania genus into two subgenera, *L.* (*Leishmania*) and *L.* (*Viannia*) for *Suprapylaria* section, and *Peripylaria* section, respectively. Intrinsic characteristics (biochemical, immunological, and molecular) of *Leishmania* were identified in the early 1970s, and were used to develop new classification systems. In the 1970s, isoenzyme electrophoresis had been widely used as a typing system and accepted as the gold standard for identification and is still a valuable tool as a reference technique for parasite characterization. Since 1980s, Adansonia phenetic classification was applied all together based on multiple similarity-weighted characters, i.e., polythetic, without any prior hypothesis. Next, phylogenetic analysis further exposed parental relationships between various *Leishmania* species. Other phenotypic classifications on the basis of isoenzymes have also been reported by (Cupolillo, Medina-Acosta, Noyes, Momen, & Grimaldi, 2000) for new world and (Le Blanq, Belehu, & Peters, 1986) for old world species(Rioux, 1990) which combined all old and new world taxa into a single classification system. Concordance between classifications was mutually validated in both extrinsic and intrinsic identification criteria.

Based on molecular analysis from several studies, a new *Leishmania* classification has been put forth that differentiates into two major phylogenetic lineages, section *Euleishmania* and *Paraleishmania* (Cupolillo et al., 2000). *Euleishmania* section constitutes four subgenera namely, *Leishmania* strain (*L. donovani*), *Viannia* strain (*L. braziliensis*), *Sauro-leishmania* strain (*L. tarentolae*) and lastly, *Leishmania enriettii* complex strain (*L. enriettii*). *Para-leishmania* section constitutes *Leishmania hertigi*, *Leishmania equatorensis*, *Leishmania deanei*, *Leishmania colombiensis*, *Leishmania herreri*, and formerly *Endotrypanum* genus *L. colombiensis* was the only pathogenic species regarding humans from this group. Evolution of *Paraleishmania* has still not been resolved hence it has been so far a polyphyletic clade within *Leishmania* genus. On the basis of available isoenzyme data, *Leishmania* genus was considered as monophyletic especially with respect to the position of *Endotrypanum* with respect to intra-erythrocyte developmental stage and divergent morphological form, trypomastigote or epimastigote, within *Paraleishmania* section. *Viannia* subgenus is confined to Neotropics, whereas subgenus presence is in both the old and new world. Fifty-three species named without any synonyms, have been documented, out of which 29 species are present in the old world and 20 species in the new world. Out of the above-recognized species only 20 species have been known to infect humans (Ritter et al., 2009) (Table 1.3).

1.8   Epidemiology

Epidemiologically, leishmaniasis is a very dynamic in nature hence transmission of the disease depends upon variability in environmental conditions, demography, human behavior, and immunogenic contour as well as economic status of affected human populations. All such factors may influence identification of cases, necessary diagnosis and treatment required as well as preventive measures employed against leishmaniasis, economically poor countries in particular. Fig. 1.1 represents reproduced data for global endemicity of leishmaniasis (WHO-reports, 2018).

1.8.1 Visceral leishmaniasis

Several nations (Kenya, India, Ethiopia, Brazil, Somalia, and Sudan) have reported around 90% cases of VL in 2015. However, more than 60 countries are endemic to VL. In both, the Indian subcontinent and east Africa have suffered from devastating epidemics. However, global occurrences of VL have declined substantially in the past decade and less than 900,000 new cases were reported in 2000 (Bogdan et al., 2000; Pandey, Pande, & Samant, 2020). India, Bangladesh, and Nepal, altogether used to have more than 50% of the global burden of VL. In 2005, it was marked as a public health problem when these countries became committed to eliminate VL by 2015, and so far, that deadline has been subsequently comprehended. The elimination target was set at less than 1 per 10,000 people/year at a district level in Nepal and sub district level in both India and Bangladesh, where such occurrence rate is well thought-out to be no longer a public health concern. However, cyclical reoccurrence, despite of appreciable decline, VL still persists (Rougeron et al., 2009). East Africa still faces the burden of VL with short, cyclical patterns of about 6 to10-year time intervals. Forced migration of nonimmune populations to endemic areas is the major hindrance for previous outbreaks (Akopyants et al., 2009). Coinfection with HIV has also contributed to elevated transmission. More than 40% patients in Ethiopia have

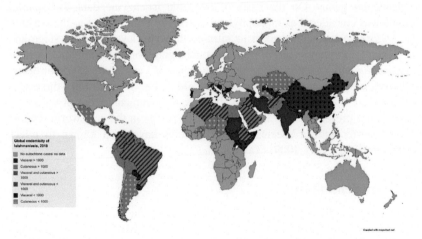

FIGURE 1.1 Global endemicity of leishmaniasis, WHO-Reports, 2018. *created by <https:// mapchart.net/world.html>.*

contributed for transmission in 2006 HIV and VL coinfection might have contributed to increased transmission (Salih et al., 2007). Endemic areas also share grounds for asymptomatic infections with a seroprevalence that range between 7% and 63% for *L. donovani* in the Indian subcontinent and 29%– 34% for *L. Infantum* in Brazilian children. Humans are the primary reservoir for VL caused by *L. donovani* in the Indian subcontinent. Transmission occurs domestically in alluvial plains of the Ganges, that with an altitude below 700 m (Mukhopadhyay et al., 2015). The encompassing areas experience heavy monsoon, relatively high humidity, 15°C–38°C temperature range, highly vegetative, and have subsoil water level (Bogdan et al., 2000). *L. donovani* transmission occurs at altitudes of more than 1000 m in hilly regions of Nepal (Das et al., 2016) and Bhutan VL is most prevalent in farming villages where mud-walled houses with earthen floors and the livestock share same roof or at close distance, thus, forms favorable ecological niche for *P. argentipes* sand-flies. Domestic dogs are primary reservoir of *L. infantum*, with a median range of 18% seroprevalence in south-western Europe (Perry et al., 2013) although other mammalian reservoirs also exist, in particular to central Asia A thorough study in Italy observed that mostly all infected dogs tend to develop symptomatic disease within two-year span (Perry et al., 2015a,b). Studies based on PCR have also proved infection up to 80% in dogs in the endemic areas showing no symptoms, of which, significant proportions were found infectious (Perry et al., 2015a,b; Kumar, Pandey, & Samant, 2020). Apart from rural areas in the Mediterranean Basin, recent VL outbreak has occurred in Spain in an urban area close to Madrid, in which wild hares served as primary reservoir (Desjeux et al., 2013). Sporadic, non-vector transmission routes have also been described in Latin America that includes congenital (Ben-Shimol et al., 2016), transfusion, organ transplants, or through laboratory accidents (Showler & Boggild, 2015). Alone in Spain, the risk of direct transmission of *L. infantum* has been reported in drug abusers that have been co-infected with HIV via needle sharing (Machado et al., 2015; Kumar, Pandey, & Samant, 2018). In patients, *Leishmania* parasites can continue to exist for decades after handling in immune-compromised individuals (Masmoudi et al., 2013) as reoccurrence of infection is possible due to post-transplant immunosuppressive therapy (compromised immunity), HIV infection or usage of immunomodulators.

1.8.2   Post-kala-azar dermal leishmaniasis

This form of dermal leishmaniasis is characterized by a derma (skin) condition that arises soon after treatment of VL caused by *L. donovani*. From the pathophysiological point of view, dermal leishmaniasis (post-kala-azar) is associated with an interferon-γ mediated immune response in host against dermal parasites. Exposure to UV-light and incomplete treatment are two major risk factors (Guerra et al., 2011), whereas some treatments direct to an elevated frequency of dermal leishmaniasis (post-kala-azar) (Kassi et al., 2008). In Asia, 5%−10% of cases of VL suffered with dermal leishmaniasis and emerges after 2−3 years posttreatment, whereas in East Africa about 50% of such cases occur typically within a year after treatment, even-though more than 85% of such lesions are self-healing (Guerra et al., 2011). However, more than 5% of patients in the India with this clinical manifestation have not reported with a previous episode of VL (Guerra et al., 2011). Patients with lesions of Post kala-azar dermal leishmaniasis typically have an effect on quality of life ahead in particular among youths (Lessa et al., 2001). Most importantly, sand-flies easily get infection through these lesions and, if left untreated, might remain for decades thus, and potentially constitute reservoirs of infection during inter-epidemic time lapses (Vargas-Inchaustegui et al., 2010).

1.8.3   Cutaneous and mucocutaneous leishmaniasis

WHO estimates approximately one million cases worldwide of CL annually with over 90% cases occur alone in Pakistan, Afghanistan, Saudi Arabia, Syria, Algeria, Brazil, Iran, and Peru (Rajasekaran & Chen, 2015) due to forced migration; the number of cases of CL cases has considerably augmented as cases imported from other countries are relatively frequent in non-endemic countries (Haldar et al., 2011). CL is caused by several old and new world leishmanial species. Prominent among the old-world species viz., *L. tropica, L. aethiopica,* and *L. major,* are endemic around the middle-eastern countries, the Mediterranean basin, the Indian subcontinent, and horn of Africa whereas the new world species viz., *L. amazonensis, L. braziliensis, Leishmania guyanensis,* and *Leishmania mexicana* are prevalent in South and Central part of the America (Freitas-Jr et al., 2012). CL parasite belongs to either of the two subgenera of *Leishmania (Viannia),* with a taxonomic variation that depends chiefly upon attachment and development sites of promastigotes in guts of sand flies (Sundar & Chakravarty, 2013). However, CL is considered as a mild appearance, but nearly 10% of infection cases reported originate via strain from *Viannia* subgenus, and develops a life-threatening and disfiguring condition known as mucocutaneous leishmaniasis. Transmission of CL is complex, both anthroponotic by *L. tropica* (zoonotic) caused by *L. aethiopica* and *L. major* and almost all new world species exists via sand flies that belong to *Phlebotomus* of the old world or by *Lutzomyia* of the new world. Populations living near crop and forest areas oror those who own dogs are major risk factors for acquiring infections via the new world species (Sundar & Chakravarty, 2015). The Syrian crisis between 2000 and 2012 represents a recent recrudescence of old-world CL where 97% of refugees acquired CL in Lebanon. An increment in CL cases is expected in the Mediterranean countries where *Phlebotomus sergenti* (vector) is widespread.

1.9 Conclusion

Leishmaniasis continues to be a serious community health problem in most developing regions of the world as epidemiologically its position is not evenly determined. The pragmatic chronological distinction with epidemiology is chiefly because of differences in the distribution of species of *Leishmania*, sand flies, as well as hosts. The evolutionary relationship between sand flies and *Leishmania* has always been tied together for leishmaniasis to flourish till modern times hence it becomes very necessary to gain precise information about the origin of both *Leishmania* species and *Phlebotominae* sand flies and also their chronological history of coevolution. However, there is an absence of a universal agreement concerning classification of *Leishmania*, in particular for defining species using defined criteria. Even though, placing *Leishmania* at subgeneric levels and the definition of "complexes" in *Leishmania* classification have gained wide acceptance since being reported by Lainson and Shaw, it still poses serious challenges in terms of the genus composition. It also becomes a necessity from epidemiological point of view about its transmission. With war and conflict zones in the Middle East, for example Syria, outburst of cutaneous form is particularly evident. Other factors such as migration, ecological disasters, and even domesticated animals indicate close association with leishmaniasis epidemics.

References

Adler, S., & Ber, M. (1941). The transmission of *Leishmania tropica* by the bite of Phlebotomus papatasi. *Indian Journal of Medical Research*, *29*, 803−809.

Akopyants, N. S., Kimblin, N., Secundino, N., Patrick, R., Peters, N., Lawyer, P., & Sacks, D. L. (2009). Demonstration of genetic exchange during cyclical development of Leishmania in the sand fly vector. *Science*, *324*(5924), 265−268.

Alvar, J., Velez, I. D., Bern, C., Herrero, M., Desjeux, P., Cano, J., ... de Boer, M. (2012). Leishmaniasis worldwide and global estimates of its incidence. *PLoS One*.

Bailly-Chaumara, H., Abonnec, E., & Pastre, J. (1971). Contribution à l'etude desphlebotomes du Maroc (Diptera: Psychodidae). Donnees faunistiques et ecologiques. *Cahiers ORSTOM. Série Entomologie Medicale et Parazitologie*, *4*, 431−460.

Ben-Shimol, S., Sagi, O., Horev, A., Avni, Y. S., Ziv, M., & Riesenberg, K. (2016). Cutaneous leishmaniasis caused by *Leishmania infantum* in Southern Israel. *Acta Parasitologica*, *61*(4), 855−858.

Bern, C., Maguire, J. H., & Alvar, J. (2008). Complexities of assessing the disease burden attributable to leishmaniasis. *PLoS Neglected Tropical Diseases*.

Boelaert, M., & Sundar, S. (2014). Leishmaniasis. In J. Farrer, P. Hotez, T. Junghanss, G. Kang, D. Lalloo, & N. J. White (Eds.), *Manson's tropical infectious diseases* (23rd ed., pp. 631−651). Philadelphia: Elsevier Saunders.

Bogdan, C., Donhauser, N., Döring, R., Röllinghoff, M., Diefenbach, A., & Rittig, M. G. (2000). Fibroblasts as host cells in latent leishmaniosis. *The Journal of Experimental Medicine*, *191* (12), 2121−2130.

Bray, R. S., Ashford, R. W., & Bray, M. A. (1973). The parasite causing cutaneous leishmaniasis in Ethiopia. *Transactions of the Royal Society of Tropical Medicine and Hygiene*, *67*, 345−348.

Caldart, E. T., Freire, R. L., Ferreira, F. P., Ruffolo, B. B., Sbeghen, M. R., Mareze, M., & Navarro, I. T. (2017). Leishmania in synanthropic rodents (*Rattus rattus*): New evidence for the urbanization of *Leishmania* (Leishmania) *amazonensis*. *Revista Brasileira de Parasitologia Veterinária*, *26*(1), 17−27.

Costa, M. A., Matheson, C., Iachetta, L., Llagostera, A., & Appenzeller, O. (2009). Ancient leishmaniasis in a highland desert of northern Chile. *PLoS One*, *4*(9).

Croan, D. G., Morrison, D. A., & Ellis, J. T. (1997). Evolution of the genus *Leishmania* revealed by comparison of DNA and RNA polymerase gene sequences. *Molecular and Biochemical Parasitology*, *89*, 149−159.

Cupolillo, E., Grimaldi, G., Jr., & Momen, H. (1994). A general classification of New World Leishmania using numerical zymotaxonomy. *The American Journal of Tropical Medicine and Hygiene*, *50*, 250−311.

Cupolillo, E., Medina-Acosta, E., Noyes, H., Momen, H., & Grimaldi, G., Jr. (2000). A revised classification for *Leishmania* and *Endotrypanum*. *Parasitology Today*, *16*, 142−144.

da Cunha, A. M., & Chagas, E. (1937). Nova espécie de protozoário do gênero *Leishmania* patogenicopara o homem. Leishmania chagas in. sp. Nota previa. *Hospital (Rio de Janeiro, Brazil)*, *11*, 3−9.

Dahroug, M. A., Almeida, A. B., Sousa, V. R., Dutra, V., Guimaraes, L. D., Soares, C. E., & de Souza, R. L. (2011). The first case report of *Leishmania* (leishmania) *chagasi* in Panthera leo in Brazil. *Asian Pacific Journal of Tropical Biomedicine*, *1*(3), 249−250.

daMatta, A. (1916). Sur les leishmanio sestegumentaires. Classification generale des leishmanioses. *Bulletin de la Société de pathologie exotique*, *9*, 494−503.

Dantas-Torres, F., Lorusso, V., Testini, G., de Paiva-Cavalcanti, M., Figueredo, L. A., Stanneck, D., et al. (2010). Detection of *Leishmania infantum* in Rhipicephalussanguineus ticks from Brazil and Italy. *Parasitology Research*, *106*, 857−860.

Das, S., et al. (2016). Chronic arsenic exposure and risk of post Kala-azar dermal leishmaniasis development in India: A retrospective cohort study. *PLoS Neglected Tropical Diseases*, *10*, e0005060.

De Araujo, V. A. L., Boite, M. C., Cupolillo, E., Jansen, A. M., & Roque, A. L. R. (2013). Mixed infection in the anteater Tamandua tetradactyla (Mammalia: Pilosa) from Para State, Brazil: *Trypanosoma cruzi*, *T. rangeli* and *Leishmania infantum*. *Parasitology*, *140*(4), 455−460.

de Oliveira Guerra., Prestes, S. R., Silveira, H., Câmara, L. I. D. A. R., Gama, P., & de Lima Ferreira, L. C. (2011). Mucosal leishmaniasis caused by Leishmania (Viannia) braziliensis and Leishmania (Viannia) guyanensis in the Brazilian Amazon. *PLoS Negl Trop Dis*, *5*(3), e980.

de Castro Ferreira, E., Pereira, A. A. S., Silveira, M., Margonari, C., Marcon, G. E. B., de Oliveira Franca, A., & Dorval, M. E. C. (2017). *Leishmania (V.) braziliensis* infecting bats from Pantanal wetland, Brazil: First records for Platyrrhinus lineatus and Artibeus planirostris. *Acta Tropica*, *172*, 217−222.

De Rezende, M. B., Herrera, H. M., Carvalho, C. M. E., Carvalho Anjos, E. A., Ramos, C. A. N., De Araujo, F. R., & de Oliveira, C. E. (2017). Detection of Leishmania spp. in bats from an area of Brazil endemic for visceral leishmaniasis. *Transboundary and Emerging Diseases*, *64*(6), e36−e42.

Desjeux, P., Ghosh, R.S., Dhalaria, P., Strub-Wourgaft, N., & Zijlstra, E.E. (2013). Report of the post kala-azar dermal leishmaniasis (PKDL) consortium meeting, New Delhi, India, 27−29 June 2012.

Donovan, C. (1903). On the possibility of the occurrence of trypanosomiasis in India. *British Medical Journal*, *2*, 79.

Edrissian, G. H., Rokni, M. B., Mohebali, M., Nateghpour, M., Mowlavi, G., & Bahadori, M. (2016). History of medical parasitology and parasitic infections in Iran. *Archives of Iranian Medicine*, *19*, 601−607.

Fernandes, A. P., Nelson, K., & Beverley, S. M. (1993). Evolution of nuclear ribosomal RNAs in kinetoplastid protozoa: Perspectives on the age and origins of parasitism. *Proceedings of the National Academy of Sciences of the United States of America, 90,* 11608–11612.

Flegontov, P., Votýpka, J., Skalický, T., Logacheva, M. D., Penin, A. A., Tanifuji, G., & Lukeš, J. (2013). Paratrypanosoma is a novel early-branching trypanosomatid. *Current Biology, 23* (18), 1787–1793.

Freitas-Junior, L. H., Chatelain, E., Kim, H. A., & Siqueira-Neto, J. L. (2012). Visceral leishmaniasis treatment: what do we have, what do we need and how to deliver it? *International Journal for Parasitology: Drugs and Drug Resistance, 2,* 11–19.

Frias, L., Leles, D., & Araujo, A. (2013). Studies on protozoa in ancient remains-A Review. *Memórias do Instituto Oswaldo Cruz, 108*(1), 1–12.

Galati, E. A. B. (2003). Classificacao de Phlebotominae. In E. R. Rangel, & R. Lainson (Eds.), *Flebotomineos do Brasil* (367, pp. 23–52). Rio de Janeiro, Brazil: Editora Fiocruz.

Galati, E. A. B. (2014). Classificação, morfologia, terminologia e identificaçao de Adultos: Bioecologia e Identificação de Phlebotominae. In E. F. Rangel, & R. Lainson (Eds.), *Flebotomíneos do Brasil* (p. 367). Río de Janeiro: Fiocruz.

Gibson, M. E. (1983). The identification of kala-azar and the discovery of *Leishmania donovani*. *Medical History, 27*(2), 203–213.

Guerra, J. A., et al. (2011). Mucosal leishmaniasis caused by *Leishmania* (Viannia) *braziliensis* and *Leishmania* (Viannia) *guyanensis* in the Brazilian Amazon. *PLoS Neglected Tropical Diseases, 5,* e980.

Haldar, A. K., Sen, P., & Roy, S. (2011). Use of antimony in the treatment of leishmaniasis: current status and future directions. *Molecular biology international, 2011.*

Hamilton, P. T., Votýpka, J., Dostálová, A., Yurchenko, V., Bird, N. H., Lukeš, J., & Perlman, S. J. (2015). Infection dynamics and immune response in a newly described Drosophila-trypanosomatid association. *MBio, 6*(5).

Handman, E., & Bullen, D. V. (2002). Interaction of Leishmania with the host macrophage. *Trends in Parasitology, 18,* 332–334.

Kamhawi, S. (2006). Phlebotomine sand flies and Leishmania parasites: Friends or foes? *Trends in Parasitology, 22,* 439–445.

Kassi, M., Kassi, M., Afghan, A. K., Rehman, R., & Kasi, P. M. (2008). Marring leishmaniasis: the stigmatization and the impact of cutaneous leishmaniasis in Pakistan and Afghanistan. *PLoS Negl Trop Dis, 2*(10), e259.

Kerr, S. F. (2000). Palaearctic origin of *Leishmania*. *Memorias do Instituto Oswaldo Cruz, 95,* 75–80.

Killick-Kendrick, R., Killick-Kendrick, M., Tang, Y., & Bastien, P. (1996). Metacyclic promastigotes of Leishmania in the salivary glands of experimentally infected phlebotomine sandflies. *Parasite, 3,* 55–60.

Kloehn, J., Saunders, E. C., O'Callaghan, S., Dagley, M. J., & McConville, M. J. (2015). Characterization of metabolically quiescent Leishmania parasites in murine lesions using heavy water labeling. *PLoS Pathog, 11*(2), e1004683.

Kumar, A., Pandey, S. C., & Samant, M. (2018). Slow pace of antileishmanial drug development. *Parasitology Open, 4*(e4), 1–11.

Kumar, A., Pandey, S. C., & Samant, M. (2020). A spotlight on the diagnostic methods of a fatal disease Visceral Leishmaniasis. *Parasite Immunol, 42*(10), e12727. Available from https://doi.org/10.1111/pim.12727.32378226.

Lainson, R. (2010). The Neotropical Leishmania species: A brief historical review of their discovery, ecology and taxonomy. *Revista Pan-Amazônica de Saúde, 1*(2), 13–32.

Le Blanq, S. M., Belehu, A., & Peters, W. (1986). Leishmania in the Old world: The distribution of L. aethiopica zymodemes. *Transactions of the Royal Society of Tropical Medicine and Hygiene, 80*, 360−366.

Leelayoova, S., Siripattanapipong, S., Hitakarun, A., Kato, H., Tan-ariya, P., Siriyasatien, P., & Mungthin, M. (2013). Multilocus characterization and phylogenetic analysis of Leishmania siamensis isolated from autochthonous visceral leishmaniasis cases, Southern Thailand. *B microbiology, 13*(1), 1−7.

Leger, N., Depaquit, J., & Gay, F. (2012). Description of the sandfly species *Chiniussamarensisn*. sp. (*Psychodidae*; Diptera) from the Philippines. *Pathogens and Global Health, 106*, 346−351.

Leishman, W. B. (1903). On the possibility of the occurrence of trypanosomiasis in India. *British Medical Journal, 1*, 1252−1254.

Lessa, H. A., Machado, P., Lima, F., Cruz, A. A., Bacellar, O., Guerreiro, J., & Carvalho, E. M. (2001). Successful treatment of refractory mucosal leishmaniasis with pentoxifylline plus antimony. *The American Journal of Tropical Medicine and Hygiene, 65*(2), 87−89.

Lewis, D. J. (1971). Phlebotomid sandflies. *Bulletin of the World Health Organization, 44*, 535−551.

Lewis, D. J. (1974). The Phlebotomid sandflies of Yemen Arab Republic. *Tropenmedizin und Parasitologie, 25*, 187−197.

Lewis, D. J. (2010). The Phlebotomine sandflies (Diptera: Psychodidae) of the Oriental Region. *Bulletin of the British Museum (Natural History), 37*, 217−343.

Lewis, D. J., & Dyce, A. (1988). Taxonomy of the Australasian *Phlebotominae* (Diptera: *Psychodidae*) with revision of genus *Sergentomyia* from the region. *Invertebrate Taxonomy, 2*(6), 755−804.

Luhe, M. (1906). Die im Bluteschmarotzenden Protozoen und ihrenachsten Verwandten. In C. Mense (Ed.), *Handbuch der Tropenkrankheiten* (Band 3, pp. 69−268). Leipzig: Verlag J.A. Barth.

Lysenko, A. J. (1971). Distribution of leishmaniasis in the Old World. *Bulletin of the World Health Organization, 44*, 515−520.

Machado, P. R., Rosa, M. E. A., Guimarães, L. H., Prates, F. V., Queiroz, A., Schriefer, A., & Carvalho, E. M. (2015). Treatment of disseminated leishmaniasis with liposomal amphotericin B. *Clinical infectious diseases, 61*(6), 945−949.

Malta, M. C. C., Tinoco, H. P., Xavier, M. N., Vieira, A. L. S., Costa, E. A., & Santos, R. L. (2010). Naturally acquired visceral leishmaniasis in non-human primates in Brazil. *Veterinary Parasitology, 169*(1-2), 193−197.

Maroli, M., Pennisi, M. G., Di Muccio, T., Khoury, C., Gradoni, L., & Gramiccia, M. (2007). Infection of sandflies by a cat naturally infected with *Leishmania infantum*. *Veterinary Parasitology, 145*(3-4), 357−360.

Maslov, D. A., Votypka, J., Yurchenko, V., & Lukes, J. (2013). Diversity and phylogeny of insect trypanosomatids: All that is hidden shall be revealed. *Trends in Parasitology, 1*, 43−52.

Masmoudi, A., Hariz, W., Marrekchi, S., Amouri, M., & Turki, H. (2013). Old World cutaneous leishmaniasis: diagnosis and treatment. *Journal of Dermatological Case Reports, 7*(2), 31.

Maspero, G. (1896). (5th ed., p. 218)*The dawn of civilization—Egypt and Chaldaea*, (1910, p. 218). London: Society for the Promotion of Christian Knowledge.

Mauricio, I. L., Howard, M. K., Stothard, J. R., & Miles, M. A. (1999). Genetic diversity in the *Leishmania donovani* complex. *Parasitology, 119*, 237−246.

Momen, H., & Cupolillo, E. (2000). Speculations on the origin and evolution of the genus *Leishmania*. *Memorias do Instituto Oswaldo Cruz, 95*, 583.

Montoya, A., de Quadros, L. P., Mateo, M., Hernandez, L., Galvez, R., Alcantara, G., & Miro, G. (2016). *Leishmania infantum* infection in Bennett's Wallabies (*Macropus rufogriseus rufogriseus*) in a Spanish wildlife park. *Journal of Zoo and Wildlife Medicine, 47*(2), 586−593.

Moreno, G., Rioux, J. A., Lanotte, G., Pratlong, F., & Serres, E. (1986). Le complex *Leishmania donovanis*. 1. Analyse enzymatique et Al., traitementnumérique. Individualisation du complexe *Leishmania infantum*. In J. A. Rioux (Ed.), *Leishmania: Taxonomieet Phylogenese. Application Éco-epidemiologiques (Colloque International du CNRS/INSERM, 1984)* (pp. 105−117). Montpellier: IMEE.

Mukhopadhyay, D., Mukherjee, S., Roy, S., Dalton, J. E., Kundu, S., Sarkar, A., & Chatterjee, M. (2015). M2 polarization of monocytes-macrophages is a hallmark of Indian post kala-azar dermal leishmaniasis. *PLoS Negl Trop Dis, 9*(10), e0004145.

Murray, H. W., Berman, J. D., Davies, C. R., & Saravia, N. G. (2005). Advances in leishmaniasis. *The Lancet., 366*(9496), 1561−1577.

Nicolle, C. (1908). Sur troiscasd'infection splénique infantile à corps de Leishman observes en Tunisie. *Archives de l'Institut Pasteur de Tunis, 3*−26.

Nowak, R. M. (1991). *Walker's mammals of the world,* . (5th ed., pp. 643−1629). (Vol. II, pp. 643−1629). Baltimore and London: The Johns Hopkins University Press.

Nowak, R. M. (1999). *Walker's mammals of the world.* Baltimore and London: John Hopkins University Press.

Noyes, H. (1998). Implications of a Neotropical origin of the genus *Leishmania. Memorias do Instituto Oswaldo Cruz, 93*, 657−661.

Oryan, A. (2015). Plant-derived compounds in treatment of leishmaniasis. *Iranian Journal of Veterinary Research, 16*(1), 1.

Pandey, S. C., Pande, V., & Samant, M. (2020). DDX3 DEAD-box RNA helicase (Hel67) gene disruption impairs infectivity of Leishmania donovani and induces protective immunity against visceral leishmaniasis. *Scientific Reports, 10*(1), 18218. Available from https://doi.org/10.1038/s41598-020-75420-y.33106577.

Perfil'ev, P. P. (1968). Phlebotomidae. Translation of Perfil'ev, 1966 Diptera: Family Phlebotomidae. *Fauna SSSR, 93*, 1−382.

Perry, M. R., Wyllie, S., Raab, A., Feldmann, J., & Fairlamb, A. H. (2013). Chronic exposure to arsenic in drinking water can lead to resistance to antimonial drugs in a mouse model of visceral leishmaniasis. *Proceedings of the National Academy of Sciences, 110*(49), 19932−19937.

Perry, M. R., et al. (2015a). Arsenic exposure and outcomes of antimonial treatment in visceral leishmaniasis patients in Bihar, India: A retrospective cohort study. *PLOS Neglected Tropical Diseases, 9*, e0003518.

Perry, M., Wyllie, S., Prajapati, V., Menten, J., Raab, A., Feldmann, J., & Fairlamb, A. (2015b). Arsenic, antimony, and Leishmania: has arsenic contamination of drinking water in India led to treatment-resistant kala-azar? *The Lancet, 385*, S80.

Poinar, G., Jr (2008). Lutzomyiaadiketis sp. n. (Diptera: *Phlebotomidae*), a vector of *Paleoleishmanianeo tropicum* sp. n. (Kinetoplastida: *Trypanosomatidae*) in Dominican amber. *Parasite Vectors, 1*, 22.

Poinar, G., Jr, & Poinar, R. (2004a). Evidence of vector-borne disease of Early Cretaceous reptiles. *Vector Borne and Zoonotic Diseases (Larchmont, N.Y.), 4*, 281−284.

Poinar, G., Jr, & Poinar, R. (2004b). *Paleoleishmania proterusn.* gen., n. sp. (Trypanosomatidae: Kinetoplastida) from Cretaceous Burmese amber. *Protist, 155*, 305−310.

Rajasekaran, R., & Chen, Y. P. (2015). Potential therapeutic targets and the role of technology in developing novel antileishmanial drugs. *Drug Discovery Today, 20*, 958−968.

Reuss, S. M., Dunbar, M. D., Calderwood Mays, M. B., Owen, J. L., Mallicote, M. F., Archer, L. L., & Wellehan, J. F., Jr (2012). Autochtonous *Leishmania siamensis* in horse, Florida, USA. *Emerging Infectious Diseases, 18*, 1545−1547.

Rioux, J. A. (1990). Taxonomy of Leishmania. Use of isoenzymes. Suggestions for a new classification. *Annales de Parasitologie Humaine et Comparee, 65*, 11−125.

Rispal, R., & Leger, N. (1998). Numerical taxonomy of Old World Phlebotominae (Diptera: Psychodidae). I. Considerations of Morphological Characters in the genus Phlebotomus Rondani & Berte. *Memorias do Instituto Oswaldo Cruz, 93*, 793−785.

Ritter, U., et al. (2009). Are neutrophils important host cells for Leishmania parasites? *Trends in Parasitology, 25*, 505−510.

Roque, A. L. R., & Jansen, A. M. (2014). Wild and synanthropic reservoirs of Leishmania species in the Americas. *International Journal for Parasitology: Parasites and Wildlife, 3*(3), 251−262.

Ross, R. (1903). Note on the bodies recently described by Leishman and Donovan. *British Medical Journal, 2*, 1261−1262.

Rougeron, V., De Meeûs, T., Hide, M., Waleckx, E., Bermudez, H., Arevalo, J., & Bañuls, A. L. (2009). Extreme inbreeding in Leishmania braziliensis. *Proceedings of the national academy of sciences, 106*(25), 10224−10229.

Russell, A. (1756). The natural history of Aleppo, and parts adjacent, with the climate, inhabitants, and diseases, particularly the plague, the methods used by Europeans for their preservation. Folding and other copperplates of Eastern customs, natural history, etc., London (pp. 262−266).

Salih, M. A., Ibrahim, M. E., Blackwell, J. M., Miller, E. N., Khalil, E. A., ElHassan, A. M., & Mohamed, H. S. (2007). IFNG and IFNGR1 gene polymorphisms and susceptibility to post-kala-azar dermal leishmaniasis in Sudan. *Genes & Immunity, 8*(1), 75−78.

Schnur, L. F. (1987). On the clinical manifestations and parasites of Old World leishmaniasis and *Leishmania tropica* causing visceral leishmaniasis. In D. T. Hart (Ed.), *Leishmaniasis: The current status and new strategies for control. NATO ASI series* (171, p. 93943).

Schodde, R., & Calaby, J. H. (1972). *The biogeography of the Australo-Papuan Bird and mammal faunas in relation to Torres Strait. Bridge and barrier: The natural and cultural history of Torres Strait* (pp. 257−300). Canberra, Australia: Australian Nat. Univ.

Shirian, S., Oryan, A., Hatam, G. R., Panahi, S., & Daneshbod, Y. (2014). Comparison of conventional, molecular, and immunohistochemical methods in diagnosis of typical and atypical cutaneous leishmaniasis. *Archives of Pathology and Laboratory Medicine, 138*(2), 235−240.

Showler, A. J., & Boggild, A. K. (2015). Cutaneous leishmaniasis in travellers: A focus on epidemiology and treatment in 2015. *Current Infectious Disease Reports, 17*, 489.

Slama, D., Haouas, N., Remadi, L., Mezhoub, H., Babba, H., & Chaker, E. (2014). First detection of *Leishmania infantum* (Kinetoplastida: *Trypanosomotidae*) in Culicoides spp. (Diptera: Ceratopogonidae). *Parasites and Vectors, 7*, 51.

Soares, I. R., Silva, S. O., Moreira, F. M., Prado, L. G., Fantini, P., Maranhao, R. D. P. A., & Palhares, M. S. (2013). First evidence of autochthonous cases of *Leishmania* (Leishmania) *infantum* in horse (*Equus caballus*) in the Americas and mixed infection of Leishmania infantum and *Leishmania* (Viannia) *braziliensis*. *Veterinary Parasitology, 197*(3-4), 665−669.

Stevens, J., & Rambaut, A. (2001). Evolutionary rate differences in trypanosomes. *Infection, Genetics and Evolution: Journal of Molecular Epidemiology and Evolutionary Genetics in Infectious Diseases, 1*, 143−150.

Sundar, S., & Chakravarty, J. (2013). Leishmaniasis: An update of current pharmacotherapy. *Expert Opinion on Pharmacotherapy, 14*, 53−63.

Sundar, S., & Chakravarty, J. (2015). An update on pharmacotherapy for leishmaniasis. *Expert Opinion on Pharmacotherapy, 16*, 237−252.

Theodor, O. (1958). Psychodidae, Phlebotominae. In E. Lindner (Ed.), *Die Fliegen der Palaearktischen Region, Psychodidae* (9, pp. 1–55). Stuttgart: E. Schweizerbart'scheVerlag.

Thomaz-Soccol, V., Lanotte, G., Rioux, J. A., Pratlong, F., Martini-Dumas, A., & Serres, E. (1993). Monophyletic origin of the genus Leishmania Ross, 1903. *Annales de Parasitologie Humaine et Comparee, 68*, 107–108.

Tsakmakidis, I, Angelopoulou, K., Dovas, C. I., Dokianakis, E, Tamvakis, A, Symeonidou, I., & Diakou, A (2017). Leishmania infection in rodents in Greece. *Tropical Medicine & International Health, 22*(12), 1523–1532.

Tuon, F. F., Neto, V. A., & Amato, V. S. (2008). *Leishmania*: Origin, evolution and future since the Precambrian. *FEMS Immunology and Medical Microbiology, 54*, 158–166.

Twining, W. (1827). Observations on diseases of the spleen particularly on the vascular engorgement of that organ common in Bengal. *Trans Med Phys Soc Bengal, 3*, 351–412.

Vargas-Inchaustegui, D. A., et al. (2010). CXCL10 production by human monocytes in response to *Leishmania braziliensis* infection. *Infection and Immunity, 78*, 301–308.

Vianna, G. (1911). Sobre uma nova especie de Leishmania (nota preliminar). *Brasil-Médico, 25*, 411.

Yakimoff, W. L., & Schokhor, N. I. (1914). Recherchessur les maladies tropicaleshumaine set animales au Turkestan. II. La leishmanio secutanée (boutond'Orient) spontanée du chien Turkestan. *Bulletin de la Société de pathologie exotique, 7*, 186–187.

Young, D. G., & Duncan, M. A. (1994). *Guide to the identification and geographic distribution of Lutzomyia sandflies in Mexico, the West Indies, Central and South America (Diptera: Psychodidae),* . *Memoirs of the American Entomological Institute* (54, p. 88). Gainesville: Associate Publishers.

Yurchenko, V. Y., Lukes, J., Jirku, M., Zeledon, R., & Maslov, D. A. (2006). *Leptomonas costaricensis sp.* n. (Kinetoplastea: *Trypanosomatidae*), a member of the novel phylogenetic group of insect trypanosomatids closely related to the genus *Leishmania*. *Parasitology, 133*, 537–546.

Zink, A. R., Spigelman, M., Schraut, B., Greenblatt, C. L., Nerlich, A. G., & Donoghue, H. D. (2006). Leishmaniasis in ancient Egypt and upper Nubia. *Emerging Infectious Diseases, 12* (10), 1616.

Chapter 2

Neoteric strategies for vector control and identification of zoonotic reservoirs

Deepa Bisht, Khushboo Dasauni and Tapan Kumar Nailwal
Department of Biotechnology, Kumaun University, Sir J C Bose Technical Campus, Bhimtal, India

2.1 Introduction

Leishmaniasis is a global spectrum of a vector carried; neglected epidemiological disease caused by parasite *Leishmania* (Alvar et al., 2012). More than 20 *Leishmania* species and around 600 species of sand flies are divided into five genera: Brumptomyia, Lutzomyia, and Warileya are found in the new world, and Sergentomyia and Phlebotomus are found in the old world and are known to transmit the parasite. It is a native disease in 97 countries and around 1 million cases are reported worldwide annually (Alemayehu & Alemayehu, 2017; Ready, 2013). Most people in endemic areas are at very high risk of transmission (WHO Leishmaniasis, 2018). It invades human and other mammalian population when flies, humans, and reservoir hosts share a similar habitat (Lemma et al., 2017). Currently some treatments are available, but due to high toxicity risk, delay in administration of drug, treatment failures, etc., they often emerge as a major problem (Kumar, Pandey, & Samant, 2018). There is no vaccine that is 100% efficient so far and overdoses of pesticides are developing resistance in sand flies, which is a major problem (Hemingway & Ranson, 2000; Pandey, Pande, & Samant, 2020). In view of the significance of leishmaniasis on human health and welfare, it is pivotal to examine the following new vector control strategies:

- introduction of *Wolbachia* into vector *Lutzomyia longipalpis* cell lines to check its effect on immune system linked expression of genes and in vitro interplay with *Leishmania infantum*;
- noninvasive sand fly−*Leishmania* model and identification of fluorescent *Leishmania tarentolae* postinfection;

Pathogenesis, Treatment and Prevention of Leishmaniasis. DOI: https://doi.org/10.1016/B978-0-12-822800-5.00007-X

- insecticide-treated cost-effective durable wall lining (ITWL) to monitor leishmaniasis;
- optimal amalgamation of control strategies and its cost-effective analysis;
- establishment of procedure for sand fly *L. longipalpis* egg microinjection;
- genetically modified insects using new tools such as CRISPR- Cas9 editing;
- metagenomic profile analysis of taxa linked with sand fly *L. longipalpis*;
- transcriptomic study of male and female wild *L. longipalpis* species of sand fly.

Animal reservoirs are of utmost importance for supporting and maintaining the life cycle of many *Leishmania* species, and it plays a significant role in transmission of sylvatic/rural infections (Alemayehu & Alemayehu, 2017). A reservoir host is defined as an agent that can spread a parasite into the next vector (Akhoundi et al., 2016; Jansen & Roque, 2010). A mammal is a *Leishmania* reservoir when it is infectious for the sand fly (Roque & Jansen, 2014) (Fig. 2.1).

Life cycle of the parasite *Leishmania* being heteroxenous shows two morphological forms; promastigote form in the gut of the sand fly and

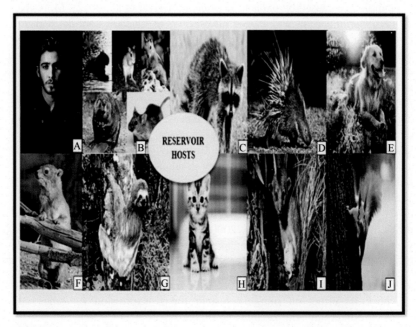

FIGURE 2.1 Reservoir hosts of human leishmaniasis: (A) humans, (B) rodents, (C) raccoon, (D) porcupines, (E) dog, (F) rock hyrax, (G) sloth, (H) cat, (I) kinkajou, and (J) red squirrel, etc. in different endemic regions of the world (Alemayehu & Alemayehu, 2017).

amastigote form present in macrophages of the mammalian host (Cox, 2009). Multifarious nature of *Leishmania* is due to temporal and regional variations. Ecological and parasitological research can determine the role of animals as potent reservoirs (Roque & Jansen, 2014; Raymond, McHugh, Witt, & Kerr, 2003). Transportability power of host species in an area depends on the availability of *Leishmania* parasite to vector which plays an immense role in transmission of the disease. Rate of transmission of the disease is higher in cities and rural urban transition zones, where wildlife and humans share their environment (Daszak, Cunningham, & Hyatt, 2001) (Fig. 2.2).

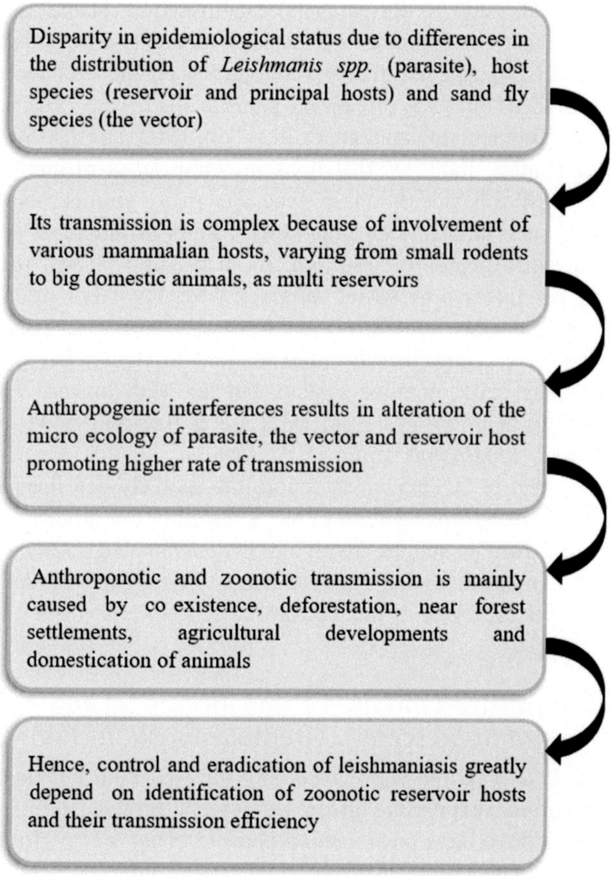

Disparity in epidemiological status due to differences in the distribution of *Leishmanis spp.* (parasite), host species (reservoir and principal hosts) and sand fly species (the vector)

Its transmission is complex because of involvement of various mammalian hosts, varying from small rodents to big domestic animals, as multi reservoirs

Anthropogenic interferences results in alteration of the micro ecology of parasite, the vector and reservoir host promoting higher rate of transmission

Anthroponotic and zoonotic transmission is mainly caused by co existence, deforestation, near forest settlements, agricultural developments and domestication of animals

Hence, control and eradication of leishmaniasis greatly depend on identification of zoonotic reservoir hosts and their transmission efficiency

FIGURE 2.2 Role of zoonotic reservoirs in transmission of leishmaniasis (Alemayehu & Alemayehu, 2017).

2.1.1 Neoteric strategies for vector control in different types of leishmaniasis

2.1.1.1 Introduction of Wolbachia *into vector* L. longipalpis *to check its effects on immune system linked gene expression and in vitro interaction studies with* L. infantum

In America sand flies of genus, *L. longipalpis* (Diptera: Psychodidae) are the main vector of visceral leishmaniasis (VL) (Ready, 2013; Sant'Anna et al., 2012). Bacteria *Wolbachia* has been used as a new tool for controlling vector transmitted diseases, by arresting the pathogen effect (De Oliveira et al., 2015; Hilgenboecker, Hammerstein, Schlattmann, Telschow, & Werren, 2008). Earlier it was used in viruses that are carried by mosquitoes, like dengue, chikungunya, and Zika and its new insertion in vectors has been potent against plasmodium (Aliota et al., 2016; Dutra et al., 2016; Moreira et al., 2009; Tan et al., 2017). Researchers established a stable infection of wMelPop-CLA and wMelstrains of genus Wolbachia into embryonic cell lines Lulo and LL-5 and its effects were studied on the immune system of the sand fly and no adverse effects on parasite load were observed. Down regulation of immune associated genes like Toll, IMD, and Jak-Stat, in comparison with control, indicates that trans infection leads to immune activation. Inducible nitric oxide synthase gene and many antimicrobial peptides response were seen in LL-5 cell line which results in failure of presence of *Wolbachi*a in early phases of infection. In succeeding phases, the sand fly cell line was not infected by wMel, although wMelPop-CLA strain was able to completely and stably infect LL-5 and Lulo cells at a lesser concentration.

Lulo cells were comparatively more tolerant to *Wolbachia strain* infection affecting the cell's immune system, but not with in vitro *L. infantum* interaction. This demonstrates Lulo cells are a fine and good system for *Wolbachia* in *L. longipalpis* strain of *Leishmania*. In this experiment they tested the prospect of *Wolbachia* infection into sand fly cell lines, as an initial step towards using this bacteria to block transmission of leishmaniasis.

In vivo and further studies involving *Wolbachia* and *Leishmania* are a new frontier that needs to be explored due to complexity of the organism and heteroxenous life cycle of the parasite.

*2.1.1.2 Noninvasive sand fly–*Leishmania model *and identification of fluorescent* L. tarentolae *postinfection*

Female flies *L. longipalpis* were artificially infected with human nonpathogenic *L. tarentolae* expressing green fluorescent protein (GFP) (Adler & Theodor, 1935). Five days postinfection parasite count was performed and a proportion of infected flies versus survival rate of infected flies was found similar. Epifluorescence inverted microscope was used to identify the presence of parasites in whole living female flies and localized green fluorescent specific area was seen in upper thorax. Evaluation of the parasite population and localized florescence in dissected flies confirms the presence of infection. Parasite population and the rate of infection were almost the same in *L. tarentolae* with GFP and wild type. A unique fact of this experiment was the observation of a particular region of fluorescence in the midgut region of the thorax in normal light, fluorescence, and the dissected gut under fluorescence microscopy (moving from left towards right) (Diaz-Albiter et al., 2018).

Further from dissection studies it was observed that a huge portion of the fly population showed florescence and flies, which do not show this feature, have no or very low proportion of parasite. This hazard free system is a modern tool to study for vector–parasite interaction. It can also be used to step up gene silencing in infected flies. This florescent model could help us understand parasite resistance in the sand fly to a greater extent and are used for many other medically important types of *Leishmania* species (Diaz-Albiter et al., 2018; Soares & Turco, 2003; Volf & Peckova, 2007).

2.1.1.3   Insecticide-treated cost-effective durable wall lining to monitor Leishmaniasis

ITWL or insecticide-treated durable wall lining is a whole modern exemplar for controlling vector-borne diseases as a potential alternate to indoor residual spraying (IRS). ITWL remains effective for many years and can be connected to inner side walls of house. This strategy overcomes first-line control strategies like IRS campaigns and long-lasting insecticidal nets (LLINs). Initial trials of ITWL resulted in higher vector mortality when combined with LLINs (Messenger & Rowland, 2017). Qualitative studies of ITWL have concluded that its cost effectiveness, artistic, and entomological efficiency are key factors for household acceptability and use. Earlier ITWL has been reported to be efficient against malaria and Chagas disease. It can interplay a key function in blocking transmission of the disease (Bern, 2015; WHO, 2010).

Management of the vector is one of the major and crucial control strategies, targeting chief resting areas of sand flies, usually with IRS (Picado, Dash, Bhattacharya, & Boelaert, 2012). In Bangladesh, India, and Nepal, ITWL was investigated and a higher number of household sand fly mortality rate and reduction in vector density was observed after a year trial (Huda et al., 2016; Mondal et al., 2016). However, there are no epidemiological termination points for concluding its assessment on VL (Messenger & Rowland, 2017).

2.1.1.4   Optimal amalgamation of control strategies and its cost-effective analysis

VL is a lethal type of leishmaniasis and requires public efforts and large scale effective eradication programs. Variability in regional, seasonal, and temperature variations are major factors to consider for strategy formulation (Stockdale & Newton, 2013). In this study, an anthroponotic VL model was used that compartmentalized human beings into [Post-kala-azar dermal leishmaniasis (PKDL)-infected, symptomatic and asymptomatic] and sand fly groups. Examination was done on infected population to know the effect of minimal control strategy combinations within a model. To mimic natural realistic situations, the role of seasonal variations on the biting rate of vector sand fly was considered as an integrable function in a period of time (Biswas, Subramanian, ELMojtaba, Chattopadhyay, & Sarkar, 2017).

Further, they mathematically analyzed the model to calculate basic reproduction number R_o and proved that if $R_o > 1$, then the population is asymptomatic and stable. If $R_o < 1$, it denotes disease-free equilibrium condition in the model. They numerically estimated this model by analyzing factors for VL cases known in the south Sudan in 2012 (Abubakar et al., 2014). They also standardized the model for predicting the number of cases in 2013 and it was comparable with actual data that was calculated at the end of the year. Basic number of reproduction R_o that was calculated in variable ecology in the south Sudan (2012) was 2.67. Use of optimum and time dependent strategy can reduce rate of vector-borne diseases like leishmaniasis in this particular time frame (Biswas et al., 2017).

In this research, they studied three types of control, that is, use of treatment of infectives, treated bed nets, and spray of insecticides and four different strategies:

1. Strategy A: In this combination of all three were used.
2. Strategy B: In this combination of two strategies, that is, treatment of infective individuals and use of treated bed nets.
3. Strategy C: In this combination of combination of two strategies, that is, spray of insecticides and use of treated bed nets.
4. Strategy D: In this combination of two strategies, that is, spray of insecticides and treatment of infective individuals.

A and D strategies performed best during the time-period of intervention. For complete elimination of disease, a long application period of combined strategies can combat the disease. These events can restart over a period of time, opposite to cutaneous leishmaniasis (CL) model which cannot show resurrection (Abubakar et al., 2014; Zamir, Zaman, & Alshomrani, 2016). The model is a precise tool for VL by including asymptomatic, symptomatic, and transient infectious types and their combination optimally as control strategies and cost-effective analysis to introduce an efficient and effective elimination program. So, this model can be very helpful for researchers, who faced the problem of partitioning of resources, to choose different control strategies with respect to the intensity of the disease (Biswas et al., 2017).

2.1.1.5   Establishment of procedure for sand fly L. longipalpis egg microinjection

Neoteric control strategies, which are being studied for vector transmitted diseases, largely depend on the potential to consistently inject eggs in the target organism. Its application in methods like *Wolbachia* mediated blocking of pathogens and use of CRISPR−Cas9 editing for genetic modification of insects. This method was used for injecting preblastoderm eggs of vector *L. longipalpis*. In order to determine efficacy of the method for focusing infection on germline of sand fly, wMel *Wolbachia* was extracted from eggs of *Drosophila melanogaster* and this bacteria was employed like a marker for injection. This procedure resulted in generation of early lines of *Wolbachia* transinfected *L. longipalpis*, displaying the ability to frame the basis for new strategies against sand flies, which includes both *Wolbachia*-based method and gene alteration (Jeffries, Rogers, & Walker, 2018).

Embryo microinjection of mosquito plays vital method as the beginning step in development of neoteric control strategies that are undergoing initial field trials. Using mosquito microinjection method *Wolbachia*-infected *Aedes* lines were created (Blagrove, Arias-Goeta, Failloux, & Sinkins, 2012; Joubert et al., 2016; Walker et al., 2011; Xi, Khoo, & Dobson, 2005). This protocol was important for successful gene manipulation of vectors (Jasinskiene, Juhn, & James, 2007) (Fig. 2.3).

Major determinants of egg microinjection techniques are physiology of eggs and its size. Other subsidiary factors include injection volume and pressure, and buffer used for pH maintenance. Different developmental phases of

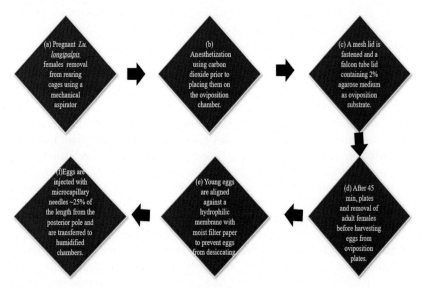

FIGURE 2.3   Important steps involved in protocol of microinjection of egg (Jeffries et al., 2018).

embryo are also vital as, younger eggs will cleave during injection while, melanized eggs with strong chorion prevents penetration of the needle.

This concludes that an egg microinjection procedure has the following elements:

1. Particular numbers of preblastoderm stage of insect eggs in a short span and,
2. Protocol for rapid injection of eggs with fertile G_o stage females (Jeffries et al., 2018).

This method had conquered the first barrier for microinjection of an egg in which young eggs of *L. longipalpis* can be harvested for microinjection. Changed protocol, derived from amalgamation of mosquito egg and *Drosophila* injection protocols, has pregnant sand fly females present with an oviposition substrate within small chambers. This resulted in rich oviposition although there is absence of a high concentration of degrading organic matter, which supports earlier research that volatiles of bacteria acts as a signal for oviposition (Peterkova-Koci, Robles-Murguia, Ramalho-Ortigao, & Zurek, 2012) instead of being directly required on oviposition surface (Jeffries et al., 2018). Tissue bent of *Wolbachia* variants in sand flies is important to determine whether development of *Leishmania* can be inhibited within the vector. As observed by (Dostálová & Volf, 2012), *Leishmania* development is restricted to the digestive tract associated with proteophosphogly and can present in anterior midgut which acts as a plug. Adherence of parasite to stomodeal valve injured the lining of chitin and resulted in regression of *Leishmania* from midgut. Hence, *Wolbachia* infections in the midgut of a sand fly, acts as a model for Drosophila *Wolbachia* variants in *Aedes aegypti* mosquitoes, which can lead to parasite inhibition (Jeffries et al., 2018; Walker et al., 2011).

2.1.1.6 Genetically modified insects using new tools such as CRISPR−Cas9 editing

The power to inject preblastoderm stage eggs provides a scope for gene level manipulation of sand flies. Successful nucleases like transcription activator-like effector nucleases frequently present interspaced short palindromic sequences (CRISPR−Cas9) in model organisms like *D. melanogaster* and has molded research into resettable gene drive systems in the wild insect population. CRISPR−Cas9 technology can be used to target all major vectors that transmit diseases (Bassett & Liu, 2014). For example, genome editing using CRISPR−Cas9 has been used for the prime vector of Zika and dengue viruses (Dostálová & Volf, 2012) and it was observed that female mosquitoes were converted into harmless (nonbiting) males (Hall et al., 2015). CRISPR−Cas9 was used to find application of transgenic gene drive systems in mosquito vectors for malaria and its ability to create aseptic female *Anopheles gambiae* with high conveyance around (> 90%) into progeny (Hammond et al., 2016; Jeffries et al., 2018).

Overall, the study details a novel procedure to alter blood fed flies and getting a high population of *L. longipalpis* eggs that are important for an egg microinjection. With this technique they proved postinfection, microinjection using *Wolbachia* like a marker in initial generations and evidence that bacteria can replicate and can be maternally inherited in *L. longipalpis*. However, low viability after injection including complexity of sand flies makes *Wolbachia* transinfected lines and gene manipulation a difficult procedure. With all these barriers, this procedure offers a new horizon to use *Wolbachia* as a biocontrol agent and for genetic manipulation of leishmaniasis vector (Bassett & Liu, 2014; Jeffries et al., 2018).

2.1.1.7 Analysis of metagenomic profile of taxa linked with sand fly L. longipalpis

Discovery of microbial community linked with vectors in specimens can aid in discovery of new methods for vector control and elimination. In this study, wild female and male *L. longipalpis* from VL location were used. Total RNA was isolated from insects and studied with unbiased high-throughput pyrosequencing, and subsequent analysis showed the presence of sequences from fungi, bacteria, protists, metazoans, and plants in Table 2.1 (McCarthy, Diambra, & Pomar, 2011). Metagenomics is a culture-independent examination of microbiota (Handelsman, 2005) aided by databases and tools of bioinformatics; an efficient approach that does not require previous knowledge of target group of organisms. Metagenomic sequencing of eukaryotic communities is mostly forbidden because of their large and complex genome sizes and coding regions (McCarthy et al., 2011; Thomas, 1971). Still, from a viewpoint, no inclusion of eukaryotes from a metagenomic analysis improves efficiency for identification of microbiota. To evade junk eukaryotic sequence, RNA sequencing data is preferred. In phlebotomine sand flies, the study associated or linked with flies refers to casual interlink because of casual environmental touch (e.g., pathogenic plant fungi spores attached to hairy surface of sand flies on sugar fed plant variety) to closer symbiotic interactions or pathogenic link (e.g., protists that effect phlebotomine or gut microbiota).

This examination revealed that sequences were of protists, bacteria, fungi, metazoans, and plants. RNA isolation and sequence amplification were key determinants of the experiment (Margulies et al., 2005). Vector sequences were very efficient and since it enabled identification of taxa around 0.00036%, the tse of RNA and mRNA was appropriate as many taxa were identified with homology (McCarthy et al., 2011). As a result, diversity of endemic and nonendemic areas of bacterial, fungal, protist, plant, and metazoan sequences in wild adult *L. longipalpis* mostly provides information on their feeding habits and behavior. It has significance in dispersal and

TABLE 2.1 Different taxa results identified by sequence homology with different databases (McCarthy et al., 2011).

Bacteria	Fungi	Protists	Metazoans	Plants
Ralstonia pickettii, Anoxybacillus flavithermus, Geobacillus kaustophilus, Streptomyces coelicolor, Propionibacterium acnes and Acinetobacter Baumannii	*Peronospora conglomerata, Cunninghamel-la bertholletiae, Mortierella verticillata and Toxicocladospo-rium Irritans*	Parasitise Diptera (*Ascogregarina taiwanensis, Psychodiellachagasi*), birds (*Eimeria tenella, Sarcocystisfalcatula, Sarcocystis cornixi*), mammals (*Cryptosporidium muris, Sarcocystis Arieticanis, Besnoitia besnoiti, Plasmodium falciparum, Plasmodium berghei*) and reptiles, birds, and mammals (*Sarcocystis sp.*)	*Homo sapiens, Gallus gallus and Anolis carolinensis*	*Elaeis guineensis, Capsicum annuum, Juglans hindsii, Artemisia annua, Brassica napus, Vitis vinifera, Solanum tuberosum, Nicotiana tabacum, Oryza sativa and Rhapidophy-lluhystrix*

transmission of this expanding disease due to its geographical location. Moreover, a larger number of species must be included to study the importance of metagenomic analysis of *L. longipalpis* results (McCarthy et al., 2011).

2.1.1.8   Transcriptomic study of male and female adult vectors of L. longipalpis *agent of VL*

An extensive transcriptomic method was used to analyze an infectious vector *L. longipalpis* in its habitat. Transcriptomic analysis shows characteristic profiles that correlated with their environment of origin. Various genes represent potential sites for vector control via RNA interference (RNAi) (McCarthy, Santini, Pimenta, & Diambra, 2013). For RNAi, dsRNA as a tool for sand fly population control, either one or in combination with other methods, putative targets were identified that affect survivorship, fecundity, and/or behavior. *L. longipalpis* transcripts linked to catalase, chitin, metabolism, GPCR, and chorion peroxidase were identified as potent targets for RNAi. Future studies will evaluate these gene targets, with special attention on avoiding effects like silencing or lethality of genes, in order to maximize the effect of specific gene silencing for the sand fly (Altschul et al., 1997; McCarthy et al., 2013) (Fig. 2.4).

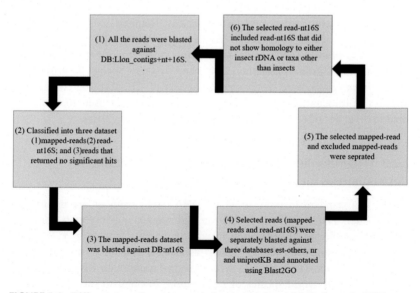

FIGURE 2.4   Different steps of sequence analysis using databases (McCarthy et al., 2013).

2.2   Identification of zoonotic reservoirs of leishmaniasis

2.2.1   Molecular assessment of *Leishmania tropica* and *Leishmania major* using nested PCR

To calculate frequency and to identify species of *Leishmania* and their reservoirs that infect humans and stray dogs, blood samples were collected from dogs and humans. Conventional polymerase chain reaction (PCR) linked with nested PCR showed presence of infection. Five dogs (1.6%) were infected by *L. tropica*, seven patients (25.9%) by *L. major* and *L. tropica* (Alanazi et al., 2019).

2.2.2   Molecular typing and isozymes analysis for species identification

A systematic evaluation of CL in Colombia was performed via molecular typing and isozyme analysis. *Leishmania* types from different sources like humans, sand flies, and other reservoirs were typed as *Leishmania brazilien-sis* 27.1% (88), *Leishmania panamensis* 61.3% (201), *Leishmania guyanensis* 0.9% (3), *Leishmania infantum Leishmania chagasi* 4% (12), *Leishmania lainsoni* 0.6% (2), *Leishmania mexicana* 2.1% (8), *Leishmania equatoriensis* 0.6% (2), *Leishmania amazonensis* 2.8% (9), and *Leishmania colombiensis* 0.6% (2) (Ramírez et al., 2016). Cyt b barcoding was performed and nine species associated with CL were detected. Genetic markers have been efficient for identification of *Leishmania*. The World Health Organization suggested MLEE (Multilocus Enzyme Electrophoresis) as the gold standard, still it is a time consuming process (Hernandez & Ramirez, 2013). Polymerase chain reaction-restriction fragment length polymorphism (PCR-RFLP) linked Heat Shock Protein (HSP) gene sequencing is an important technique for species typing (Auwera, Dujardin, 2015) and two new species *L. braziliensis* and *L. panamensis* were discovered as agents of CL. Cytb barcoding with MLST (Multilocus Sequence Typing) studies were also used to determine genetic diversity of an unknown species (Ramírez et al., 2016).

2.2.3   High resolution melting and multilocus enzyme electrophoresis for identification of species

MLEE is a standard method, in which DNA-based methods are used popularly (Dedet, 2002). PCR amplification and sequencing of Cyt b gene, are effective for species identification in wild varieties (Hernandez & Ramirez, 2013). High resolution melting (HRM) assay is a systematic procedure that targets HSP70 and ITS1. Primers were designed along with HRM analysis to discover six new world species of *Leishmania*. In order to finalize the algorithm, 35 natural isolates were studied which were obtained from mammals, human cases, and vectors. Genotyping assay allowed detection of *Leishmania* species (*L. infantum, L. mexicana, L. amazonensis, L. brazilien-sis, L. panamensis,* and *L. guyanensis*) based on standard types (Hernandez et al., 2014).

HRM is widely used in genotyping of fungi, bacteria protozoan parasites, and vertebrates (Hernandez et al., 2014; Higuera, Guhl, & Ramírez, 2013) and can be used for genotyping and detection of *Leishmania* variants (Myint et al., 2008). In conclusion, HRM assay is a powerful, quick and replicable technique that allows correct genotyping, less labor, and wide applications in different areas of molecular epidemiological studies (Hernandez et al., 2014).

2.3 Conclusion

Vector control strategies were very efficient in the past for controlling diseases like leishmaniasis. But mismanagement, low funded programs, and factors like ecology, insecticide resistance, and the increasing population are huge problems. So, the solution to this problem is effective implementation and finding novel tools and researches for vector and reservoir host control and management. This chapter summarized the neoteric control strategies like using *Wolbachia*, genetic level modification of insects, analysis taxa, creation of fluorescent model of sand fly and *Leishmania*, ITWL, and transcriptomic approach, etc. *Leishmania* reservoirs identification techniques such HRM, PCRs, nested PCRs, MLEE, and isozyme-based analysis were also discussed (Wilson et al., 2020).

Leishmaniasis research is of paramount importance for eco-epidemiological studies and requires standardized reservoir identification methods for eradication of leishmaniasis (Hernandez & Ramirez, 2013). The need of the hour is to discover novel vector control strategies and neoteric methods to identify zoonotic reservoirs and their transmissibility power. We should encourage scientific research communities to study leishmaniasis in order to fully validate surveillance and control tools at a continental level.

References

Abubakar, A., Ruiz-Postigo, J. A., Pita, J., Lado, M., Ben-Ismail, R., Argaw, D., & Alvar, J. (2014). Visceral leishmaniasis outbreak in South Sudan 2009−2012: Epidemiological assessment and impact of a multisectoral response. *PLoS Neglected Tropical Diseases, 8*(3).

Adler, S., & Theodor, O. (1935). Investigation on Mediterranean kala azar X- A note on Trypanosoma platydactyli and Leishmania tarentolæ. *Proceedings of the Royal Society of London. Series B-Biological Sciences, 116*(801), 543−544.

Akhoundi, M., Kuhls, K., Cannet, A., Votýpka, J., Marty, P., Delaunay, P., & Sereno, D. (2016). A historical overview of the classification, evolution, and dispersion of Leishmania parasites and sandflies. *PLoS Neglected Tropical Diseases, 10*(3).

Alanazi, A. D., Rahi, A. A., Ali, M. A., Alyousif, M. S., Alanazi, I. O., Mahmoud, M. S., & Alouffi, A. S. (2019). Molecular detection and phylogenetic analysis of Leishmania major in stray dogs in Riyadh Province, Saudi Arabia. *Tropical Biomedicine, 36*(2), 315−323.

Alemayehu, B., & Alemayehu, M. (2017). Leishmaniasis: a review on parasite, vector and reservoir host. *Health Science Journal, 11*(4), 1.

Aliota, M. T., Walker, E. C., Yepes, A. U., Velez, I. D., Christensen, B. M., & Osorio, J. E. (2016). The wMel strain of Wolbachia reduces transmission of chikungunya virus in Aedes aegypti. *PLoS Neglected Tropical Diseases, 10*(4).

Altschul, S. F., Madden, T. L., Schäffer, A. A., Zhang, J., Zhang, Z., Miller, W., & Lipman, D. J. (1997). Gapped BLAST and PSI-BLAST: A new generation of protein database search programs. *Nucleic Acids Research, 25*(17), 3389−3402.

Alvar, J., Vélez, I. D., Bern, C., Herrero, M., Desjeux, P., Cano, J., & WHO Leishmaniasis Control Team. (2012). Leishmaniasis worldwide and global estimates of its incidence. *PLoS One, 7*(5).

Bassett, A., & Liu, J. L. (2014). CRISPR/Cas9 mediated genome engineering in Drosophila. *Methods, 69*(2), 128−136.

Bern, C. (2015). Chagas' disease. *New England Journal of Medicine, 373*(5), 456−466.

Biswas, S., Subramanian, A., ELMojtaba, I. M., Chattopadhyay, J., & Sarkar, R. R. (2017). Optimal combinations of control strategies and cost-effective analysis for visceral leishmaniasis disease transmission. *PLoS One, 12*(2).

Blagrove, M. S., Arias-Goeta, C., Failloux, A. B., & Sinkins, S. P. (2012). Wolbachia strain wMel induces cytoplasmic incompatibility and blocks dengue transmission in Aedes albopictus. *Proceedings of the National Academy of Sciences, 109*(1), 255−260.

Cox, F. E. (Ed.), (2009). *Modern parasitology: A textbook of parasitology.* John Wiley & Sons.

Daszak, P., Cunningham, A. A., & Hyatt, A. D. (2001). Anthropogenic environmental change and the emergence of infectious diseases in wildlife. *Acta Tropica, 78*(2), 103−116.

De Oliveira, C. D., Gonçalves, D. D. S., Baton, L. A., Shimabukuro, P. H. F., Carvalho, F. D., & Moreira, L. A. (2015). Broader prevalence of Wolbachia in insects including potential human disease vectors. *Bulletin of Entomological Research, 105*(3), 305−315.

Dedet, J. P. (2002). Currentstatus of epidemiology of leishmaniases. In Leishmania (pp. 1-10). Springer, Boston, MA.

Diaz-Albiter, H. M., Regnault, C., Alpizar-Sosa, E. A., McGuinness, D., Barrett, M., & Dillon, R. J. (2018). Non-invasive visualisation and identification of fluorescent Leishmania tarentolae in infected sand flies. *Wellcome Open Research,* 3.

Dostálová, A., & Volf, P. (2012). Leishmania development in sand flies: Parasite-vector interactions overview. *Parasites & Vectors, 5*(1), 276.

Dutra, H. L. C., Rocha, M. N., Dias, F. B. S., Mansur, S. B., Caragata, E. P., & Moreira, L. A. (2016). Wolbachia blocks currently circulating Zika virus isolates in Brazilian Aedes aegypti mosquitoes. *Cell Host & Microbe, 19*(6), 771−774.

Hall, A. B., Basu, S., Jiang, X., Qi, Y., Timoshevskiy, V. A., Biedler, J. K., & Sharakhov, I. V. (2015). A male-determining factor in the mosquito Aedes aegypti. *Science, 348*(6240), 1268−1270.

Hammond, A., Galizi, R., Kyrou, K., Simoni, A., Siniscalchi, C., Katsanos, D., & Burt, A. (2016). A CRISPR-Cas9 gene drive system targeting female reproduction in the malaria mosquito vector Anopheles gambiae. *Nature Biotechnology, 34*(1), 78−83.

Handelsman, J. (2005). Metagenomics: Application of genomics to uncultured microorganisms. *Microbiology and Molecular Biology Reviews, 69*(1), 195-195.

Hemingway, J., & Ranson, H. (2000). Insecticide resistance in insect vectors of human disease. *Annual Review of Entomology, 45*(1), 371−391.

Hernandez, C., & Ramirez, J. D. (2013). Molecular diagnosis of vector-borne parasitic diseases. *Air & Water Borne Diseases, 2*, 1−10.

Hernandez, C., Alvarez, C., González, C., Ayala, M. S., Leon, C. M., & Ramírez, J. D. (2014). Identification of six New World Leishmania species through the implementation of a High-Resolution Melting (HRM) genotyping assay. *Parasites & Vectors, 7*(1), 501.

Higuera, S. L., Guhl, F., & Ramírez, J. D. (2013). Identification of Trypanosoma cruzi Discrete Typing Units (DTUs) through the implementation of a High-Resolution Melting (HRM) genotyping assay. *Parasites & Vectors, 6*(1), 112.

Hilgenboecker, K., Hammerstein, P., Schlattmann, P., Telschow, A., & Werren, J. H. (2008). How many species are infected with Wolbachia? a statistical analysis of current data. *FEMS Microbiology Letters, 281*(2), 215−220.

Huda, M. M., Kumar, V., Das, M. L., Ghosh, D., Priyanka, J., Das, P., & Mondal, D. (2016). Entomological efficacy of durable wall lining with reduced wall surface coverage for strengthening visceral leishmaniasis vector control in Bangladesh, India and Nepal. *BMC Infectious Diseases, 16*(1), 539.

Jansen, A. M., & Roque, A. L. R. (2010). Dostic and wild mammalian reservoirs. In J. Telleria, & M. Tibayrenc (Eds.), *American trypanosomiasis: Chagas disease one hundred years of research*.

Jasinskiene, N., Juhn, J., & James, A. A. (2007). Microinjection of A. aegypti embryos to obtain transgenic mosquitoes. *JoVE (Journal of Visualized Experiments), 5*, e219.

Jeffries, C. L., Rogers, M. E., & Walker, T. (2018). Establishment of a method for Lutzomyia longipalpis sand fly egg microinjection: The first step towards potential novel control strategies for leishmaniasis. *Wellcome Open Research, 3*.

Joubert, D. A., Walker, T., Carrington, L. B., De Bruyne, J. T., Kien, D. H. T., Hoang, N. L. T., & O'Neill, S. L. (2016). Establishment of a Wolbachia superinfection in Aedes aegypti mosquitoes as a potential approach for future resistance management. *PLoS Pathogens, 12*(2).

Kumar, A., Pandey, S. C., & Samant, M. (2018). Slow pace of antileishmanial drug development. *Parasitology Open, 4*(4), 1−11.

Lemma, W., Bizuneh, A., Tekie, H., Belay, H., Wondimu, H., Kassahun, A., & Hailu, A. (2017). Preliminary study on investigation of zoonotic visceral leishmaniasis in endemic foci of Ethiopia by detecting Leishmania infections in rodents. *Asian Pacific Journal of Tropical Medicine, 10*(4), 418−422.

Margulies, M., Egholm, M., Altman, W. E., Attiya, S., Bader, J. S., Bemben, L. A., & Dewell, S. B. (2005). Genome sequencing in microfabricated high-density picolitre reactors. *Nature, 437*(7057), 376−380.

McCarthy, C. B., Diambra, L. A., & Pomar, R. V. R. (2011). Metagenomic analysis of taxa associated with Lutzomyia longipalpis, vector of visceral leishmaniasis, using an unbiased high-throughput approach. *PLoS Neglected Tropical Diseases, 5*(9).

McCarthy, C. B., Santini, M. S., Pimenta, P. F., & Diambra, L. A. (2013). First comparative transcriptomic analysis of wild adult male and female Lutzomyia longipalpis, vector of visceral leishmaniasis. *PLoS One, 8*(3).

Messenger, L. A., & Rowland, M. (2017). Insecticide-treated durable wall lining (ITWL): Futureprospects for control of malaria and other vector-borne diseases. *Malaria Journal, 16* (1), 213.

Mondal, D., Das, M. L., Kumar, V., Huda, M. M., Das, P., Ghosh, D., & Chowdhury, R. (2016). Efficacy, safety and cost of insecticide treated wall lining, insecticide treated bed nets and indoor wall wash with lime for visceral leishmaniasis vector control in the Indian sub-continent: A multi-country cluster randomized controlled trial. *PLoS Neglected Tropical Diseases, 10*(8).

Moreira, L. A., Iturbe-Ormaetxe, I., Jeffery, J. A., Lu, G., Pyke, A. T., Hedges, L. M., & Hugo, L. E. (2009). A Wolbachia symbiont in Aedes aegypti limits infection with dengue, Chikungunya, and Plasmodium. *Cell, 139*(7), 1268−1278.

Myint, C. K., Asato, Y., Yamamoto, Y. I., Kato, H., Bhutto, A. M., Soomro, F. R., & Katakura, K. (2008). Polymorphisms of cytochrome b gene in Leishmania parasites and their relation to types of cutaneous leishmaniasis lesions in Pakistan. *The Journal of Dermatology, 35*(2), 76−85.

Pandey, S. C., Pande, V., & Samant, M. (2020). DDX3 DEAD-box RNA helicase (Hel67) gene disruption impairs infectivity of Leishmania donovani and induces protective immunity against visceral leishmaniasis. *Scientific Reports, 10*(1), 18218. Available from https://doi.org/10.1038/s41598-020-75420-y.

Peterkova-Koci, K., Robles-Murguia, M., Ramalho-Ortigao, M., & Zurek, L. (2012). Significance of bacteria in oviposition and larval development of the sand fly Lutzomyia longipalpis. *Parasites & Vectors, 5*(1), 145.

Picado, A., Dash, A. P., Bhattacharya, S., & Boelaert, M. (2012). Vector control interventions for visceral leishmaniasis elimination initiative in South Asia, 2005-2010. *The Indian Journal of Medical Research, 136*(1), 22.

Ramírez, J. D., Hernández, C., León, C. M., Ayala, M. S., Flórez, C., & González, C. (2016). Taxonomy, diversity, temporal and geographical distribution of Cutaneous Leishmaniasis in Colombia: A retrospective study. *Scientific Reports, 6*, 28266.

Raymond, R. W., McHugh, C. P., Witt, L. R., & Kerr, S. F. (2003). Temporal and spatial distribution of Leishmania mexicana infections in a population of Neotoma micropus. *Memórias do Instituto Oswaldo Cruz, 98*(2), 171−180.

Ready, P. D. (2013). Biology of phlebotomine sand flies as vectors of disease agents. *Annual Review of Entomology, 58*.

Roque, A. L. R., & Jansen, A. M. (2014). Wild and synanthropic reservoirs of Leishmania species in the Americas. *International Journal for Parasitology: Parasites and Wildlife, 3*(3), 251−262.

Sant'Anna, M. R., Darby, A. C., Brazil, R. P., Montoya-Lerma, J., Dillon, V. M., Bates, P. A., & Dillon, R. J. (2012). Investigation of the bacterial communities associated with females of Lutzomyia sand fly species from South America. *PLoS One, 7*(8).

Soares, R. P., & Turco, S. J. (2003). Lutzomyia longipalpis (Diptera: psychodidae: phlebotominae): a review. *Anais da Academia Brasileira de Ciências, 75*(3), 301−330.

Stockdale, L., & Newton, R. (2013). A review of preventative methods against human leishmaniasis infection. *PLoS Neglected Tropical Diseases, 7*(6).

Tan, C. H., Wong, P. J., Li, M. I., Yang, H., Ng, L. C., & O'Neill, S. L. (2017). wMel limits zika and chikungunya virus infection in a Singapore Wolbachia-introgressed Ae. aegypti strain, wMel-Sg. *PLoS Neglected Tropical Diseases, 11*(5), e0005496.

Thomas, C. A., Jr (1971). The genetic organization of chromosomes. *Annual Review of Genetics, 5*(1), 237−256.

Van der Auwera, G., & Dujardin, J. C. (2015). Species typing in dermal leishmaniasis. *Clinical Microbiology Reviews, 28*(2), 265−294.

Volf, P., & Peckova, J. (2007). Sand flies and Leishmania: Specific versus permissive vectors. *Trends in Parasitology, 23*(3), 91.

WHO Leishmaniasis (2018).<https://www.who.int/leishmaniasis/en/> Accessed 1.04.20.

Walker, T. J. P. H., Johnson, P. H., Moreira, L. A., Iturbe-Ormaetxe, I., Frentiu, F. D., McMeniman, C. J., & Lloyd, A. L. (2011). The w Mel Wolbachia strain blocks dengue and invades caged Aedes aegypti populations. *Nature*, *476*(7361), 450−453.

WHO Expert Committee on the Control of the Leishmaniases. Meeting, & World Health Organization. (2010). *Control of the Leishmaniases: Report of a meeting of the who expert committee on the control of Leishmaniases*, Geneva, 22−26 March 2010 (Vol. 949). World Health Organization.

Wilson, A. L., Courtenay, O., Kelly-Hope, L. A., Scott, T. W., Takken, W., Torr, S. J., & Lindsay, S. W. (2020). The importance of vector control for the control and elimination of vector-borne diseases. *PLoS Neglected Tropical Diseases*, *14*(1), e0007831.

Xi, Z., Khoo, C. C., & Dobson, S. L. (2005). Wolbachia establishment and invasion in an Aedes aegypti laboratory population. *Science*, *310*(5746), 326−328.

Zamir, M., Zaman, G., & Alshomrani, A. S. (2016). Sensitivity analysis and optimal control of Anthroponotic Cutaneous Leishmania. *PLoS One*, *11*(8).

Chapter 3

Recent advances in the diagnostic methods of Leishmaniasis

Prashant Khare and Utkarsha Sahu
Department of Microbiology, All India Institute of Medical Sciences, Bhopal, India

3.1 Introduction

Leishmaniasis, is a protozoan disease caused by the parasite *Leishmania* which belongs to the *Trypanosomatidae* family. They are mainly characterized by the presence of kinetoplast mitochondrial DNA (Sharma & Singh, 2008). The disease is widely distributed globally which covers around 97 countries including Asia, Africa, Europe, and America (Steverding, 2017). Leishmaniasis is present mainly in three forms viz., Visceral Leishmaniasis (VL), Cutaneous Leishmaniasis (CL), and Mucocutaneous Leishmaniasis (MCL) (Thakur, Joshi, & Kaur, 2020). Among them VL is the most fatal form of Leishmaniasis. In India, VL is the most prevalent in the eastern region of the country, mainly west Bengal, Jharkhand, Uttar Pradesh, and Bihar (Thakur et al., 2018). Bihar is the most effected state with 90% of the VL cases were reported (Perry et al., 2013). *Leishmania* parasite has two hosts, sand flies and mammals and it has two forms; the flagellated promastigotes and round, tiny shaped amastigotes (Sunter & Gull, 2017). The several clinical manifestations happen due to the involvement of *Leishmania* species. The therapeutic and prophylactic approaches are not satisfactory to cure this disease (Kumar, Pandey, & Samant, 2018; Murray, 2001). Thus diagnosis of Leishmaniasis is an important step for successful eradication and mainly depends on clinical signs, laboratory diagnosis, parasitological or serological confirmation, and by molecular confirmation (Kumar, Pandey, & Samant, 2020a, 2020b; Thakur et al., 2020). Since the symptoms occur during *Leishmania*, infection is pretty much similar to a variety of other infections that could lead to a misdiagnosis hence high sensitivity and high specificity tests are required (Chappuis et al., 2007).

Pathogenesis, Treatment and Prevention of Leishmaniasis. DOI: https://doi.org/10.1016/B978-0-12-822800-5.00002-0
45

Laboratory and parasitological diagnosis are still considered to be the gold standard due to economic values and high specificity. These tests mainly depend on identification of *Leishmania* parasites through a microscope from the tissue aspirates of lymph nodes, bone marrow, and spleen (Sundar & Rai, 2002). However, it has several disadvantages; due to it being an invasive painful procedure as it needs biopsy of affected organs which may lead to the possibility of bleeding. Also there are few concerns related with variation of sensitivity for different types of samples (De Ruiter et al., 2014). Various serological tests are being used for identification of *Leishmania* parasite in clinical practices that are mainly based on antibody/antigen detection (Sundar & Rai, 2002). Serological assays are widely used in endemic areas of *Leishmania* infections. These methods are sensitive, convenient, and affordable. They are known such as latex agglutination test (LAT), indirect fluorescent antibody test (IFAT), direct agglutination test (DAT), enzyme-linked immunosorbent assay (ELISA), immunoblotting and immunochromatographic test (ICT) like rK39 strip-based assay, however they have a few disadvantages: (1) they can't detect relapses condition after cure, (2) cross-reactivity observed with closely related species, (3) antibody titers in endemic contacts as well as in asymptomatic patients, and (4) less accuracy reported in *Leishmania*−HIV coinfection patients. Molecular methods have come up a new challenging tool for *Leishmania* diagnosis and are currently being used due to various limitations observed in conventional methods (Sundar & Singh, 2018). These molecular approaches are capable of detecting nucleic acid of parasites even in lesser numbers, addressing traditional assay's limitations (Verweij & Stensvold, 2014). Various methods of nucleic acid detection have been developed that can target both DNA and RNA. So far, various molecular methods viz. polymerase chain reaction (PCR), quantitative polymerase chain reaction (QPCR), Nucleic Acid Sequence Based Amplification (NASBA), Loop-Mediated Isothermal Amplification (LAMP), Random Amplified Polymorphic DNA (RAPD)/Amplified Fragment Length Polymorphism (AFLP), and MICROARRAY have been developed and proven with their high sensitivity and specificity for the detection of *Leishmania* parasite even a few weeks ahead of clinical manifestation or disease pathology. Here in this chapter we are discussing the updated knowledge of available diagnostic tools and their limitations for detection of *Leishmania* parasite.

3.2 Laboratory diagnosis

3.2.1 Microscopic examination

Microscopic examination is a well-established old tool used for the identification of *Leishmania* parasite. Identification of the amastigote form of the *Leishmania* parasite, microscopically from the tissue aspirates of spleen, bone marrow, or lymph nodes is still considered suitable for *Leishmania* diagnosis. Due to its high specificity, high sensitivity, and the ability to detect the parasite load, the technique is advantageous now days (Siddig, Ghalib, Shillington, & Petersen, 1988). However, the procedure is invasive and involves high risk for internal bleeding during splenic aspiration and is also not compatible in the field setting because of the requirement of slides/reagents. It also requires a well-trained microscopist for an accurate diagnosis. Another way to diagnose is the culture of parasites isolated from tissue aspirates, however it is restricted to major referral labs because it's tedious and an expensive procedure. Several advancements have been made in this area such as isolation of *Leishmania* by microculture method (Allahverdiyev et al., 2005), application of buffy coat, and peripheral blood mononuclear cells isolation taken from the patient's blood for the diagnosis of *Leishmania* (Maurya et al., 2010).

3.2.2   Culture characteristics

The sensitivity for *Leishmania* parasite identification could be improved by various culture methods. The promastigotes form of *Leishmania* parasite can be grown in artificial culture medium (Sundar & Rai, 2002). Various culture media are currently being used viz. bemonophasic (M199, Grace's medium and Schneider's insect medium) or diphasic (Novy-McNeal Nicolle medium and Tobies medium), Roswell Park Memorial Institute (RPMI) 1640 (Gibco BRL, Grand Island, NY) (Pandey, Pande, & Samant, 2020), and M199 medium containing 20% fetal calf serum to boost up parasite growth (Sundar et al., 2001). Hockmeyer's medium, modified form of Schneider's culture medium containing 30% heat-inactivated fetal calf serum with penicillin and streptomycin antibiotics, is very easy to use and effective for diagnosis of VL, however, it is expensive (Hockmeyer, Kager, Rees, & Hendricks, 1981). The pH and temperature play a crucial role for the growth of *Leishmania* parasite. The culture should be kept at 26°C−28°C for splenic/bone marrow aspirates (BMAs) up to 4 weeks before being discarded as negative. Contamination in parasite culture or in the culture media can be treated and avoided by adding penicillin (200 IU/mL) and streptomycin (200 μg/mL) to the medium (for bacteria), as well as 5-flucytosine (500 μg/mL) (as an antimycotic agent) (Claborn, 2010). In the case of amastigotes *in vitro* culture, various macrophages adherent cells are being used, for example, P388D and J774G8 or they can be grown in human peripheral blood monocytes (Grogl, Daugirda, Hoover, Magill, & Berman, 1993). For *in vivo* maintenance of *Leishmania* parasites, the golden hamster is the widely accepted animal model for maintaining *Leishmania donovani* complex (Bray). It can be infected via many routes, however the intracardiac route is the most preferred one. Both forms of parasites, amastigotes and promastigotes, can be used to infect the hamster. Due to morphologically similarity, the species level of identification of *Leishmania* complex is difficult, although few methods are in the process such as cellulose acetate electrophoresis (Kreutzer et al., 1993), DAT with species-specific monoclonal antibodies (Jaffe & Sarfstein, 1987), minicircle kinetoplast DNA (kDNA)(Maurya et al., 2010; Sacks et al., 1995), and analysis of released antigenic factors (Ilg, Stierhof, Wiese, Mcconville, & Overath, 1994). Moreover, if the parasite load is less, the mini and microculture techniques are useful because of being economical, easy to handle, and require only a small volume of culture medium (Boggild et al., 2008). While in the case of amastigotes, identification needs considerable training and expertise. Overall, culturing parasites for their identification and diagnosis is time consuming and requires expensive equipment, but still they are in clinical practice.

3.3 Serological diagnosis

Due to various limitations of laboratory diagnosis, serological methods were developed. These techniques rely on detection of antibodies in the serum of *Leishmania* patients. Earlier crude or total antigens were used for the identification of *Leishmania*-specific antibodies, however recombinant antigens have good sensitivity and specificity and now are incorporated in immunological diagnosis. Currently recombinant antigens, a kinesin-related protein, rK39, has shown better results and has been accepted widely in the form of immunochromatographic strip test for the rapid, easy to operate *Leishmania* diagnosis (Srividya, Kulshrestha, Singh, & Salotra, 2012).

3.3.1 Indirect fluorescent antibody test

This test depicts promising sensitivity and specificity (77%−100%) for *Leishmania* diagnosis (Boelaert et al., 2004; Iqbal et al., 2002) due to less cross-reactivity with trypanosomal sera promastigote forms of *Leishmania* and should be used for the diagnosis of Leishmaniasis (Badaro, Reed, & Carvalho, 1983). The low titer of antibodies observed in the sera of patients after the treatment clearly indicates a probable relapse. Mostly the antibody response is in the early course of infection and reaches to undetectable up to 9 months after the infection (Singh & Sivakumar, 2003). For this type of test a well-equipped fluorescence microscope is needed.

3.3.2 ELISA

ELISA have been used and played an important role in *Leishmania* diagnosis. Various Leishmanial antigens/proteins have been reported to generate antibody-mediated humoral immune responses in *Leishmania* patients, including ribosomal proteins, surface antigens, histones, kinesin-related proteins, and nuclear proteins, hence showing their diagnostic potential. rK39 along with other kinesin-related proteins such as KRP42, K26, K9, and

KE16 have been validated for their immunodiagnostic potential by ELISA (Mohapatra, Singh, Sen, Bharti, & Sundar, 2010; Sivakumar, Sharma, Chang, & Singh, 2006; Takagi et al., 2007). The amastigote-specific protein (A2) and amastin were also found to induce an antibody response and have shown sensitivity in different regions (Carvalho, Charest, & Tavares, 2002; Ghedin et al., 1997; Rafati et al., 2006). The molecular chaperones known as heat-shock proteins (HSPs) such as HSP70 and HSP83 and also histone proteins H2A, H2B, H3, and H4 which are conserved throughout the evolutionary process have also shown their potential for the diagnosis of Leishmaniasis (Amorim, Carrington, Miles, Barker, & De Almeida, 1996; Perez-Alvarez, Larreta, Alonso, & Requena, 2001). Humoral immune response is also observed against few antigens such as lipid-binding proteins and 9-O-acetylated sialic acid (Bandyopadhyay et al., 2004; Maache et al., 2005). The biggest disadvantage of serological diagnosis is to distinguish between past infections with asymptomatic cases due to the presence of antibodies during the course of time, even after the treatment. Hence a combinatorial approach is needed which can distinguish between asymptomatic and cured Leishmaniasis patients.

3.3.3   Western blotting or immunoblotting

Western blotting or immunoblotting assay is broadly used for the accurate *Leishmania* diagnosis. This is based on the conjugation of immobilized protein/antigen with respective antibodies. Proteins are isolated after the lysis of promastigotes or amastigotes forms of *Leishmania* parasite and then separated on SDS-PAGE. To make separated protein immobilized, they are electro transferred onto a polyvinylidene fluoride or nitrocellulose membrane and finally probed with patient's sera in different dilutions. The technique is more sensitive as compared to IFAT and ELISA and offers meticulous antibody responses against several Leishmanial proteins. It is also a great tool for the diagnosis of *Leishmania*−HIV coinfections (Cota, De Sousa, Demarqui, & Rabello, 2012; Mary, Lamouroux, Dunan, & Quilici, 1992; Santos-Gomes, Gomes-Pereira, Campino, Araujo, & Abranches, 2000). The major limitation of this technique is that it is not cost effective and has a cumbersome process.

3.3.4   Direct agglutination test/latex agglutination test

DAT is an easy to implement, broadly relevant technique having high sensitivity (around 90%−100%) and specificity (95%−100%) and has been applicable for the past two decades (El Harith, El Mutasim, Mansour, Fadil Mustafa, & Arvidson, 2003; El Mutasim, Mansour, Abass, Hassan, & El Harith, 2006; Jacquet et al., 2006; Sreenivas et al., 2002). The assay can be performed with serum, plasma, and also urine samples, indicating its suitability in both laboratory application and field area (Bhattarai, Auwera, & Khanal, 2009; Chappuis, Rijal, & Jha, 2006; Mandal et al., 2008; Oliveira, Pedras, De Assis, & Rabello, 2009; Sundar et al., 2007). LAT, such as KAtex test, is used to identify non-protein antigens of *Leishmania* in urine samples engaging latex beads which are presensitized *L. donovani* antigen antibodies (El-Safi et al., 2003; Vilaplana et al., 2004). This assay is mainly used and developed for rapid diagnosis and can detect anti-*Leishmania* antibodies generated against the A2 protein of amastigote form. It also has been found to detect crude antigens of the promastigote form from an Iranian strain of *L. infantum*. In another study having comparison with the DAT, showed the sensitivity of human sera tested with DAT yielded 88.4% while the specificity reported around 93.5% on A2-LAT amastigote (Akhoundi et al., 2013; Ghatei, Hatam, Hossini, & Sarkari, 2009). LAT has more sensitivity in the comparison with DAT and it was observed around 88.4% while specificity was 93.5% (Akhoundi et al., 2013). In another study, kala-azar LAT (Katex) was evaluated and has shown the sensitivity was average, that is, 75%, however specificity was observed 100% resulting in restrictions of the use of KAtex due to less sensitivity (Salam et al., 2012). Currently, this test is suitable for the *Leishmania* diagnosis where no antibody production is reported. Furthermore, the LAT is simple, rapid, easy to perform, inexpensive, and reliable a screening test. Recently so many efforts have been made for the advancement of this technique, due to its feasibility in developing countries (Srivastava, Dayama, Mehrotra, & Sundar, 2011).

3.3.5   Immunochromatographic

The ICT is mainly a strip-based test and currently being broadly accepted due to its usage in field area. rK39 antigen (39 amino-acid-repeat recombinant Leishmanial antigen from *Leishmania chagasi*) has been widely used in the past few years. It is a membrane-based qualitative test where rK39 antigen is impregnated with nitrocellulose strips. This test basically identifies the antibodies generated against K 39 antigens in patient's sera. The rK39 strips sensitivity and specificity various among different populations. It has been reported in India that sensitivity was 100% and specificity was 93%−98% (Sundar, Pai, Sahu, Kumar, & Murray, 2002; Sundar, Reed, Singh, Kumar, & Murray, 1998), while in the case of Brazil the sensitivity was 90% and specificity was 100% however in the Mediterranean area the 100% sensitivity and specificity was observed (Otranto, Paradies, Sasanelli, Spinelli, & Brandonisio, 2004). However, in southern Europe, it was found that 71.4% of the cases of VL; in Sudan, rK39 IC showed a sensitivity of 67% (Zijlstra et al., 2001). These variations in sensitivity could be observed due to differences in ethnicity. Furthermore, this is the only assay that has proven to be used in the field area in a rapid manner of testing with its acceptable specificity and sensitivity and also gives reproducible results.

3.3.6   Antigen detection

Earlier reports have shown the use of Leishmanial antigens for the *Leishmania* diagnosis. The 72−75 kDa and 123 kDa, two fractions of polypeptide were found in the urine of kala-azar patients (De Colmenares et al., 1995). In another study published by 2002, Sarkari et al. described heat stable antigens that are carbohydrate-based in a urine ranging from 5 to 20 kDa, of VL patients (Sarkari, Chance, & Hommel, 2002). In another report, a heat-stable and low molecular weight carbohydrate Leishmanial antigen, has been identified in the urine sample of VL patients confirmed by an agglutination test. The sensitivity of both fractions were found 60%−71% and specificity was 79%−94% respectively (Boelaert et al., 2004).

3.4   Molecular diagnosis

The discovery of molecular methods (Tlamcani, 2016) has evolved due to certain constraints and limitations in the conventional parasitological and serological techniques for the diagnosis of Leishmaniasis (De Paiva-Cavalcanti et al., 2015). Molecular assays are suggested nowadays specially for CL due to their high accuracy and rapid results (Azizi, Soltani, & Alipour, 2012). Molecular methods of diagnosis for Leishmaniasis become an alternative method of diagnosis due to their safety, feasibility, and reproducibility worldwide.

3.4.1   Polymerase chain reaction

PCR is an early and main detection technique that offers very rapid results that are reliable and sensitive for the diagnosis of *Leishmania* infection. Several targets or genes of interest were identified and validated for human and canine VL diagnosis. It mainly involves kDNA (Cortes, Rolão, Ramada, & Campino, 2004; Maurya et al., 2005; Salotra et al., 2001); ribosomal RNA genes (Lachaud et al., 2000; Srivastava, Mehrotra, Tiwary, Chakravarty, & Sundar, 2011); internal transcribed spacer regions (Mauricio, Stothard, & Miles, 2004; Schönian, et al., 2003); genomic repeats (Kuhls et al., 2007); miniexon-derived RNA (med RNA) genes, glycoprotein 63 (gp63) gene locus (Guerbouj et al., 2001; Quispe Tintaya et al., 2004); and the β-tubulin gene region (Akman L et al., 2000; Dey & Singh, 2007). The conventional PCR methods are still promising due to several advancements such as (1) early parasite detection even before any pathologies or clinical signs; (2) can be used in different clinical substances viz. urine, peripheral blood, serum, bone marrow, lymph node, and skin, etc.; (3) analysis of biopsy samples, formalin-fixed tissue, skin biopsy, and Giemsa-stained of BMAs is possible through PCR; and (4) monitoring of the parasite load with PCR.

3.4.2   Q-PCR

Q-PCR or real-time PCR is a useful molecular tool for quantitation and rapid identification of *Leishmania* parasite. This technique relies upon evaluation of fluorescent signals produced during target amplification. SYBR green-based Q-PCR assay is widely used for detection and *Leishmania* parasites load in VL and post-kala-azar dermal Leishmaniasis (PKDL) clinical samples using kDNA specific primers (Verma et al., 2010). This is also used by multiplex to determine bacterial and *Leishmania* coinfection from blood/BMA (Selvapandiyan et al., 2005; Selvapandiyan et al., 2008). Q-PCR multiplexing using two-cysteine proteinase (CPB) isogene can detect *L. donovani* complex within the species and intraspecies groups (Quispe Tintaya et al., 2004). Although this data suggests the importance of real-time PCR for accurate and rapid diagnosis of *Leishmania*. However, it requires well-equipped laboratories and regents which is very expensive and big hurdle for developing or low-income countries. More advancement is still needed. A very sensitive *Leishmania*-specific PCR known as oligochromatographic test (*Leishmania* OligoC-test) is now validated and established which mainly targets a short sequence within the *Leishmania* 18S rRNA gene (Basiye et al., 2010; Deborggraeve et al., 2008; Saad et al., 2010).

3.4.3   Nucleic acid sequence-based amplification

NASBA is a transcription-based amplification and isothermal complex method created to determine the RNA target (Van Der Meide et al., 2008). It has mainly two modifications viz. quantitative-NASBA (QT-NASBA) and paired with oligochromatography (NASBA-OC). Viability of *Leishmania* parasite is required for the assessment drug efficacy and expecting outcomes after treatment (Reithinger & Dujardin, 2007). Recently reports suggest that QT-NASBA can be used to detect 100-fold lower parasite load than detected by normal PCR. They observed sensitivity was 97.5% and specificity was 100%, respectively (Van Der Meide et al., 2008). This is the only isothermal amplification technique that uses RNA as a starting material; however, presence of ribonuclease contamination limits its applicability (Zanoli & Spoto, 2013). QT-NASBA has been successfully adopted in the case of visceral Leishmaniasis for the quantification parasites after treatment (De Vries et al., 2006; Van Der Meide et al., 2008; Van Der Meide, Schoone, & Faber, 2005) while NASBA-OC is used to a better tool to identify active disease and can also be used as a test for a cure (Basiye et al., 2010; Saad et al., 2010).

3.4.4   RAPD/AFLP

Randomly amplified polymorphic DNA (RAPD)

RAPD is involved in the amplification of DNA by PCR using arbitrary short primer. These short sequence primers can be used for any genetic material of an organism even with an unknown target sequence. RAPD can be used alone or with the combination with some other techniques to validate the differences that occur at intraspecific and interspecific *Leishmania* species (Botilde et al., 2006). This method has been used for identification of *Leishmania tropica*, a causative agents for CL in Iran. Although for getting accurate specificity; it requires pure Leishmanial DNA and optimum PCR conditions (Akhoundi et al., 2017).

Amplified fragment length polymorphism (AFLP)

AFLP is more advanced technique compare to RAPD for identification of variations in strains or closely related species (Kumar et al., 2010). Basically, it's a combination of RAPD and RFLP. Firstly, restriction enzymes are used for the digestion of genomic DNA followed by selective PCR amplification of digested fragments. This is a very more reproducible, sensitive, and convenient method for identification of polymorphic DNA fragments of an unknown sequence in *Leishmania* species. (Kumar et al., 2010). AFLP is widely used for phylogenetic analysis and in genetics of many organisms (Bensch, Åkesson, 2005). Recently Kumar et al. showed genetic variations between *Leishmania major* and *L. tropica* (Kumar et al., 2010). In another study, AFLP is used to characterize genetic diversity between *Leishmania panamensis* and *Leishmania guyanens* which is isolated from Panamanian CL patients (Restrepo et al., 2013).

3.4.5 Loop-mediated isothermal amplification

Recently Loop-mediated isothermal amplification (LAMP) of DNA has emerged as a novel tool for the diagnosis of Leishmaniasis (Adams, Schoone, Ageed, Safi, & Schallig, 2010; Notomi, Okayama, & Masubuchi, 2000) under isothermal conditions. Since the reaction happens in isothermal conditions, hence no thermal cycle is required. This method is highly specific (requires six primers), more economical, fast and requires no specific equipment. Moreover, the reagents used for LAMP assay do not require cold chain due to stability at room temperature (Takagi et al., 2009). In this method RNA is used in amplification process and increases its sensitivity (Adams et al., 2010). This assay was used in patients with suffering from PKDL and VL and observed to have good sensitivity of 96.4%−98.5% in blood samples of VL, 96.8%−98.5% in samples of tissue biopsy and 96.8% for PKDL cases (Verma et al., 2013). In another study in the Sudan, a specificity of 99.01% and sensitivity of 100% was depicted (Mukhtar et al., 2018).

3.4.6 Microarray

DNA microarray is a technology that utilizes base-pairing (A-T and G-C for DNA; A-U and G-C for RNA) mechanism to monitor and identify a large number of single nucleotide polymorphisms on a single chip of an organism genome. In this method the samples to be analyzed are arranged in a sequence to provide a medium for examination of known and unknown DNA samples allowing complementary base-pairing which can detect the unknown sample automatically (Govindarajan, Duraiyan, Kaliyappan, & Palanisamy, 2012). This method can be utilized for detection of gene sequence and checking of their expression level as well. In addition to this it can be widely employed in parasitology research for identification of drug targets, vaccine candidates, and marker genes (Pandey, Kumar, & Samant, 2020; Kumar et al., 2020a, 2020b).

3.4.6.1 Parasite development and life cycle

Variations in expression of genes during different stages of parasite life cycle could be estimated by transcriptional profiling, thus providing a new tool to study parasite development. Genes involved in initial development of parasite and during later stages can be recognized by gene expression patterns after exposure to the number of developmental stimulates like malnourishment and drug treatment. However, the major drawback of this technique is the ability to produce satisfactory amounts and quantities of RNA for analysis. Also, the complexity of attaining the desired quality and quantity of RNA is under a development. In bigger scale *in vitro* parasite culture this problem could be addressed by using parasites-based phase-specific molecular markers for selectively differentiation. However, the other manipulation such as RNA preparation should be minimal to avoid the changes in gene expression (Kumar et al., 2020a, 2020b).

3.4.6.2 Host responses to infection

Host parasite interactions are crucial for parasitology studies. The host gene array complements to the parasite gene array and studying the host cell undergoing infection, transcription profiling, growth latency, and mortality gives a clear idea about the development and survival of parasites in the host cell. These interactions can be explored by three ways: (1) Understanding and establishment of parasite infection in the host cell and initiation of an immune response; (2) Induction of immune responses stimulated by parasite; (3) Determining if the host transcripts facilitate the host or the parasite. The closely connected genes may have some difficulty. It should be assured that the signal detected is not because of cross-hybridization between host DNA printed on the microarray and parasite transcripts. The ribosomal protein genes are the among the ones that are highly conserved, hence hybridization could occur between them (Diehn et al., 2000). The host genes controlled during parasitic infection are broadly divided into three different categories: pro-host genes that increases host survival, pro-parasite genes which increases the survival of parasite, and the bystander genes that are regulated during regulation of first two genes. Microarray-based tests are based on the involvement of transcripts and pathways that offer several reporter assays, supporting in the detection of these factors (Boothroyd, Blader, Cleary, & Singh, 2003).

3.4.6.3   Vaccine target identification

Exploring the potential vaccine target and development of vaccine against *Leishmania* parasite is the leading objective of *Leishmania* research. The *Leishmania* genes transcriptional activity can be studied using GeneChip arrays under *in vivo* conditions. Also, the rarely expressing but potentially important genes could be identified by these arrays. DNA/gene/genome chip, Biochip, gene array, oligonucleotide-based DNA arrays, etc., are well described and established DNA microarray technology. Various steps are involved in the design and for successful operation of a DNA microarray experiment to study the parasite gene expression profile (Bumgarner, 2013). The use of microarray technique has made for a better advancement of the identification and validation of biomarker/target against Leishmaniasis. It is also contributing in better diagnostic and prognostic tools as well as for the identification of novel therapeutic targets. Hence, microarrays of *Leishmania* genes have provided better understanding toward molecular biotechnology which can reduce the agony resulting from *Leishmania* infection (Kumar et al., 2020b).

3.5   Conclusion

The management of *Leishmania* infection is very important, due to the lack of good prophylactic and therapeutic measures. The complete cure is only possible once the disease is diagnosed accurately and during the early course of infection. As per the World Health Organization recommendations, an ideal diagnostic test must be sensitive, specific, easy to use, and have low cost values so that it can reach to poverty-stricken populations. Diagnostic assays giving false-negative test could lead to a fatal outcome while false-positive test results could induce side effect of drugs prescribed by physicians. Hence accurate diagnosis is on demand VL for the cure of parasitic *Leishmania* infection. The currently available parasitological methods and serological assays have their specific merits and demerits. The PCR-based molecular assays are more specific, sensitive, and up to the mark for the correct diagnosis of *Leishmania* infection however due to high cost, need of equipment, reagents, and technical expertise they are vulnerable and more challenging to developing or low-income countries of endemic regions. In conclusion, due to various limitations in all diagnostic assays, at least two assays should be performed with different time intervals for the confirmation of the Leishmaniasis or *Leishmania* infection. Furthermore, invention of new diagnostic tools is necessary for the complete elimination of this deadly disease.

References

Adams, E. R., Schoone, G. J., Ageed, A. F., Safi, S. E., & Schallig, H. D. (2010). Development of a reverse transcriptase loop-mediated isothermal amplification (LAMP) assay for the sensitive detection of *Leishmania* parasites in clinical samples. *The American Journal of Tropical Medicine and Hygiene, 82*(4), 591–596.

Akhoundi, B., Mohebali, M., Shojaee, S., Jalali, M., Kazemi, B., Bandehpour, M., et al. (2013). Rapid detection of human and canine visceral Leishmaniasis: Assessment of a latex agglutination test based on the A2 antigen from amastigote forms of *Leishmania* infantum. *Experimental Parasitology, 133*(3), 307–313.

Akhoundi, M., Downing, T., Votypka, J., Kuhls, K., Lukes, J., Cannet, A., et al. (2017). *Leishmania* infections: Molecular targets and diagnosis. *Molecular Aspects of Medicine, 57*, 1–29.

Akman L., A. H., Wang, R. Q., et al. (2000). Multi-site DNA polymorphism analyses of *Leishmania* isolates define their genotypes predicting clinical epidemiology of Leishmaniasis in a specific region. *The Journal of Eukaryotic Microbiology, 47*(6), 545–554.

Allahverdiyev, A. M., Bagirova, M., Uzun, S., Alabaz, D., Aksaray, N., Kocabas, E., et al. (2005). The value of a new microculture method for diagnosis of visceral Leishmaniasis by using bone marrow and peripheral blood. *The American Journal of Tropical Medicine and Hygiene, 73*(2), 276–280.

Amorim, A. G., Carrington, M., Miles, M. A., Barker, D. C., & De Almeida, M. L. (1996). Identification of the C-terminal region of 70 kDa heat shock protein from *Leishmania* (Viannia) braziliensis as a target for the humoral immune response [published correction appears in Cell Stress Chaperones. *Cell Stress and Chaperones, 1*(3), 177–187.

Azizi, K., Soltani, A., & Alipour, H. (2012). Molecular detection of *Leishmania* isolated from cutaneous Leishmaniasis patients in Jask County, Hormozgan Province, Southern Iran, 2008. *Asian Pacific Journal of Tropical Medicine, 5*(7), 514–517.

Badaro, R., Reed, S. G., & Carvalho, E. M. (1983). Immunofluorescent antibody test in American visceral Leishmaniasis: Sensitivity and specificity of different morphological forms of two *Leishmania* species. *The American Journal of Tropical Medicine and Hygiene, 32*(3), 480–484.

Bandyopadhyay, S., Chatterjee, M., Pal, S., Waller, R. F., Sundar, S., Mcconville, M. J., et al. (2004). Purification, characterization of O-acetylated sialoglycoconjugates-specific IgM, and development of an enzyme-linked immunosorbent assay for diagnosis and follow-up of indian visceral Leishmaniasis patients. *Diagnostic Microbiology and Infectious Disease, 50*(1), 15–24.

Basiye, F. L., Mbuchi, M., Magiri, C., Kirigi, G., Deborggraeve, S., Schoone, G. J., et al. (2010). Sensitivity and specificity of the *Leishmania* OligoC-TesT and NASBA-oligochromatography for diagnosis of visceral Leishmaniasis in Kenya. *Tropical Medicine and International Health, 15*(7), 806–810.

Bensch, S., & Åkesson, M. (2005). Ten years of AFLP in ecology and evolution: Why so few animals? *Molecular Ecology, 14*(10), 2899–2914.

Bhattarai, N. R., Auwera, G. V. D., Khanal, B., et al. (2009). PCR and direct agglutination as *Leishmania* infection markers among healthy Nepalese subjects living in areas endemic for Kala-Azar. *Tropical Medicine and International Health, 14*(4), 404–411.

Boelaert, M., Rijal, S., Regmi, S., Singh, R., Karki, B., Jacquet, D., et al. (2004). A comparative study of the effectiveness of diagnostic tests for visceral Leishmaniasis. *The American Journal of Tropical Medicine and Hygiene, 70*(1), 72–77.

Boggild, A. K., Miranda-Verastegui, C., Espinosa, D., Arevalo, J., Martinez-Medina, D., Llanos-Cuentas, A., et al. (2008). Optimization of microculture and evaluation of miniculture for the isolation of *Leishmania* parasites from cutaneous lesions in Peru. *The American Journal of Tropical Medicine and Hygiene*, *79*(6), 847−852.

Boothroyd, J. C., Blader, I., Cleary, M., & Singh, U. (2003). DNA microarrays in parasitology: Strengths and limitations. *Trends in Parasitology*, *19*(10), 470−476.

Botilde, Y., Laurent, T., Quispe Tintaya, W., Chicharro, C., Canavate, C., Cruz, I., et al. (2006). Comparison of molecular markers for strain typing of *Leishmania* infantum. *Infection, Genetics and Evolution*, *6*(6), 440−446.

Bray, R.S. Experimental Leishmaniasis of mammals. In Peters, W., & Killick-Kendrick R. (eds.) *The* Leishmaniasis *in biology and medicine*, (Vol. 1, pp. 425-464.), New York, NY, Academic Press.

Bumgarner, R. E. (2013). Overview of DNA microarrays: Types, applications, and their future. *Current Protocols in Molecular Biology*, *101*, 22.21.21-22.21.11.

Carvalho, F. A., Charest, H., Tavares, C. A., et al. (2002). Diagnosis of American visceral Leishmaniasis in humans and dogs using the recombinant *Leishmania* donovani A2 antigen. *Diagnostic Microbiology and Infectious Disease*, *43*(4), 289−295.

Chappuis, F., Rijal, S., Jha, U. K., et al. (2006). Field validity, reproducibility and feasibility of diagnostic tests for visceral Leishmaniasis in rural Nepal. *Tropical Medicine and International Health*, *11*(1), 31−40.

Chappuis, F., Sundar, S., Hailu, A., Ghalib, H., Rijal, S., Peeling, R. W., et al. (2007). Visceral Leishmaniasis: what are the needs for diagnosis, treatment and control? *Nature reviews. Microbiology*, *5*(11), 873−882.

Claborn, D. M. (2010). The biology and control of Leishmaniasis vectors. *Journal of Global Infectious Diseases*, *2*(2), 127−134.

Cortes, S., Rolão, N., Ramada, J., & Campino, L. (2004). PCR as a rapid and sensitive tool in the diagnosis of human and canine Leishmaniasis using *Leishmania* donovani s.l.-specific kinetoplastid primers. *Transactions of the Royal Society of Tropical Medicine and Hygiene*, *98*(1), 12−17.

Cota, G. F., De Sousa, M. R., Demarqui, F. N., & Rabello, A. (2012). The diagnostic accuracy of serologic and molecular methods for detecting visceral Leishmaniasis in HIV infected patients: meta-analysis. *PLoS Neglected Tropical Diseases*, *6*(5), e1665.

De Colmenares, M., Portus, M., Riera, C., Gallego, M., Aisa, M. J., Torras, S., et al. (1995). Short report: Detection of 72-75-kD and 123-kD fractions of *Leishmania* antigen in urine of patients with visceral Leishmaniasis. *The American Journal of Tropical Medicine and Hygiene*, *52*(5), 427−428.

De Paiva-Cavalcanti, M., De Morais, R. C., Pessoa, E. S. R., Trajano-Silva, L. A., Gonçalves-De-Albuquerque Sda, C., Tavares Dde, H., et al. (2015). *Leishmania*ses diagnosis: An update on the use of immunological and molecular tools. *Cell & Bioscience*, *5*, 31.

De Ruiter, C. M., Van Der Veer, C., Leeflang, M. M., Deborggraeve, S., Lucas, C., & Adams, E. R. (2014). Molecular tools for diagnosis of visceral Leishmaniasis: systematic review and meta-analysis of diagnostic test accuracy. *Journal of Clinical Microbiology*, *52*(9), 3147−3155.

De Vries, P. J., Van Der Meide, W. F., Godfried, M. H., Schallig, H. D., Dinant, H. J., & Faber, W. R. (2006). Quantification of the response to miltefosine treatment for visceral Leishmaniasis by QT-NASBA. *Transactions of the Royal Society of Tropical Medicine and Hygiene*, *100*(12), 1183−1186.

Deborggraeve, S., Laurent, T., Espinosa, D., Van Der Auwera, G., Mbuchi, M., Wasunna, M., et al. (2008). A simplified and standardized polymerase chain reaction format for the diagnosis of Leishmaniasis. *The Journal of Infectious Diseases*, *198*(10), 1565−1572.

Dey, A., & Singh, S. (2007). Genetic heterogeneity among visceral and post-Kala-Azar dermal Leishmaniasis strains from eastern India. *Infection, Genetics and Evolution, 7*(2), 219−222.

Diehn, M., Eisen, M., Botstein, D., et al. (2000). Large-scale identification of secreted and membrane-associated gene products using DNA microarrays. *Nature Genetics, 25*, 58−62.

El Harith, A., El Mutasim, M., Mansour, D., Fadil Mustafa, E., & Arvidson, H. (2003). Use of glycerol as an alternative to freeze-drying for long-term preservation of antigen for the direct agglutination test. *Tropical Medicine and International Health, 8*(11), 1025−1029.

El Mutasim, M., Mansour, D., Abass, E. M., Hassan, W. M., & El Harith, A. (2006). Evaluation of a glycerol-preserved antigen in the direct agglutination test for diagnosis of visceral Leishmaniasis at rural level in eastern Sudan. *Journal of Medical Microbiology, 55*(pt 10), 1343−1347.

El-Safi, S. H., Abdel-Haleem, A., Hammad, A., El-Basha, I., Omer, A., Kareem, H. G., et al. (2003). Field evaluation of latex agglutination test for detecting urinary antigens in visceral Leishmaniasis in Sudan. *Eastern Mediterranean Health Journal, 9*(4), 844−855.

Ghatei, M. A., Hatam, G. R., Hossini, M. H., & Sarkari, B. (2009). Performance of latex agglutination test (KAtex) in diagnosis of visceral Leishmaniasis in Iran. *Iranian Journal of Immunology: IJI, 6*(4), 202−207.

Ghedin, E., Zhang, W. W., Charest, H., Sundar, S., Kenney, R. T., & Matlashewski, G. (1997). Antibody response against a *Leishmania* donovani amastigote-stage-specific protein in patients with visceral Leishmaniasis. *Clinical and Diagnostic Laboratory Immunology, 4*(5), 530−535.

Govindarajan, R., Duraiyan, J., Kaliyappan, K., & Palanisamy, M. (2012). Microarray and its applications. *Journal of Pharmacy & Bioallied Sciences, 4*(Suppl 2), S310−S312.

Grogl, M., Daugirda, J. L., Hoover, D. L., Magill, A. J., & Berman, J. D. (1993). Survivability and infectivity of viscerotropic *Leishmania* tropica from Operation Desert Storm participants in human blood products maintained under blood bank conditions. *The American Journal of Tropical Medicine and Hygiene, 49*(3), 308−315.

Guerbouj, S., Victoir, K., Guizani, I., Seridi, N., Nuwayri-Salti, N., Belkaid, M., et al. (2001). Gp63 gene polymorphism and population structure of *Leishmania* donovani complex: Influence of the host selection pressure? *Parasitology, 122*(Pt 1), 25−35.

Hockmeyer, W. T., Kager, P. A., Rees, P. H., & Hendricks, L. D. (1981). The culture of *Leishmania* donovani in Schneider's insect medium: its value in the diagnosis and management of patients with visceral Leishmaniasis. *Transactions of the Royal Society of Tropical Medicine and Hygiene, 75*(6), 861−863.

Ilg, T., Stierhof, Y. D., Wiese, M., Mcconville, M. J., & Overath, P. (1994). Characterization of phosphoglycan-containing secretory products of *Leishmania*. *Parasitology, 108*, S63−S71.

Iqbal, J., Hira, P. R., Saroj, G., Philip, R., Al-Ali, F., Madda, P. J., et al. (2002). Imported visceral Leishmaniasis: Diagnostic dilemmas and comparative analysis of three assays. *Journal of Clinical Microbiology, 40*(2), 475−479.

Jacquet, D., Boelaert, M., Seaman, J., Rijal, S., Sundar, S., Menten, J., et al. (2006). Comparative evaluation of freeze-dried and liquid antigens in the direct agglutination test for serodiagnosis of visceral Leishmaniasis (ITMA-DAT/VL). *Tropical Medicine and International Health, 11* (12), 1777−1784.

Jaffe, C. L., & Sarfstein, R. (1987). Species-specific antibodies to *Leishmania* tropica (minor) recognize somatic antigens and exometabolites. *Journal of Immunology, 139*(4), 1310−1319.

Kreutzer, R. D., Grogl, M., Neva, F. A., Fryauff, D. J., Magill, A. J., & Aleman-Munoz, M. M. (1993). Identification and genetic comparison of *Leishmania*l parasites causing viscerotropic and cutaneous disease in soldiers returning from Operation Desert Storm. *The American Journal of Tropical Medicine and Hygiene, 49*(3), 357−363.

Kuhls, K., Keilonat, L., Ochsenreither, S., Schaar, M., Schweynoch, C., Presber, W., & Schönian, G. (2007). Multilocus microsatellite typing (MLMT) reveals genetically isolated populations between and within the main endemic regions of visceral Leishmaniasis. *Microbes and Infection*, *9*(3), 334−343.

Kumar, A., Boggula, V. R., Misra, P., Sundar, S., Shasany, A. K., & Dube, A. (2010). Amplified fragment length polymorphism (AFLP) analysis is useful for distinguishing *Leishmania* species of visceral and cutaneous forms. *Acta Tropica*, *113*(2), 202−206.

Kumar, A., Pandey, S. C., & Samant, M. (2018). Slow pace of anti*Leishmania*l drug development. *Parasitology Open*, *4*(4), 1−11.

Kumar, A., Pandey, S. C., & Samant, M. (2020a). A spotlight on the diagnostic methods of a fatal disease Visceral Leishmaniasis. *Parasite Immunology*, e12727.

Kumar, A., Pandey, S. C., & Samant, M. (2020b). DNA-based microarray studies in visceral Leishmaniasis: Identification of biomarkers for diagnostic, prognostic and drug target for treatment. *Acta Tropica*105512.

Lachaud, L., Dereure, J., Chabbert, E., Reynes, J., Mauboussin, J. M., Oziol, E., Dedet, J. P., & Bastien, P. (2000). Optimized PCR using patient blood samples for diagnosis and follow-up of visceral Leishmaniasis, with special reference to AIDS patients. *Journal of Clinical Microbiology*, *38*(1), 236−240.

Maache, M., Azzouz, S., Diaz De La Guardia, R., Alvarez, P., Gil, R., De Pablos, L. M., et al. (2005). Host humoral immune response to *Leishmania* lipid-binding protein. *Parasite Immunology*, *27*(6), 227−234.

Mandal, J., Khurana, S., Dubey, M. L., Bhatia, P., Varma, N., & Malla, N. (2008). Evaluation of direct agglutination test, rk39 Test, and ELISA for the diagnosis of visceral Leishmaniasis. *The American Journal of Tropical Medicine and Hygiene*, *79*(1), 76−78.

Mary, C., Lamouroux, D., Dunan, S., & Quilici, M. (1992). Western blot analysis of antibodies to *Leishmania* infantum antigens: potential of the 14-kD and 16-kD antigens for diagnosis and epidemiologic purposes. *The American Journal of Tropical Medicine and Hygiene*, *47*(6), 764−771.

Mauricio, I. L., Stothard, J. R., & Miles, M. A. (2004). *Leishmania* donovani complex: genotyping with the ribosomal internal transcribed spacer and the mini-exon. *Parasitology*, *128*(Pt 3), 263−267.

Maurya, R., Mehrotra, S., Prajapati, V. K., Nylen, S., Sacks, D., & Sundar, S. (2010). Evaluation of blood agar microtiter plates for culturing *Leishmania* parasites to titrate parasite burden in spleen and peripheral blood of patients with visceral Leishmaniasis. *Journal of Clinical Microbiology*, *48*(5), 1932−1934.

Maurya, R., Singh, R. K., Kumar, B., Salotra, P., Rai, M., & Sundar, S. (2005). Evaluation of PCR for diagnosis of Indian kala-azar and assessment of cure. *Journal of Clinical Microbiology*, *43*(7), 3038−3041.

Mohapatra, T. M., Singh, D. P., Sen, M. R., Bharti, K., & Sundar, S. (2010). Compararative evaluation of rK9, rK26 and rK39 antigens in the serodiagnosis of Indian visceral Leishmaniasis. *Journal of Infection in Developing Countries*, *4*(2), 114−117.

Mukhtar, M., Ali, S., Boshara, S., Albertini, A., Monnerat, S., Bessell, P., et al. (2018). Sensitive and less invasive confirmatory diagnosis of visceral Leishmaniasis in Sudan using loop-mediated isothermal amplification (LAMP). *PLoS Neglected Tropical Diseases*, *12*, e0006264.

Murray, H. W. (2001). Clinical and experimental advances in treatment of visceral Leishmaniasis. *Antimicrobial Agents and Chemotherapy*, *45*(8), 2185−2197.

Notomi, T., Okayama, H., Masubuchi, H., Yonekawa, T., Watanabe, K., Amino, N., & Hase, T. (2000). Loop-mediated isothermal amplification of DNA. *Nucleic Acids Research*, *28*(12), E63.

Oliveira, E., Pedras, M. J., De Assis, I. E., & Rabello, A. (2009). Improvement of direct agglutination test (DAT) for laboratory diagnosis of visceral Leishmaniasis in Brazil. *Transactions of the Royal Society of Tropical Medicine and Hygiene, 103*(12), 1279–1281.

Otranto, D., Paradies, P., Sasanelli, M., Spinelli, R., & Brandonisio, O. (2004). Rapid immunochromatographic test for serodiagnosis of canine Leishmaniasis. *Journal of Clinical Microbiology, 42*(6), 2769–2770.

Pandey, S. C., Kumar, A., & Samant, M. (2020). Genetically modified live attenuated vaccine: A potential strategy to combat visceral leishmaniasis. *Parasite Immunology*, e12732.

Pandey, S. C., Pande, V., & Samant, M. (2020). DDX3 DEAD-box RNA helicase (Hel67) gene disruption impairs infectivity of *Leishmania donovani* and induces protective immunity against visceral leishmaniasis. *Scientific Reports, 10*(1), 1–10.

Perez-Alvarez, M. J., Larreta, R., Alonso, C., & Requena, J. M. (2001). Characterisation of a monoclonal antibody recognising specifically the HSP70 from *Leishmania. Parasitology Research, 87*(11), 907–910.

Perry, D., Dixon, K., Garlapati, R., Gendernalik, A., Poche, D., & Poche, R. (2013). Visceral Leishmaniasis prevalence and associated risk factors in the saran district of Bihar, India, from 2009 to July of 2011. *The American Journal of Tropical Medicine and Hygiene, 88*(4), 778–784.

Quispe Tintaya, K. W., Ying, X., Dedet, J. P., Rijal, S., De Bolle, X., & Dujardin, J. C. (2004). Antigen genes for molecular epidemiology of Leishmaniasis: Polymorphism of cysteine proteinase B and surface metalloprotease glycoprotein 63 in the *Leishmania* donovani complex. *The Journal of Infectious Diseases, 189*(6), 1035–1043.

Rafati, S., Hassani, N., Taslimi, Y., Movassagh, H., Rochette, A., & Papadopoulou, B. (2006). Amastin peptide-binding antibodies as biomarkers of active human visceral Leishmaniasis. *Clinical and Vaccine Immunology: CVI, 13*(10), 1104–1110.

Reithinger, R., & Dujardin, J. C. (2007). Molecular diagnosis of Leishmaniasis: Current status and future applications. *Journal of Clinical Microbiology, 45*(1), 21–25.

Restrepo, C. M., De La Guardia, C., Sousa, O. E., Calzada, J. E., Fernandez, P. L., & Lleonart, R. (2013). AFLP polymorphisms allow high resolution genetic analysis of American Tegumentary Leishmaniasis agents circulating in Panama and other members of the *Leishmania* genus. *PLoS ONE, 8*(9), e73177.

Saad, A. A., Ahmed, N. G., Osman, O. S., Al-Basheer, A. A., Hamad, A., Deborggraeve, S., et al. (2010). Diagnostic accuracy of the *Leishmania* OligoC-TesT and NASBA-Oligochromatography for diagnosis of Leishmaniasis in Sudan. *PLoS neglected tropical diseases, 4*(8), e776.

Sacks, D. L., Kenney, R. T., Kreutzer, R. D., Jaffe, C. L., Gupta, A. K., Sharma, M. C., et al. (1995). Indian kala-azar caused by *Leishmania* tropica. *Lancet, 345*(8955), 959–961.

Salam, M. A., Khan, M. G., Bhaskar, K. R., Afrad, M. H., Huda, M. M., & Mondal, D. (2012). Peripheral blood buffy coat smear: A promising tool for diagnosis of visceral Leishmaniasis. *Journal of Clinical Microbiology, 50*(3), 837–840.

Salotra, P., Sreenivas, G., Pogue, G. P., Lee, N., Nakhasi, H. L., Ramesh, V., et al. (2001). Development of a species-specific PCR assay for detection of *Leishmania* donovani in clinical samples from patients with kala-azar and post-kala-azar dermal Leishmaniasis. *Journal of Clinical Microbiology, 39*(3), 849–854.

Santos-Gomes, G., Gomes-Pereira, S., Campino, L., Araujo, M. D., & Abranches, P. (2000). Performance of immunoblotting in diagnosis of visceral Leishmaniasis in human immunodeficiency virus-*Leishmania* sp.-coinfected patients. *Journal of Clinical Microbiology, 38*(1), 175–178.

Sarkari, B., Chance, M., & Hommel, M. (2002). Antigenuria in visceral Leishmaniasis: Detection and partial characterisation of a carbohydrate antigen. *Acta Tropica, 82*(3), 339−348.

Schönian, G., Nasereddin, A., Dinse, N., Schweynoch, C., Schallig, H. D. F. H., Presber, W., & Jaffe, C. L. (2003). PCR diagnosis and characterization of *Leishmania* in local and imported clinical samples. *Diagnostic Microbiology and Infectious Disease, 47*(1), 349−358.

Selvapandiyan, A., Duncan, R., Mendez, J., Kumar, R., Salotra, P., Cardo, L. J., et al. (2008). A *Leishmania* minicircle DNA footprint assay for sensitive detection and rapid speciation of clinical isolates. *Transfusion, 48*(9), 1787−1798.

Selvapandiyan, A., Stabler, K., Ansari, N. A., Kerby, S., Riemenschneider, J., Salotra, P., et al. (2005). A novel semiquantitative fluorescence-based multiplex polymerase chain reaction assay for rapid simultaneous detection of bacterial and parasitic pathogens from blood. *The Journal of Molecular Diagnostics, 7*(2), 268−275.

Sharma, U., & Singh, S. (2008). Insect vectors of *Leishmania*: Distribution, physiology and their control. *Journal of Vector Borne Diseases, 45*(4), 255−272.

Siddig, M., Ghalib, H., Shillington, D. C., & Petersen, E. A. (1988). Visceral Leishmaniasis in the Sudan: comparative parasitological methods of diagnosis. *Transactions of the Royal Society of Tropical Medicine and Hygiene, 82*(1), 66−68.

Singh, S., & Sivakumar, R. (2003). Recent advances in the diagnosis of Leishmaniasis. *Journal of Postgraduate Medicine, 49*(1), 55−60.

Sivakumar, R., Sharma, P., Chang, K. P., & Singh, S. (2006). Cloning, expression, and purification of a novel recombinant antigen from *Leishmania* donovani. *Protein Expression and Purification, 46*(1), 156−165.

Sreenivas, G., Ansari, N. A., Singh, R., Raju, B. V., Bhatheja, R., Negi, N. S., et al. (2002). Diagnosis of visceral Leishmaniasis: Comparative potential of amastigote antigen, recombinant antigen and PCR. *British Journal of Biomedical Science, 59*(4), 218−222.

Srivastava, P., Dayama, A., Mehrotra, S., & Sundar, S. (2011). Diagnosis of visceral Leishmaniasis. *Transactions of the Royal Society of Tropical Medicine and Hygiene, 105*(1), 1−6.

Srivastava, P., Mehrotra, S., Tiwary, P., Chakravarty, J., & Sundar, S. (2011). Diagnosis of Indian visceral Leishmaniasis by nucleic acid detection using PCR. *PLoS One, 6*(4), e10493.

Srividya, G., Kulshrestha, A., Singh, R., & Salotra, P. (2012). Diagnosis of visceral Leishmaniasis: Developments over the last decade. *Parasitology Research, 110*(3), 1065−1078.

Steverding, D. (2017). The history of Leishmaniasis. *Parasites & Vectors, 10*(1), 82.

Sundar, S., & Rai, M. (2002). Laboratory diagnosis of visceral Leishmaniasis. *Clinical and Diagnostic Laboratory Immunology, 9*(5), 951−958.

Sundar, S., & Singh, O. P. (2018). Molecular diagnosis of Visceral Leishmaniasis. *Molecular Diagnosis & Therapy, 22*(4), 443−457.

Sundar, S., Pai, K., Kumar, R., Pathak-Tripathi, K., Gam, A. A., Ray, M., et al. (2001). Resistance to treatment in Kala-azar: Speciation of isolates from northeast India. *The American Journal of Tropical Medicine and Hygiene, 65*(3), 193−196.

Sundar, S., Pai, K., Sahu, M., Kumar, V., & Murray, H. W. (2002). Immunochromatographic strip-test detection of anti-K39 antibody in Indian visceral Leishmaniasis. *Annals of Tropical Medicine and Parasitology, 96*(1), 19−23.

Sundar, S., Reed, S. G., Singh, V. P., Kumar, P. C., & Murray, H. W. (1998). Rapid accurate field diagnosis of Indian visceral Leishmaniasis. *Lancet, 351*(9102), 563−565.

Sundar, S., Singh, R. K., Bimal, S. K., Gidwani, K., Mishra, A., Maurya, R., et al. (2007). Comparative evaluation of parasitology and serological tests in the diagnosis of visceral

Leishmaniasis in India: A phase III diagnostic accuracy study. *Tropical Medicine and International Health*, *12*(2), 284−289.

Sunter, J., & Gull, K. (2017). Shape, form, function and *Leishmania* pathogenicity: From textbook descriptions to biological understanding. *Open Biology*, *7*(9).

Takagi, H., Islam, M. Z., Itoh, M., Islam, A. U., Saifuddin Ekram, A. R., Hussain, S. M., et al. (2007). Short report: Production of recombinant kinesin-related protein of *Leishmania* donovani and its application in the serodiagnosis of visceral Leishmaniasis. *The American Journal of Tropical Medicine and Hygiene*, *76*(5), 902−905.

Takagi, H., Itoh, M., Islam, M. Z., Razzaque, A., Ekram, A. R., Hashighuchi, Y., et al. (2009). Sensitive, specific, and rapid detection of *Leishmania* donovani DNA by loop-mediated isothermal amplification. *The American Journal of Tropical Medicine and Hygiene*, *81*(4), 578−582.

Thakur, L., Singh, K. K., Shanker, V., Negi, A., Jain, A., Matlashewski, G., et al. (2018). Atypical Leishmaniasis: A global perspective with emphasis on the Indian subcontinent. *PLoS Neglected Tropical Diseases*, *12*(9), e0006659.

Thakur, S., Joshi, J., & Kaur, S. (2020). Leishmaniasis diagnosis: An update on the use of parasitological, immunological and molecular methods. *Journal of Parasitic Diseases*, *44*(2), 253−272.

Tlamcani, Z. (2016). Visceral Leishmaniasis: An update of laboratory diagnosis. *Asian Pacific Journal of Tropical Disease*, *6*(7), 505−508.

Van Der Meide, W., Guerra, J., Schoone, G., Farenhorst, M., Coelho, L., Faber, W., et al. (2008). Comparison between quantitative nucleic acid sequence-based amplification, real-time reverse transcriptase PCR, and real-time PCR for quantification of *Leishmania* parasites. *Journal of Clinical Microbiology*, *46*(1), 73−78.

Van Der Meide, W. F., Schoone, G. J., Faber, W. R., et al. (2005). Quantitative nucleic acid sequence-based assay as a new molecular tool for detection and quantification of *Leishmania* parasites in skin biopsy samples. *Journal of Clinical Microbiology*, *43*(11), 5560−5566.

Verma, S., Avishek, K., Sharma, V., Negi, N., Ramesh, V., & Salotra, P. (2013). Application of loop-mediated isothermal amplification assay for the sensitive and rapid diagnosis of visceral Leishmaniasis and post-kala-azar dermal Leishmaniasis. *Diagnostic Microbiology and Infectious Disease*, 75.

Verma, S., Kumar, R., Katara, G. K., Singh, L. C., Negi, N. S., Ramesh, V., et al. (2010). Quantification of parasite load in clinical samples of Leishmaniasis patients: IL-10 level correlates with parasite load in visceral Leishmaniasis. *PLoS One*, *5*(4), e10107.

Verweij, J. J., & Stensvold, C. R. (2014). Molecular testing for clinical diagnosis and epidemiological investigations of intestinal parasitic infections. *Clinical Microbiology Reviews*, *27*(2), 371−418.

Vilaplana, C., Blanco, S., Dominguez, J., Gimenez, M., Ausina, V., Tural, C., & Muñoz, C. (2004). Noninvasive method for diagnosis of visceral Leishmaniasis by a latex agglutination test for detection of antigens in urine samplesc. *Journal of Clinical Microbiology*, *42*(4), 1853−1854.

Zanoli, L. M., & Spoto, G. (2013). Isothermal amplification methods for the detection of nucleic acids in microfluidic devices. *Biosensors (Basel)*, *3*(1), 18−43.

Zijlstra, E. E., Nur, Y., Desjeux, P., Khalil, E. A., El-Hassan, A. M., & Groen, J. (2001). Diagnosing visceral Leishmaniasis with the recombinant K39 strip test: Experience from the Sudan. *Tropical Medicine and International Health*, *6*(2), 108−113.

Chapter 4

Recent advances on computational approach towards potential drug discovery against leishmaniasis

Tushar Joshi[1,2], Priyanka Sharma[3], Tanuja Joshi[2], Shalini Mathpal[1,2], Satish Chandra Pandey[4], Anupam Pandey[5] and Subhash Chandra[2]
[1]Department of Biotechnology, Kumaun University, Sir J C Bose Technical Campus, Bhimtal, India, [2]Department of Botany, Kumaun University, SSJ Campus, Almora, India, [3]Department of Botany, Kumaun University, DSB Campus, Nainital, India, [4]Cell and Molecular Biology Laboratory, Department of Zoology, Kumaun University, SSJ Campus, Almora, India, [5]ICAR-Directorate of Coldwater Fisheries Research, Nainital, India

4.1 Introduction

Leishmaniasis is a complex disease that is caused by several species of *Leishmania* genus. The leishmaniasis disease symptoms range in severity from cutaneous and mucocutaneous lesions to the chronic visceral form, resulting in death if not treated properly. This disease has been reported in 98 countries, and 85 out of them are developing or emerging countries. Leishmaniasis is a vector born disease that is mostly transmitted to the host by the sand fly which is why it is difficult to control at the level of a vector (Kumar, Pandey, & Samant, 2020a, 2020b). The control of leishmaniasis is carried out by giving chemotherapy to patients. For treating leishmaniasis, several potential drugs are available in the market, including amphotericin B, pentamidine, miltefosine, sodium stibogluconate, and paromomycin allopurinol, and sitamaquine (Croft & Coombs, 2003). Unfortunately, the prevalence of parasites becoming resistant to the first-line drug, that is, pentavalent antimony (SbV), increases great health concerns worldwide (Kumar, Pandey, & Samant, 2018; Kumar et al., 2020a,b). Another main issue in leishmaniasis is that the restricted range of medication choices and the harmful effects are (Oliveira et al., 2011; Sundar & Chakravarty, 2010) increasing the mortality rate and several studies have reported that there are decreases in efficacy, resistance, and toxicity against these drugs (Kumar et al., 2018). Besides, there are records of medication failures due to enhanced parasite tolerance to the first medication of choice, that is, antimonials (Goyeneche-Patino, Valderrama, Walker, & Saravia, 2008). Moreover, there is a lack of effective vaccines to control leishmaniasis by immunization (Pandey, Kumar, & Samant, 2020). Therefore there is a need to research the investigation of potential compounds and vaccine candidates that may be effective in the control of leishmaniasis (Pandey, Pande, & Samant, 2020). Many proteins as drug targets have been reported based on their known function, expression level, and localization to discover an anti-leishmaniasis drug (Dhami, Pandey, Shah, Bisht, & Samant, 2020; Pandey, Dhami, et al., 2019; Pandey, Jha, Kumar, & Samant, 2019). These targets are involved in critical metabolic processes in the parasite. For example, Topoisomerases, kinases proteins localized and targeted to lysosomes, are potential *Leishmania* drug targets (Carrero-Lerida, Perez-Moreno, Castillo-Acosta, Ruiz-Perez, & Gonzalez-Pacanowska, 2009; Das, Ganguly, & Majumder, 2008; de Azevedo & Soares, 2009; Libusova, Sulimenko, Sulimenko, Hozǎk, & Draber, 2004). Among them, protein kinases protein has been researched for a long time for their function in growth, apoptosis, and differentiation and cell responses.

Currently, the massive availability of genomic sequences of pathogenic organisms, protein 3D structures, protein expression databases, drug databases, omics databases, metabolome, and proteome, along with the development of novel computational techniques, present unique opportunities to discover novel and potential drug candidates based on specific molecular targets. The computational method in drug designing, discovery, and development processes achieves rapid exploration, implementation, and admiration. Usually, introducing a new drug in a market is typically a very complicated, risky, and expensive process in terms of time, money, and human resources. Generally, drug development takes around 10–14 years, and the cost of drug development is more than 1 billion dollars of capital in total (Daina et al., 2017). Hence, for reducing time, cost and risk are borne factors, Computer-Aided Drug Design (CADD) process is widely used to discover a new drug candidate. It has been found that by using CADD approaches, we can reduce the expense of drug discovery and production up to 50% (Xiang, Cao, Fan, Chen, & Mo, 2012). Usually, CADD is based on many software programs to find hit to lead. Leads are further optimized and evaluated in laboratory conditions before reaching the drug in the market.

Therefore computational approaches are valuable and essential tools for drug discovery and development processes. Various open-source and proprietary computational tools are available to help the researchers for the identification and investigation of new molecules (Brogi, 2019). These computational techniques include structure-based methods primarily molecular docking studies, molecular dynamics (MD) simulations] and ligand-based approaches such as ligand similarity, ligand-based pharmacophore, three-dimensional quantitative structure−activity relationship (3D QSAR) models, and machine learning (ML) approaches (Kapetanovic, 2008; Talele, Khedkar, & Rigby, 2010) (Fig. 4.1). In addition, sets of extraction strategies are used to remove undesirable compounds based on harmful physicochemical, pharmacokinetics, and toxicity properties and to enrich the drug-like compound data (Bielska et al., 2011).

Since leishmaniasis is a neglected disease that mainly occurs in the developing world, it is not being addressed properly because the pharma companies argue that the production of the new drug is so expensive and high risk to invest in low return neglected diseases. Thus the lack of drug research and development for neglected diseases requires extreme demand to be cured in developing and emerging countries. This chapter discusses the various computational approaches to pay attention to researchers to develop new drugs against leishmanial disease, which will encourage the public and private companies to take the initiative to create unique and useful drug candidates against leishmaniasis.

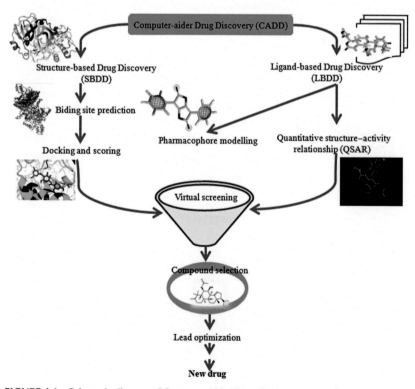

FIGURE 4.1   Schematic diagram of Computer-Aided Drug Design.

4.2 Structure-based drug design

The structure-based drug design (SBDD) method is widely used to screen a large data set. Various computational approaches serve as a powerful tool to speed up the development of drugs, including different screening procedures, combinatorial chemistry, and calculations properties such as absorption, distribution, metabolism, excretion, and toxicity (ADMET) (Batool, Ahmad, & Choi, 2019) (Fig. 4.2). In SBDD, to discover new drug candidates, the molecular target's 3D structure is required (Imam & Gilani, 2017). Apart from protein structure, a data set of unknown molecules is also necessary to conduct SBDD. Usually, it's used to dock the large databases of small molecules or fragments of compounds into the target protein's active sites. These compounds are then ranked by the various scoring function, mostly based on electrostatic and steric interactions with the protein's binding site.

SBDD efforts have contributed to discovering novel molecules for both well-established and newly developed drug targets in *Leishmania* spp. One example is the pteridinereductase 1 (PTR1) enzyme that is involved in the pteridine salvage pathway and folate metabolism and is a validated target for drug discovery against leishmaniasis (Ong, Sienkiewicz, Wyllie, & Fairlamb, 2011). This enzyme has been used for designing novel inhibitors that

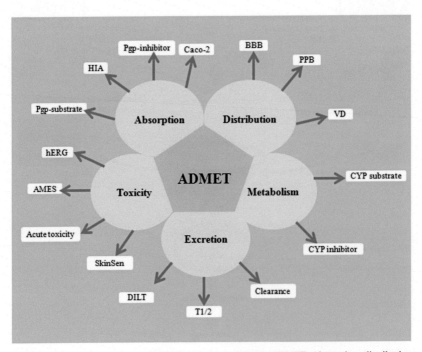

FIGURE 4.2 Main features in ADMET properties of drugs. *ADMET*, Absorption, distribution, metabolism, excretion, and toxicity.

combine the features of dihydropyrimidine and chalcone derivatives using SBDD techniques (Rashid et al., 2016). Another example is discovering the inhibitor of Type 2 NADH dehydrogenase (NDH2), a mitochondrial enzyme that catalyzes the electron transfer from NADH to ubiquinone using SBDD. Hence it is an emerging drug target in leishmaniasis drug discovery (Marreiros et al., 2017). A recent report by Stevanović et al., 2018 developed a 3D structure using the homology model of the NDH2 enzyme and conducted a pharmacophore-based virtual screening (VS) to find novel *Leishmania* (*L.*) *infantum* NDH2 inhibitors. Therefore SBDD is a method of computing commonly used by pharmaceutical firms and scientists. There are many medicines commercially available that have been identified by SBDD. There are following processes under SBDD.

4.2.1 Target protein

The essential process in the SBDD method is the identification and validation of target proteins (Grant, 2009). The 3D structures of all therapeutically essential proteins are experimentally evaluated by integrative structure biology approaches such as NMR, X-ray crystallography, or cryo-electron microscopy but if a protein structure is not available, the 3D structure of proteins are used to model by in silico methods. Up to date, the total 72 resolve 3D structures of *Leishmania* spp. have been submitted in RCSB-PDB (Research Collaboratory for Structural Bioinformatics-Protein data bank) database. Many of these proteins can be used as a receptor to find novel drugs against leishmaniasis. Apart from these structures, some essential drug targets of *Leishmania* species are not present in protein databank. To resolve this problem, homology modeling approach is one of the excellent and most reliable techniques in computational biology as it builds 3D structures of a protein based on the knowledge of 3D structures of homologous proteins having >40% similarity (Song, Lim, & Tong, 2009).

4.2.2 Virtual screening: a lead identification approach

VS is a computational technique applied to identify lead molecules using a huge and diverse collection of chemical compounds library. VS is an essential technique for developing lead compounds as it is faster, more cost-efficient, and less resource-intensive in comparison to an experimental approach such as high-throughput screening (Kitchen, Decornez, Furr, & Bajorath, 2004; Shoichet, 2004). In VS, libraries of various types of drug-like or lead-like molecules are screened computationally against the well-known 3D structures of target proteins. The filtering of molecules libraries is provided by docking approach, where compounds are evaluated based on their binding affinity (Phatak, Stephan, & Cavasotto, 2009; Shoichet, 2004). In recent study, Maia et al. (2020) used VS techniques against leishmaniasis. VS techniques have been traditionally subdivided into two major approaches:

1. Ligand-based screening
2. Receptor-based screening

In the ligand-based screening techniques the descriptors of known actives and sometimes inactive molecules are applied to obtain other compounds of interest from a database library by employing similar search techniques or by seeking a common substructure, pharmacophore, or shape parameters in the active set. In structure-based (or receptor-based) screening techniques the library of compounds database are docked into a binding site or over the entire surface of receptor, then graded using one or more scoring functions. In the study, Pandey, Kumbhar, Sundar, Kunwar, and Prajapati (2016) used structure-based VS against leishmaniasis by targeting trypanothione reductase enzyme as an inhibitor.

4.2.3 Molecular docking

Molecular docking is a popular and effective method in SBDD because it determines the conformation and binding of molecules within the active site of the target with high precision (Meng, Zhang, Mezei, & Cui, 2011). It is a type of computational modeling that involves the interaction of two or more molecules to give the binding affinity. This approach can be used to study important molecular mechanisms such as a ligand-binding pose and intermolecular interactions of complex stability. Moreover, docking analysis calculate and predict the energies and rank of the binding molecules via various score functions (Huang & Zou, 2010).

4.2.3.1 Types of docking

1. Rigid docking, here both small molecule and the receptor are considered as rigid.
2. Flexible ligand docking, here the receptor is kept rigid, but the molecule is considered as flexible; and
3. Flexible docking, here both receptor and ligand flexibility is considered.

Rigid receptor/flexible ligand model algorithms are being used most frequently in docking analysis. The essential docking techniques that are widely used are Monte Carlo, genetic algorithm, fragment-based and MD. Various computational tools that are mostly applied for high throughput docking of a huge library of compounds include AutoDockVina, DOCK, FlexX, GOLD, and ICM. Further results of docking are evaluated by MD simulations.

4.2.4 Molecular dynamics simulations

MD is a physics-based modeling technique developed in the late 1950s (McCammon, Gelin, & Karplus, 1977), that attempts to solve this restriction by using basic assumptions based on Newtonian physics to simulate atomic motion, that offers extensive knowledge on atomic and molecular variations and substance conformational changes. This approach is used to characterize the patterns, strengths, and properties of protein behavior, drug-receptor interactions, molecular solvation, conformational changes that proteins or molecules may undergo different conditions, and other activities that require the systematic assessment of molecular properties in dynamic molecular models. The molecular dynamics simulation method is offering its role in discovering new drugs against Leishmaniasis. Several studies have found new drugs against Leishmaniasis and other diseases by using simulation techniques (de Mattos Oliveira et al., 2018; Sharma, Joshi, Joshi, Chandra, & Tamta, 2020; Shinde, Mol, Jamdar, & Singh, 2014). Various researchers have used molecular docking and MD simulation techniques to discover potential drugs against leishmaniasis (Pandey, Dhami, et al., 2019; Pandey, Jha, et al., 2019; Shinde et al., 2014; Vadloori, Sharath, Prabhu, & Maurya, 2018).

4.2.5 De novo drug design

De novo drug design is an iterative process that used the three-dimensional structure of the receptor to design newer molecules. This involves determining the structure of the lead target complexes and designing the lead changes using molecular modeling tools. It can also be used to design new chemical classes of compounds that provide alternatives to the target using a template or scaffold, which is chemically different from the previously classified leads (Jain & Agrawal, 2004).

Basically, a stochastic technique is applied for de novo design techniques, and it is essential to address the search space information in the design algorithm. Positive and negative, two types of designs are being used in this technique. In the former design, a search is limited to the particular areas of chemical space with a higher chance of discovering hits that have necessary characteristics. In contrast, in the negative mode the search parameters are predefined to avoid the detection of false positives (Richardson & Richardson, 1989). Different techniques of de novo drug design are following.

1. Receptor-based de novo drug design,
2. Ligand-based de novo drug design,
3. Fragment-based de novo design.

4.2.5.1 Receptor-based de novo drug design

In receptor-based design, the consistency of the structures of the target protein and correct knowledge of its active site in protein are essential since the necessary compounds are constructed by fitting the segment into the receptor binding site. This method may be done through computational tools or by cocrystallization of the molecules with the receptor (Schneider & Fechner, 2005). Two types of methods in receptor-based design: building blocks, either atoms or fragments such as single rings, amines, and hydrocarbons are joined together to make a complete chemical molecule or simply by increasing a molecule from a single unit.

4.2.5.2 Ligand-based de novo drug design

In the absence of a 3D structure of the target protein, new active molecules can still be formulated when the activity data of a collection of defined molecules are available (Wang et al., 2018). These data typically come from the analysis of structure—activity relationship analysis or screening campaigns and represent the basis of a ligand-based design approach. A typical pharmacophore is described from a group of active compounds and used to generate novel compounds that share similar properties. The main advantage of the ligand-based design approach is that there is no need for crystalline data at hand. Crystallography such as G protein-coupled receptors makes it an ideal method to challenge biological targets. Calculation tools that basically apply for ligand-based de novo drug design approaches are namely: TOPAS, SYNOPSIS, and DOGS (Hartenfeller et al., 2012; Vinkers et al., 2003).

4.2.5.3 Fragment-based de novo design

Fragment-based de novo design creates new compounds using the entire chemical space. Fragment anchoring can occur at the binding site of receptors by using (1) the outside-in approach and (2) the inside-out approach. In the outside-in approach, building blocks are mostly positioned across the binding site of proteins, which develops inward. In the course of the inside-out approach, the building blocks are mainly positioned to the common binding site of protein and built outward (Kalyaanamoorthy & Chen, 2011).

4.3 Ligand-based drug discovery

The main alternative technique of SBDD is ligand-based drug discovery (LBDD) methods. LBDD approach is an alternative protocol where the structure of potential drug target is unknown and prediction of this structure by using homology modeling or structure prediction is challenging or undesirable (Loew, Villar, & Alkorta, 1993; Mason, Good, & Martin, 2001). The LBDD strategy requires the calculation of known molecules to bind with a protein of interest. This approach carried out with a set of reference molecules that derived from known molecules to connect with the target of interest and calculate their 2D or 3D structures. These molecules are represented in such a manner that the physicochemical characteristics are most essential for their required interactions, while the additional information is discarded that is not applicable for the interactions. This approach is considered an indirect method for drug discovery, which does not require knowledge of the target structure. Nevertheless, this strategy depends on the interpretation of small compounds that bind to the interested target. Pharmacophore modeling, molecular similarity approaches and QSAR modeling are some popular LBDD techniques (Vanommeslaeghe et al., 2010).

Two basic approaches of LBDD are (1) choosing compounds based on chemical similarities to known active ingredients by means of some calculation of similarities or (2) building a QSAR model forecasting biological activity from a chemical structure of molecules. The difference between these two methods is that the latter weighs the features of the chemical structure of molecules according to their effects on the biological behavior of interest, whereas the former does not. These techniques are applied in silico screening for novel molecules for the biological activity of interest, hit-to-lead and lead-to-drug optimization, and DMPK/ADMET properties. The LBDD is based on a similar property principle published by Johnson and Maggiora (1990), which stated that structurally similar molecules have similar properties. LBDD approaches may also be applied when the 3D structure of the receptor is unknown. Besides, active molecules that are identified by ligand-based virtual high-throughput screening (LB-vHTS) approach are often more reliable than those identified in SB-vHTS (Stumpfe et al., 2010). In a recent study, Bhowmik et al. (2020) carried out a ligand-based VS and they used Sphingosine as a reference drug (known inhibitor of DNA primase protein of *Leishmania* (*L.*) *donovani*) for screening the compounds from zinc database. Further screened compounds were subjected to molecular docking and dynamic simulation techniques against molecular targets of *L. donovani*.

4.3.1 Pharmacophore modelling

Pharmacophore is a molecular framework that defines the necessary components that are responsible for the biological activity of compounds. Pharmacophore models are developed when structural knowledge about the drug target is minimal or not understood and models are developed by using the structural properties of active ligands that bind to the target (Lin, 2000). This binding site information can also be used in creating pharmacophore models when the target 3D structure information is available (Yang, 2010). The most commonly used features for describing pharmacophore maps are defined are hydrogen bond acceptors and donors, acidic and basic groups, aliphatic hydrophobic moieties, and aromatic hydrophobic moieties (Vanommeslaeghe et al., 2010). Features for pharmacophore matching are commonly introduced as spheres of a specific resistance radius (Wolber & Langer, 2008). This technique has also been used in the VS of drugs and small molecules from huge databases (Langer & Krovat, 2003; Sharma et al., 2020). There are many programs such as DISCO, GASP, and catalysta designed to identify and produce pharmacophore models. It has been reported that GASP and catalysta perform better than DISCO in reproducing the pharmacophore models (Patel, Gillet, Bravi, & Leach, 2002). Many researchers have applied pharmacophore modeling to identify potent inhibitors of *L. donovani* and *Leishmania major* (Chauhan & Poddar, 2019; de Mattos Oliveira et al., 2018).

4.4   Quantitative structure–activity relationship

QSAR models define the mathematical relationship between structural characteristics and target response of a group of molecules (Zhang et al., 2011). The classic QSAR is known as the Hansch–Fujita method and includes the interaction with the biological behavior of different mechanical, hydrophobic, and steric elements. In the 1960s, Hansch and Fujita (1964) and others began to develop QSAR models using various molecular properties like physical, chemical, and biological, focused on providing computational estimates for the bioactivity of compounds. In 1964 Free & Wilson, 1964 developed a mathematical model relating the presence of several chemical substituents to biological activity (each type of chemical group was assigned an activity contribution), and the two methods were later combined to create the Hansch/Free-Wilson method (Tmej et al., 1998).

The QSAR-based drug discovery's general workflow is first to accumulate a community of active and inactive compounds and then create mathematical descriptors that define the physicochemical and structural properties of compounds. Then, a model is constructed that determines the correlation between those descriptors and their experimental operation, optimizing the power of prediction. Finally, this model is used to forecast the behavior of a library of test compounds encoded with the same descriptors. Consequently, the efficacy of QSAR relies not only on the consistency of the initial collection of active/inactive compounds but also on the choice of descriptors and the ability to create a significant mathematical relationship.

In QSAR model set, several values may be used to measure the activity of a drug molecule. The most widely used values are inhibition constant (K_i) and half-maximal inhibitory concentration (IC_{50}). Unlike the pharmacophore models, QSAR models can be used to measure the positive or negative effects of characteristics of a drug molecule to its activity. QSAR techniques have been used successfully on several drug targets such as carbonic anhydrase, thrombin, and renin (Gupta & Kumaran, 2005; Kontogiorgis, Hadjipavlou, & Litina, 2003). In classical or 2D QSAR methods, the biological activity is associated with physical and chemical properties such as electronic hydrophobic and steric properties of molecules (Hansch & Fujita, 1964). Quantum chemical properties are also used in more advanced 3D

QSAR approaches, in addition to the physical and geometric characteristics of active drug molecules. QSAR models for membrane systems have also been developed recently (Adl, Zein, & Hassanien, 2016). QSAR studies can be developed to identify new antileishmanial drugs. In the study of Bernal and Schmidt (2019) QSAR modeling was used for the set of compounds and checked their antileishmanial activity by using a genetic algorithm as a primary variable selection tool and multiple linear regressions as statistical analysis. This technique has not been used in sufficient quantity against leishmaniasis. Further, many researchers can prefer QSAR techniques and can be used against leishmaniasis to find novel drugs.

4.5   Quantum mechanics/molecular mechanics

The quantum mechanics/molecular mechanics (QM/MM) is the first appearance in 1976 and this method has been widely used to study the chemical reactions of enzymes, which is often the focus of drug discovery programs. In principle, a fundamental understanding of the enzymatic mechanism should help researchers to develop a potent enzyme inhibitor or a new drug (Lodola & De Vivo, 2012). QM and MM combine to form the QM/MM method, commonly used when operating macromolecules (Cramer, 2004). In the QM/MM study of enzymatic mechanisms, the binding region of the active site is defined according to the appropriate QM level. The MM Force field is used to generally describe the majority of the system (most of the enzyme and the solvent), which is not directly involved in the process, but which affect the reaction through nonbinding interactions.

QM methods (e.g., molecular orbital or density functional mathematics) can be used to study the occurrence of molecular systems with hundreds of atoms. QM methods allow one to accurately calculate the internal energy and describe the range of complex interactions seen between a protein and a ligand including hydrogen bonds (H-Bonds) between 1.2 and 1.5 Å, which are usually observed within the energy-absorbing proteins, strong H-bonds ($1.5-2.2$ Å) such as NH$-$O/N, OH$-$O/N, weak H-bonds such as CH$-$O and CH$-$N ($\sim 2.0-3.0$ Å), $\pi-\pi$ stacking (edge to face or parallel displaced), to cation$-\pi$ interactions (Grimme, 2008; Meyer, Castellano, & Diederich, 2003; Rozas, 2006). Presenting a typical complex protein model using only reasonable QM levels is not feasible, but compromise solutions exist, including a range of hybrid QM/MM methods are linear scaling semiempirical, and ab initio methods (Claeyssens et al., 2006; Dixon & Merz, 1996). Hybrid simulations of QM/MM) greatly expanded the complexity of the most massive structures of quantum mechanical calculations by splitting the problem into two parts, each of which is approached with numerous computational techniques. The amount of the system that contributes directly to chemical reactions, such as catalysis, includes the active site, surface fractions, and direct amino acid residue participation, and is controlled by simulation of the

QM stage. The rest portion of the protein that is not directly involved in the reaction and generally comprises a vast number of atoms is made using compounds molecules in the biomolecular Force (FF) field. These various QM/MM approaches have advantages and drawbacks, often depending on the type of enzyme and reaction under analysis. The most common QM/MM methods are Car—Parrinello/Molecular Mechanics MD, empirical valence bond method, the cluster model, and QM/MM MD Methods (Car & Parrinello, 1985; Sousa, Fernandes, & Ramos, 2012; Warshel, 1978). QM/MM method also has not been used in sufficient quantity against leishmaniasis only one study found that the QM/MM mechanism is used to develop imipramine analogs as leads against trypanothione reductase of *Leishmania* parasites (Pandey et al., 2016).

4.6 Artificial intelligence in drug development

Artificial intelligence (AI) is the simulation of computers' human intelligence processes. The process involves obtaining information, developing rules for using data, making approximate or accurate conclusions, and self-correcting. AI has recently been developed as an essential component of the medical care industry. In drug development, AI has changed the way or target detection methods for treating diseases. This was possible because genetics information was integrated; Biochemical properties and targeting pathway (Wang, Feng, Huang, Wang, & Cheng, 2017). AI is also used in the discovery of small drug-like molecules about the use of chemical space. Chemical space offers the stage for new and high-quality molecules to be identified so the possible organic molecules can be enumerated computationally (Reymond, Deursen, Bluma, & Ruddigkeit, 2010). AI systems can reduce feature rates and R&D costs by reducing the number of synthesized compounds tested in vitro or in vivo (Okafo & Sikosek, 2018). AI also contains a subfield called ML, which uses statistical methods with the ability to learn and read with or without being explicitly programmed (Bishop, 2013; Lee et al., 2017). An additional ML subfield called deep learning (DL) uses artificial neural networks (ANNs) that adapt and learn from the vast amount of experimental data (Grys et al., 2017; Lee et al., 2017).

4.6.1 Machine learning in drug discovery

ML is an AI technology that allows systems ability, to learn and develop automatically from experience without being directly programmed. ML focuses on developing computer systems that can access the data and use it for their learning. ML algorithms are also revolutionizing drug discovery in the pharmaceutical industry. The integration of ML algorithms is an automated way to find out new compounds by analyzing, studying, and interpreting large-scale pharmaceutical data.

ML can improve several stages of the drug discovery process:

- The first but most important phases involved in the design of the chemical structure.
- Investigation of drug side effects— both in basic diagnostic research and clinical trials, where many biomedical data are produced. ML may promote the discovery of new patterns in such results.

The success of ML has been demonstrated in classification, generative modeling, and reinforcement learning (RL). The different fields of ML are supervised learning, unsupervised learning, and RL (Fig. 4.3).

4.6.1.1   Supervised learning

Supervised learning approaches are applied to built training models to forecast future values of data types or continuous variables; supervised learning approaches are used to train a model on existing relationships of input and output data such that future outcomes for new inputs can be expected. Supervised learning is learning where we teach or train a machine using well-written data which means that some information is already tagged with the correct answer. Subsequently, the machine is given a new set of examples (data) so that the supervised learning algorithm analyzes the training data (set of training examples) and produces the correct result from the

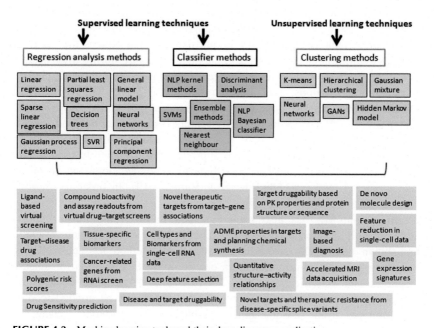

FIGURE 4.3   Machine learning tools and their drug discovery applications.

labeled data. Future results are standard models or results of data partitioning or understanding of dynamic regression.

4.6.1.2 Unsupervised learning

Unsupervised approaches are used to build models that permit data integration in a user-unspecified way. Its unsupervised learning consists of computer training with information that is not identified or labeled and helps the algorithm to operate without any instruction on that information. Here the function of the machine is to combine random data according to similarities, patterns, and differences without previous data training. The unsupervised learning method identifies hidden patterns or structures within the input data and uses these to aggregate data in meaningful ways.

4.6.1.3 Reinforcement learning

RL is a type of ML. Unlike supervised learning and unsupervised learning, RL doesn't learn from data, instead, it learns from experimenting. To model drug design that RL can be applied for de nova drug design of molecules with desired properties, two separate models are combined (1) a generative model which is responsible for generating novel molecules, and (2) a (molecular) property prediction model which is responsible for predicting the user-specified property of molecules.

ML has many uses in the clinic, such as target recognition and confirmation, drug design and development, recognition of biomarkers and disease diagnostic pathology and therapy prognosis. ML also utilizes the relationship between biological activity and chemical structure during drug design. Structural prediction of biological targets (protein structure, binding pocket, transmembrane regions, and phosphorylation and glycosylation sites) and QSAR models, pharmacophore models, molecular docking analysis, and ranking/scoring functions in similarity searches—can be applied and statistically checked by ML techniques (Lo, Rensi, Torng, & Altman, 2018). In associate with drug discovery, these approaches are frequently used within the healthcare setting, and can contribute to major developments in precision medicine (Norgeot, Glicksberg, & Butte, 2019). In order to improve clinical trial outcomes and refine the method of clinical trial eligibility determination, ML has also been extended to electronic health reports and real-world evidence (Esteva et al., 2019). For example, new research has shown that DNNs are a highly successful method for automatically collecting valuable information from electronic medical records for disease diagnosis and classification (Yang, 2010). In understanding disease and improving therapy, especially in neuroscience, ML can be applied to data now coming from sensors and wearable materials (Mohr, Zhang, & Schueller, 2017).

4.6.2 Deep learning in drug designing

DL approach has been extensively used in recent years due to their various successful results in computer vision, speech recognition, and bioinformatics (Lee et al., 2017; Min, Lee, & Yoon, 2017). The term DL refers to a category of algorithms for ML consisting of several data processing layers. DL algorithms find efficient readings of input data at multiple pull rates (LeCun, Bengio, & Hinton, 2015). Deep neural networks (DNNs) are ANN approaches that have various types of hidden layers. In a sense, DNNs are regarded as a group of DL algorithms. DNNs transform the low-level input features into more and more complex features in each subsequent layer. Neural networks (NN) represent a supervised neurology-inspired ML technique that is frequently used and successfully to address issues such as speech and image recognition ANNs are ML algorithms that act as brain neurons: receive multiple input signals and generate an activation response by calculating the sum of sounds for nonlinear input and then transmitting the output signal to the following connected neurons (Van & Bohte, 2018). In the ANN, the processing nodes are entirely or indirectly interconnected. From the input nodes, input entries are taken and converted into hidden nodes into output nodes where the output values are analyzed. The ANN preparation is performed iteratively to prepare the network by back-propagation techniques (Dreyfus, 1973). With the rapid eruption of "big data" of chemicals from combinations and HTS, ML strategies have been a crucial method for drug producers to collect chemical knowledge from vast compound databases to construct drugs rationally. With typical QSAR methods, large volumes of data, velocity, variety, and veracity classification are not possible. ML models are more accurate than a broad input model of data. DL is in high demand, becoming the data-hungry ML algorithm for processing and exploring big data. The DL methods are versatile, as opposed to other ML approaches. The first DL-based platform for structure-based small molecule drug research, Atom Wise, has helped to reliably and reliably develop new possible medicines for 27 disease targets. DNN is used for the simulation of substances with the same number of molecular properties. DNNs can accommodate thousands of descriptors without overfitting and feature selection issues in an optimal way due to the number of nodes and hidden layers, relative to the conventional ANN approach. The Tox21 dataset consisting of 12,000 compounds for 12 high-throughput toxicity assays is given by Mayr et al.'s multitasking DNN process. The estimation of computational toxicity of the descriptors of molecules and drugs was provided in those datasets. In DL techniques, such descriptors are used to predict the toxicity of chemicals (Mayr, Klambauer, Unterthiner, & Hochreiter, 2016). New molecule fingerprints or libraries with modeled pharmacokinetic characteristics of potential drugs can also be developed by using DL and these libraries can also be used for VS of large dataset (Hughes, Miller, & Swamidass, 2015).

The application of AI techniques for drug discovery against leishmaniasis has not been used widely by researchers. Several datasets against various molecular targets of *L. donovani* are available from databases like CHEMBL and PubChem, which can be exploited for the construction of machine models as training set to find out novel drugs against leishmaniasis. Few studies are available in which ML techniques have been applied against leishmaniasis to predict the biological activity of novel compounds against leishmaniasis (Balmaseda, Socarrás, & Castillo-Garit, 2019; Castillo-Garit et al., 2018; Jamal & Scaria, 2013).

4.7 Conclusion

The present chapter discusses an update in silico techniques for drug discovery against leishmaniasis. Although efficient drugs are available for the treatment of leishmaniasis due to toxicity and side effects of these drugs there is a need to develop new drugs to cure leishmaniasis. Hence, the described computational techniques are essential tools in modern time as they reduce the time and cost required in the course of drug discovery. Computational techniques use the principle of information science and data science for knowledge discovery. Some of the methods like VS, molecular docking, and MD simulation have been already reported for drug discovery against leishmaniasis disease. Still, some methods such as QM/MM and AI techniques are not being used very much. However, they can be adapted easily for leishmaniasis for the exploitation of large available data coming from different research laboratories at very high speed from all over the world. Therefore these new methods should be used by researchers for discovering new drugs so that they can find and develop anti-leishmaniasis potent medicines. These new techniques can open many new possibilities to find novel drugs against leishmaniasis as well as other diseases.

References

Adl, A., Zein, M., & Hassanien, A. E. (2016). PQSAR. *Expert Systems with Applications: An International Journal, 54*(C).

Balmaseda, N. F., Socarrás, S. R., & Castillo-Garit, J. A. (2019). Machine learning techniques and the identification of new potentially active compounds against Leishmania infantum. *International Conference on Multidisciplinary Sciences, 4.*

Batool, M., Ahmad, B., & Choi, S. (2019). A structure-based drug discovery paradigm. *International Journal of Molecular Sciences, 20*(11).

Bernal, F. A., & Schmidt, T. J. (2019). A comprehensive QSAR study on antileishmanial and antitrypanosomal cinnamate ester analogues. *Molecules, 24*(23).

Bhowmik, D., Jagadeesan, R., Rai, P., Nandi, R., Gugan, K., & Kumar, D. (2020). Evaluation of potential drugs against leishmaniasis targeting catalytic subunit of Leishmania donovani nuclear DNA primase using ligand based virtual screening, docking and molecular dynamics approaches. *Journal of Biomolecular Structure & Dynamics, 1−15.*

Bielska, E., Lucas, X., Czerwoniec, A., Kasprzak, J. M., Kaminska, K. H., & Bujnicki, J. M. (2011). Virtual screening strategies in drug design − Methods and applications. *BioTechnologia, 92,* 249−264.

Bishop, C. M. (2013). Model-based machine learning. *Philosophical Transactions. Series A, Mathematical, Physical, and Engineering Sciences, 371*(1984)20120222.

Brogi, S. (2019). Computational approaches for drug discovery. *Molecules, 24*(17).

Car, R., & Parrinello, M. (1985). Unified approach for molecular dynamics and density-functional theory. *Physical Review Letters, 55,* 2471−2474.

Carrero-Lerida, J., Perez-Moreno, G., Castillo-Acosta, V. M., Ruiz-Perez, L. M., & Gonzalez-Pacanowska, D. (2009). Intracellular location of the early steps of the isoprenoid biosynthetic pathway in the trypanosomatids Leishmania major and Trypanosoma brucei. *International Journal for Parasitology, 39*(3), 307−314.

Castillo-Garit, J. A., Flores-Balmaseda, N., Alvarez, O., Pham-The, H., Perez-Donate, V., Torrens, F., et al. (2018). Computational identification of chemical compounds with potential activity against Leishmania amazonensis using nonlinear machine learning techniques. *Current Topics in Medicinal Chemistry, 18*(27), 2347−2354.

Chauhan, N., & Poddar, R. (2019). In silico pharmacophore modeling and simulation studies for searching potent antileishmanials targeted against Leishmania donovani nicotinamidase. *Computational Biology and Chemistry, 83*107150.

Claeyssens, F., Harvey, J. N., Manby, F. R., Mata, R. A., Mulholland, A. J., Ranaghan, K. A., et al. (2006). High-accuracy computation of reaction barriers in enzymes. *Angewandte Chemie International Edition, 45,* 6856−6859.

Cramer, C.J. (2004). *Essentials of computational chemistry: theories and models.* New York.

Croft, S. L., & Coombs, G. H. (2003). Leishmaniasis--Current chemotherapy and recent advances in the search for novel drugs. *Trends in Parasitology, 19*(11), 502−508.

Daina, A., Blatter, M. C., Baillie, G. V., Palagi, P. M., Marek, D., Xenarios, I., et al. (2017). Drug design workshop: A web-based educational tool to introduce computer-aided drug design to the general public. *Journal of Chemical Education, 94*(3), 335−344.

Das, B. B., Ganguly, A., & Majumder, H. K. (2008). DNA topoisomerases of Leishmania: The potential targets for anti-leishmanial therapy. *Advances in Experimental Medicine and Biology, 625,* 103−115.

de Azevedo, W. F., Jr., & Soares, M. B. (2009). Selection of targets for drug development against protozoan parasites. *Current Drug Targets, 10*(3), 193−201.

de Mattos Oliveira, L., Araujo, J. S. C., Bacelar Costa Junior, D., Santana, I. B., Duarte, A. A., Leite, F. H. A., et al. (2018). Pharmacophore modeling, docking and molecular dynamics to identify Leishmania major farnesyl pyrophosphate synthase inhibitors. *Journal of Molecular Modeling, 24*(11), 314.

Dhami, D. S., Pandey, S. C., Shah, G. C., Bisht, M., & Samant, M. (2020). In vitro antileishmanial activity of the essential oil from Agrimonia pilosa. *National Academy Science Letters,* 1−4.

Dixon, S. L., & Merz, K. M. (1996). Semiempirical molecular orbital calculations with linear system size scaling. *The Journal of Chemical Physics, 104,* 6643−6649.

Dreyfus, S. (1973). The computational solution of optimal control problemswith time lag. *IEEE Transactions on Automatic Control, 18,* 383−385.

Esteva, A., Robicquet, A., Ramsundar, B., Kuleshov, V., DePristo, M., Chou, K., et al. (2019). A guide to deep learning in healthcare. *Nature Medicine, 25*(1), 24−29.

Free, S. M., & Wilson, J. W. (1964). A mathematical contribution to structure-activity studies. *J Med Chem, 7,* 395−399. Available from https://doi.org/10.1021/jm00334a001.

Goyeneche-Patino, D. A., Valderrama, L., Walker, J., & Saravia, N. G. (2008). Antimony resistance and trypanothione in experimentally selected and clinical strains of Leishmania panamensis. *Antimicrobial Agents and Chemotherapy*, *52*(12), 4503−4506.

Grant, M. A. (2009). Protein structure prediction in structure-based ligand design and virtual screening. *Combinatorial Chemistry & High Throughput Screening*, *12*(10), 940−960.

Grimme, B. (2008). Do special noncovalent p-p stacking interactions really exist. *Angewandte Chemie International Edition*, *47*, 3430−3434.

Grys, B. T., Lo, D. S., Sahin, N., Kraus, O. Z., Morris, Q., Boone, C., et al. (2017). Machine learning and computer vision approaches for phenotypic profiling. *The Journal of Cell Biology*, *216*(1), 65−71.

Gupta, S. P., & Kumaran, S. (2005). A quantitative structure−activity relationship study on some aromatic/heterocyclic sulfonamides and their charged derivatives acting as carbonic anhydrase inhibitors. *Journal of Enzyme Inhibition and Medicinal Chemistry*, *20*(3), 251−259.

Hansch, C., & Fujita, T. (1964). p-σ-π analysis. A method for the correlation of biological activity and chemical structure. *Journal of the American Chemical Society*, *86*(8), 1616−1626.

Hartenfeller, M., Zettl, H., Walter, M., Rupp, M., Reisen, F., Proschak, E., et al. (2012). DOGS: Reaction-driven de novo design of bioactive compounds. *PLoS Computational Biology*, *8* (2), e1002380.

Huang, S. Y., & Zou, X. (2010). Advances and challenges in protein-ligand docking. *International Journal of Molecular Sciences*, *11*(8), 3016−3034.

Hughes, T. B., Miller, G. P., & Swamidass, S. J. (2015). Modeling epoxidation of drug-like molecules with a deep machine learning network. *ACS Central Science*, *1*(4), 168−180.

Imam, S. S., & Gilani, S. J. (2017). Computer aided drug design: A novel loom to drug discovery. *Organic and Medicinal Chemistry*, *1*(4), 1−6.

Jain, S. K., & Agrawal, A. (2004). De novo drug design: An overview. *Indian Journal of Pharmaceutical Sciences*, *66*(6), 721−728.

Jamal, S., & Scaria, V. (2013). Cheminformatic models based on machine learning for pyruvate kinase inhibitors of Leishmania mexicana. *BMC Bioinformatics*, *14*, 329.

Johnson, M. A., & Maggiora, G. M. (1990). *Concepts and applications of molecular similarity*. New York: Wiley.

Kalyaanamoorthy, S., & Chen, Y. P. (2011). Structure-based drug design to augment hit discovery. *Drug Discovery Today*, *16*(17-18), 831−839.

Kapetanovic, I. M. (2008). Computer-aided drug discovery and development (CADDD): In silico-chemico-biological approach. *Chemico-Biological Interactions*, *171*(2), 165−176.

Kitchen, D. B., Decornez, H., Furr, J. R., & Bajorath, J. (2004). Docking and scoring in virtual screening for drug discovery: Methods and applications. *Nature Reviews. Drug Discovery*, *3* (11), 935−949.

Kontogiorgis, C., Hadjipavlou, -, & Litina, D. (2003). Quantitative structure -- activity relationships (QSARs) of thrombin inhibitors: Review, evaluation and comparative analysis. *Current Medicinal Chemistry*, *10*(7), 525−577.

Kumar, A., Pandey, S. C., & Samant, M. (2018). Slow pace of antileishmanial drug development. *Parasitology Open*, *4*(4), 1−11.

Kumar, A., Pandey, S. C., & Samant, M. (2020a). A spotlight on the diagnostic methods of a fatal disease Visceral Leishmaniasis. *Parasite Immunology*, e12727.

Kumar, A., Pandey, S. C., & Samant, M. (2020b). DNA-based microarray studies in visceral leishmaniasis: Identification of biomarkers for diagnostic, prognostic and drug target for treatment. *Acta Tropica*105512.

Langer, T., & Krovat, E. M. (2003). Chemical feature-based pharmacophores and virtual library screening for discovery of new leads. *Current Opinion in Drug Discovery and Development, 6*(3), 370−376.

LeCun, Y., Bengio, Y., & Hinton, G. (2015). Deep learning. *Nature, 521*(7553), 436−444.

Lee, J. G., Jun, S., Cho, Y. W., Lee, H., Kim, G. B., Seo, J. B., et al. (2017). Deep learning in medical imaging: General overview. *Korean Journal of Radiology, 18*(4), 570−584.

Libusova, L., Sulimenko, T., Sulimenko, V., Hozak, P., & Draber, P. (2004). Gamma-tubulin in Leishmania: Cell cycledependent changes in subcellular localization and heterogeneity of its isoforms. *Experimental Cell Research, 295*(2), 375−386.

Lin, S. K. (2000). Pharmacophore perception, development and use in drug design. *Molecules, 5*(7), 987−989.

Lo, Y. C., Rensi, S. E., Torng, W., & Altman, R. B. (2018). Machine learning in chemoinformatics and drug discovery. *Drug Discovery Today, 23*(8), 1538−1546.

Lodola, A., & De Vivo, M. (2012). The increasing role of QM/MM in drug discovery. *Advances in Protein Chemistry and Structural Biology, 87*, 337−362.

Loew, G. H., Villar, H. O., & Alkorta, I. (1993). Strategies for indirect computer-aided drug design. *Pharmaceutical Research, 10*(4), 475−486.

Maia, M. D. S., Silva, J., Nunes, T. A. L., Sousa, J. M. S., Rodrigues, G. C. S., Monteiro, A. F. M., et al. (2020). Virtual screening and the in vitro assessment of the antileishmanial activity of lignans. *Molecules, 25*(10).

Marreiros, B. C., Sena, F. V., Sousa, F. M., Oliveira, A. S. F., Soares, Cu. M., Batista, A. P., et al. (2017). Structural and Functional insights into the catalytic mechanism of the Type II NADH:quinone oxidoreductase family. *Scientific Reports, 7*(1), 42303.

Mason, J. S., Good, A. C., & Martin, E. J. (2001). 3-D pharmacophores in drug discovery. *Current Pharmaceutical Design, 7*(7), 567−597.

Mayr, A., Klambauer, G. n, Unterthiner, T., & Hochreiter, S. (2016). DeepTox: Toxicity prediction using deep learning. *Frontiers in Environmental Science, 3*(80).

McCammon, J. A., Gelin, B. R., & Karplus, M. (1977). Dynamics of folded proteins. *Nature, 267*(5612), 585−590.

Meng, X. Y., Zhang, H. X., Mezei, M., & Cui, M. (2011). Molecular docking: A powerful approach for structure-based drug discovery. *Current Computer-Aided Drug Design, 7*(2), 146−157.

Meyer, E. A., Castellano, R. K., & Diederich, F. (2003). Interactions with aromatic rings in chemical and biological recognition. *Angewandte Chemie International Edition, 42*, 1210−1250.

Min, S., Lee, B., & Yoon, S. (2017). Deep learning in bioinformatics. *Briefings in Bioinformatics, 18*(5), 851−869.

Mohr, D. C., Zhang, M., & Schueller, S. M. (2017). Personal sensing: Understanding mental health using ubiquitous sensors and machine learning. *Annual Review of Clinical Psychology, 13*, 23−47.

Norgeot, B., Glicksberg, B. S., & Butte, A. J. (2019). A call for deep-learning healthcare. *Nature Medicine, 25*(1), 14−15.

Okafo, G., & Sikosek, T. (2018). Adapting drug discovery to artificial intelligence. *Drug Target Review*, 50−52.

Oliveira, L. F., Schubach, A. O., Martins, M. M., Passos, S. L., Oliveira, R. V., Marzochi, M. C., et al. (2011). Systematic review of the adverse effects of cutaneous leishmaniasis treatment in the New World. *Acta Tropica, 118*(2), 87−96.

Ong, H. B., Sienkiewicz, N., Wyllie, S., & Fairlamb, A. H. (2011). Dissecting the metabolic roles of pteridine reductase 1 in Trypanosoma brucei and Leishmania major. *The Journal of Biological Chemistry, 286*(12), 10429−10438.

Pandey, R. K., Kumbhar, B. V., Sundar, S., Kunwar, A., & Prajapati, V. K. (2016). Structure-based virtual screening, molecular docking, ADMET and molecular simulations to develop benzoxaborole analogs as potential inhibitor against Leishmania donovani trypanothione reductase. *Journal of Receptor and Signal Transduction Research, 37*(1), 60−70.

Pandey, R. K., Verma, P., Sharma, D., Bhatt, T. K., Sundar, S., & Prajapati, V. K. (2016). High-throughput virtual screening and quantum mechanics approach to develop imipramine analogues as leads against trypanothione reductase of leishmania. *Biomedicine and Pharmacotherapy, 83*, 141−152.

Pandey, S. C., Dhami, D. S., Jha, A., Shah, G. C., Kumar, A., & Samant, M. (2019). Identification of *trans-2-cis-8*-Matricaria-ester from the essential oil of *Erigeron multiradiatus* and evaluation of its antileishmanial potential by in vitro and in silico approaches. *ACS Omega, 4*(11), 14640.

Pandey, S. C., Jha, A., Kumar, A., & Samant, M. (2019). Evaluation of antileishmanial potential of computationally screened compounds targeting DEAD-box RNA helicase of *Leishmania donovani*. *International Journal of Biological Macromolecules, 121*, 480−487.

Pandey, S. C., Kumar, A., & Samant, M. (2020). Genetically modified live attenuated vaccine: A potential strategy to combat visceral leishmaniasis. *Parasite Immunology*, e12732.

Pandey, S. C., Pande, V., & Samant, M. (2020). DDX3 DEAD-box RNA helicase (Hel67) gene disruption impairs infectivity of Leishmania donovani and induces protective immunity against visceral leishmaniasis. *Sci Rep, 10*(1), 18218. Available from https://doi.org/10.1038/s41598-020-75420-y.

Patel, Y., Gillet, V. J., Bravi, G., & Leach, A. R. (2002). A comparison of the pharmacophore identification programs: Catalyst, DISCO and GASP. *Journal of Computer-Aided Molecular Design, 16*(8-9), 653−681.

Phatak, S. S., Stephan, C. C., & Cavasotto, C. N. (2009). High-throughput and in silico screenings in drug discovery. *Expert Opinion on Drug Discovery, 4*(9), 947−959.

Rashid, U., Sultana, R., Shaheen, N., Hassan, S. F., Yaqoob, F., Ahmadm, M. J., et al. (2016). Structure based medicinal chemistry-driven strategy to design substituted dihydropyrimidines as potential antileishmanial agents. *European Journal of Medicinal Chemistry, 115*, 230−244.

Reymond, J. L., Deursen, R. V., Bluma, L. C., & Ruddigkeit, L. (2010). Chemical space as a source for new drugs. *Medicinal Chemistry Communication, 1*(1), 30−38.

Richardson, J. S., & Richardson, D. C. (1989). The de novo design of protein structures. *Trends in Biochemical Sciences, 14*(7), 304−309.

Rozas, I. (2006). On the nature of hydrogen bonds: an overview on computational studies and a word about patterns. *Physical Chemistry Chemical Physics, 9*, 2782−2790.

Schneider, G., & Fechner, U. (2005). Computer-based de novo design of drug-like molecules. *Nature Reviews. Drug Discovery, 4*(8), 649−663.

Sharma, P., Joshi, T., Joshi, T., Chandra, S., & Tamta, S. (2020). In silico screening of potential antidiabetic phytochemicals from Phyllanthus emblica against therapeutic targets of type 2 diabetes. *Journal of Ethnopharmacology, 248*112268.

Shinde, S., Mol, M., Jamdar, V., & Singh, S. (2014). Molecular modeling and molecular dynamics simulations of GPI 14 in Leishmania major: Insight into the catalytic site for active site directed drug design. *Journal of Theoretical Biology, 351*, 37−46.

Shoichet, B. K. (2004). Virtual screening of chemical libraries. *Nature, 432*(7019), 862−865.

Song, C. M., Lim, S. J., & Tong, J. C. (2009). Recent advances in computer-aided drug design. *Briefings in Bioinformatics, 10*(5), 579−591.

Sousa, S. F., Fernandes, P. A., & Ramos, M. J. (2012). Computational enzymatic catalysis clarifying enzymatic mechanisms with the help of computers. *Physical Chemistry Chemical Physics*, *14*, 12431−12441.

Stevanović, S., Perdih, A., Senćanski, M., Glišić, S., Duarte, M., Tomás, A. M., & Solmajer, T. (2018). In Silico Discovery of a Substituted 6-Methoxy-quinalidine with Leishmanicidal Activity in Leishmania infantum. *Molecules*, *23*(4), 772. Available from https://doi.org/10.3390/molecules23040772.

Stumpfe, D., Bill, A., Novak, N., Loch, G., Blockus, H., & Geppert, H. (2010). Targeting multifunctional proteins by virtual screening: Structurally diverse cytohesin inhibitors with differentiated biological functions. *ACS Chemical Biology*, *5*(9), 839−849.

Sundar, S., & Chakravarty, J. (2010). Antimony toxicity. *International Journal of Environmental Research and Public Health*, *7*(12), 4267−4277.

Talele, T. T., Khedkar, S. A., & Rigby, A. C. (2010). Successful applications of computer aided drug discovery: Moving drugs from concept to the clinic. *Current Topics in Medicinal Chemistry*, *10*(1), 127−141.

Tmej, C., Chiba, P., Huber, M., Richter, E., Hitzler, M., Schaper, K. J., & Ecker, G. (1998). A combined Hansch/Free-Wilson approach as predictive tool in QSAR studies on propafenone-type modulators of multidrug resistance. *Archiv der Pharmazie (Weinheim)*, *331*, 233−240.

Vadloori, B., Sharath, A. K., Prabhu, N. P., & Maurya, R. (2018). Homology modelling, molecular docking, and molecular dynamics simulations reveal the inhibition of Leishmania donovani dihydrofolate reductase-thymidylate synthase enzyme by Withaferin-A. *BMC Research Notes*, *11*(1), 246.

Van, G. M., & Bohte, S. (2018). *Artificial neural networks as models of neural information processing*. Lausanne Switzerland: Frontiers Media SA.

Vanommeslaeghe, K., Hatcher, E., Acharya, C., Kundu, S., Zhong, S., Shim, J., et al. (2010). CHARMM general force field: A force field for drug-like molecules compatible with the CHARMM all-atom additive biological force fields. *Journal of Computational Chemistry*, *31*(4), 671−690.

Vinkers, H. M., de Jonge, M. R., Daeyaert, F. F., Heeres, J., Koymans, L. M., van Lenthe, J. H., et al. (2003). SYNOPSIS: SYNthesize and OPtimize System in Silico. *Journal of Medicinal Chemistry*, *46*(13), 2765−2773.

Wang, Q., Feng, Y., Huang, J., Wang, T., & Cheng, G. (2017). A novel framework for the identification of drug target proteins: Combining stacked auto-encoders with a biased support vector machine. *PLoS One*, *12*(4), e0176486.

Wang, Y., Zhao, H., Brewer, J. T., Li, H., Lao, Y., Amberg, W., et al. (2018). De novo design, synthesis, and biological evaluation of 3,4-disubstituted pyrrolidine sulfonamides as potent and selective glycine transporter 1 competitive inhibitors. *Journal of Medicinal Chemistry*, *61*(17), 7486−7502.

Warshel, A. (1978). Energetics of enzyme catalysis. *Proceedings of the National Academy of Sciences of the United States of America*, *75*, 5250−5254.

Wolber, G., & Langer, T. (2008). LigandScout: 3-D pharmacophores derived from protein-bound ligands and their use as virtual screening filters. *Journal of Chemical Information and Modeling*, *45*, 160−169.

Xiang, M., Cao, Y., Fan, W., Chen, L., & Mo, Y. (2012). Computer-aided drug design: Lead discovery and optimization. *Combinatorial Chemistry & High Throughput Screening*, *15*(4), 328−337.

Yang, S. Y. (2010). Pharmacophore modeling and applications in drug discovery: Challenges and recent advances. *Drug Discovery Today*, *15*(11-12), 444–450.

Zhang, S., Cao, Z., Tian, H., Shen, G., Ma, Y., Xie, H., et al. (2011). SKLB1002, a novel potent inhibitor of VEGF receptor 2 signaling, inhibits angiogenesis and tumor growth in vivo. *Clinical Cancer Research*, *17*(13), 4439–4450.

Chapter 5

DNA microarray analysis of *Leishmania* parasite: strengths and limitations

Satish Chandra Pandey[1], Saurabh Gangola[2], Saurabh Kumar[3], Prasenjit Debborma[4], Deep Chandra Suyal[5], Arjita Punetha[6], Tushar Joshi[7], Pankaj Bhatt[8] and Mukesh Samant[1]

[1]*Cell and Molecular Biology Laboratory, Department of Zoology, Kumaun University, SSJ Campus, Almora, India,* [2]*School of Agriculture, Graphic Era Hill University, Bhimtal, India,* [3]*Division of Crop Research, ICAR-Research Complex for Eastern Region, Patna, India,* [4]*School of Agriculture, Graphic Era Hill University, Dehradun, India,* [5]*Department of Microbiology, Akal College of Basic Sciences, Eternal University, Baru Sahib, Sirmaur, India,* [6]*Department of Environmental Science, GBPUAT, Pantnagar, India,* [7]*Department of Botany, Kumaun University, SSJ Campus, Almora, India,* [8]*Integrative Microbiology Research Centre, South China Agricultural University, Guangzhou, China*

5.1 Introduction

Leishmaniasis is a tropical and subtropical human disease caused by around 20 species of an intracellular protozoan parasite, *Leishmania*. Leishmaniasis is endemic in Asia, Africa, the Americas, and the Mediterranean region which globally causes annual 1.5−2 million new cases and more than 70,000 deaths every year (Torres-Guerrero, Quintanilla-Cedillo, Ruiz-Esmenjaud, & Arenas, 2017). Therefore, World Health Organization has characterized leishmaniasis as one of the seven most important tropical diseases with a potentially fatal outcome. Flagellated protozoon, *Leishmania* is a digenetic endoparasite, completing its life cycle in two different hosts, viz., a mammalian host and insect vectors. Human transmission of *Leishmania* is associated with the bite of over 90 species of female sandflies, belonging to the genus *Phlebotomus* and *Lutzomyia*. In sandfly, *Leishmania* lives as a promastigote forms and in mammalian host as amastigote forms, therefore exhibiting dimorphism. Different species of *Leishmania* are reported to cause a wide spectrum of diseases like cutaneous, mucocutaneous, or visceral leishmaniasis (VL), but their clinical manifestation mainly depends on the immunity of the host. *L. major* and *L. braziliensis* causes nonfatal chronic cutaneous lesions and mucocutaneous leishmaniasis, respectively. While, fatal visceralizing leishmaniasis is

Pathogenesis, Treatment and Prevention of Leishmaniasis. DOI: https://doi.org/10.1016/B978-0-12-822800-5.00003-2

caused by *L. donovani* in the Indian subcontinent, *L. infantum* in Mediterranean basin and *L. chagasi* in Brazil (Torres-Guerrero et al., 2017).

Many drugs have been used for the treatment of leishmaniasis, but pentavalent antimonials are the most effective treatment available (Monzote, 2009). However, increasing resistance to pentavalent antimonials is a major concern as this drug is considered as the drug of last resort for leishmaniasis (Dhami, Pandey, Shah, Bisht, & Samant, 2020; Kumar, Pandey, & Samant, 2018; Pandey et al., 2019; Pandey, Jha, Kumar, & Samant, 2019). Intensive research is also going on to develop an effective vaccine that would provide protection against all types of leishmaniasis (Mohammed et al., 2020; Pandey, Kumar, & Samant, 2020). Therefore, there is an immense need to understand the parasite biology and host-parasite interactions in more depth for *Leishmania* (Kumar, Pandey, & Samant, 2020a,b). Although, advancement in DNA sequencing technology has already revolutionized the study of *Leishmania* by sequencing all the major species, in depth knowledge of gene expression pattern inside the primary and intermediate host is still limited. Therefore, DNA microarray could be the potential tool to study gene expression in Leishmaniasis.

DNA microarray is a collection of microscope probes attached on solid surface used for high-throughput expression analysis, pathogens detection, and comparative genomic hybridization studies (Martinez et al., 2015; Prasad, Hasan, Grouchy, & Gartia, 2019). DNA microarray enables the gene expression monitoring of thousands of genes simultaneously. Initial experiments on use of labeled DNA probe for expression analysis were reported in 1970, but the first article on the use of DNA microarray for expression analysis was published in 1995 by Schena, Shalon, Davis, & Brown (1995). Since then several advancements in DNA microarray technology paved its use for gene expression profiling, pathogen detection and typing, SNP detection, and CGH.

Previously, DNA microarray has been used for comparative gene expression profiling of amastigote form of *L. major*, *L. infantum*, and *L. Braziliensis* (Rochette et al., 2008). Besides expression analysis, DNA microarray has also been used for rapid and accurate detection and genotyping of various pathogenic diseases like epidemic hemorrhagic fever, leptospirosis, malaria, schistosomiasis, cholera, hemorrhagic colitis. Highly accurate and reliable microarray platform for determination of several blood protozoan species including *Leishmania* has already been developed (Chen et al., 2016). Therefore DNA microarray technology has huge potential in studying *Leishmania* biology and identification of novel drug targets to combat fatal VL.

5.2 Type of DNA microarray

DNA microarray can be divided into three types based on the mode of preparation.

1. The spotted array on glass,
2. Self-assembled arrays,
3. In situ synthesized arrays.

5.2.1 The spotted array on glass

This is the simplest form of microarray in which DNA is physically deposited from DNA containing solution into on a 1" × 3" poly-L-lysine coated glass microscope slide with the help of slotted pins. Hybridization can be detected by linking probe with fluorescent or radioactive labels.

5.2.2 Self-assembled arrays

In this type of microarray, different DNA probes are synthesized in different small polystyrene beads and deposited on the wells present in end of a pitted glass surface or fiber optic array thus creating random assembled array. For decoding of each bead, hybridization and detection of short fluorescently labeled oligonucleotide is performed in sequential manner.

5.2.3 In situ synthesized arrays

In this type of array, a short single strand of DNA is synthesized on 5-in. square quartz wafers through chemical synthesis mainly by photolithography. These DNA probes in oligonucleotide arrays are generally short length of about 25 bp. These arrays are mostly used in expression analysis, genotyping, and sequencing.

5.3 cDNA microarray versus oligonucleotide microarray

cDNA microarray was first developed by Patrick Brown in 1995 (Schena et al., 1995). For this microarray preparation, probes (PCR amplified gene) are spotted on poly-L-lysine coated slide with the help of robotic pins. Length of the oligonucleotide probe in $_c$DNA microarray usually varies from 100 to 1000 bp. For expression studies, mRNA is isolated from the sample, converted into cDNA, labeled with fluorophore during mRNA to cDNA conversion, followed by hybridization with the probe present in glass slides.

On the other hand, oligonucleotide microarray was first introduced by Stephen Fodor and colleagues in 1991 (Niemitz, 2007) which was based on in situ chemical synthesis. Further advancement of technology leads to development of GeneChips which is high density oligonucleotide-based DNA arrays. In this, short single strand of DNA is synthesized on 5-inch square quartz wafers through photolithography (Hughes & Shoemaker, 2001). These DNA probes in oligonucleotide arrays are generally short length of about 25 bp. This type of microarray is more fast, specific, and reproducible than the cDNA microarray thus preferred for expression analysis, genotyping, and sequencing.

5.4 DNA microarrays: a technique to boost molecular parasitology research

DNA microarray is an advanced biotechnological technique that can be used for several applications, viz., genotyping, gene expression profiling, transcription factor binding assays, etc. It is a lab-on-chip technique comprises of thousands of microscopic DNA spots attached to a solid surface. This technique involves several branches of the sciences, that is, biology, molecular biology, biochemistry, biophysics, bioinformatics, genetics, chemistry, computer science, and mathematics, which collectively makes it accurate and reliable. Similar to other molecular techniques, DNA microarray has both advantages as well as disadvantages (Kumar et al., 2020a,b). However, it is considered as an accurate, cost effective, sensitive, and reliable technique, especially under high sample size conditions. The methodological part of this technique can be divided into two portions—dry lab and wet lab (Miller & Tang, 2009).

The term "dry lab" refers to part of bioinformatics technology, and the "wet lab" is related to the laboratory experiments. Redesign, experimental printing, bimolecular labeling, hybridization re-imaging, and scanning are important steps of DNA microarray. The probe designing is an in silico approach that is accomplished by using appropriate softwares and databases. It comes under dry lab. On the other hand, wet lab includes spotting of the probe, labeling of target, hybridization and identification.

It is generally taken as fact that many genes and their associated RNA/proteins act in a complicated and coordinated manner in a given parasite that creates the mystery of acute and chronic infection such as VL. Orthodox molecular biology approaches, however, typically operad on the concept of one gene discovery by one experiment. This implies that the throughput is quite small and it is difficult to obtain the entire image of the function gene in a specific pathogen. DNA microarray has fascinated enormous interests in molecular parasitologists over the past few years. Such a high-throughput technique aims to track the entire genome on a single chip so that, among multiple genes simultaneously, investigators can have a clearer understanding of host–pathogen interactions (Patino & Ramirez, 2017). DNA microarray is frequently used in the field of parasitology. It can be used to study parasitic life cycle and development, analyzing host responses towards infection, target identification for drug and vaccine development, diagnostics, and screening of biomarkers. It has been used in detection and genotyping of several clinically important parasites, viz., *Plasmodium, Toxoplasma*, and *Trypanosoma* (Duncan et al., 2004). Some investigators have used it for rapid detection of several *Plasmodium* species (*P. falciparum, P. malariae, P. ovale*, and *P. vivax*) (Hong, Edel, & Demello, 2009). In the case of *Leishmania*, this technique has widely been used for studying pathogencity and identifying diagnostic biomarkers. Alonso, Larraga, and Alcolea (2018) have used it for analyzing genome of *Leishmania* spp. (Alonso et al., 2018). Furthermore, gene expression profiling of *L. donovani* (Yadav, Chandra, &

TABLE 5.1 Steps in the development and implementation of a DNA microarray in parasite biology (Kumar et al., 2020a,b).

Steps	Design and inference
1. DNA type (Probe)	Small oligos, cDNAs, whole parasite DNA on a chip
2. Fabrication	Placing probes on the chip with the help of Photolithography, pipetting, drop-touch, piezoelectric
3. Sample preparation (target)	cDNA, mRNA fluorescently labeled
4. Assays	Hybridization, long, short, ligase, electrophoresis, MS, PCR, flow cytometry
5. Readout	Fluorescence, probeless, electronic
6. Informatics	Robotics control, Image processing, DBMS, bioinformatics, data mining, Softwares

Saha, 2016) and *L. major* (Akopyants et al., 2004) has been studied thoroughly using DNA microarray. Furthermore, it has been successfully used for identifying the karyotypic variations among drug-resistant parasites (Van den Kerkhof, Sterckx, Leprohon, Maes, & Caljon, 2020). DNA microarray has also been explored for detection of fish associated parasites (El Deen, Zaki, & Fawzi, 2018). Biochip, DNA/gene/genome chip, DNA arrays based on oligonucleotides, gene array, etc. are terminology used in the literature to define the technology of DNA microarrays. For gene expression analysis of the parasite, there are many steps in the formulation and construction of a DNA microarray experiment (Bumgarner, 2013). These strategies have been summarized in Table 5.1 and strategies should have investigated at each step. After analyzing *Leishmania* parasite microarray data, we were able to obtain diagnostic, prognostic, and therapeutic target information which would be crucially important for future directions of molecular parasitology.

5.5 Link between microarray and identification of diagnostics/prognostics biomarkers and therapeutic targets in leishmaniasis

The main setback in leishmaniasis chemotherapy is drug resistance. To study this resistance phenotype against drug, DNA microarray is considered as suitable technique for RNA expression profiling. DNA microarray is a perfect tool to unravel the mRNA levels through quantification ultimately leading to a discovery of novel drug targets. It is also utilized for various other applications where high-throughput is required (Clarke, te Poele, & Workman, 2004). Moreover, this special technique is helpful in recognizing precise species as well as strain-specific biomarkers which can be useful in diagnosis and identifying the drug-resistant *Leishmania*. Furthermore, exploring the mechanism of action of drugs and their resistance nature has been successfully studied by DNA microarray technique (Brazas & Hancock, 2005; Wilson et al., 1999). In *Leishmania* DNA microarray have been used extensively for different aspects, viz., construction of clone libraries, targeted PCR fragments, whole genome analysis, and selected 70-mer oligonucleotides, etc. (Leprohon, Légaré, Girard, Papadopoulou, & Ouellette, 2006; Saxena et al., 2007; Singh et al., 2007). Drug resistance in *Leishmania* has been studied by using targeted microarray (El Fadili et al., 2005; Guimond et al., 2003).

Whole genome sequencing of *Leishmania* including other related accomplishments in several parasites have created an important source for available genomic database. It is well understood that the development of targeted drug or vaccine for *Leishmania* is a challenging as well as a daunting task (Pritchard et al., 2003). In this scenario, DNA microarray technique become the foremost diagnostic tool employed for drug or vaccine discovery (Wang & Cheng, 2006).

Revelation of biochemical pathways and target identification for new drug or any novel therapeutics in Leishmaniasis has been achieved by global gene expression profiling. Promastigotes and amastigotes are two different stages found in *Leishmania* which leads to important antigenic diversity. DNA microarray study could give insight looks to this diversity through gene expression profiling resulting in identifying effective targets. Changes in morphology and physiology of *Leishmania* during the transmission from sandfly to human alter the expression of various genes. Global gene expression profiling has been utilized to recognize the molecular phenomenon related to *Leishmania* amastigote stage. In contrast, DNA microarray technique has been used for last few years to study the gene expression behavior in *Leishmania*. Many genes involved in drug resistance were identified through gene expression profiling of both wild and mutant *Leishmania* (Guimond et al., 2003). Therefore, DNA microarray technique could be used proficiently to recognize the drug resistance characteristics of *Leishmania* strains as well as susceptible strains as it can distinguish both upregulated and downregulated genes. Furthermore, microarray can be useful to study the procyclic and metacyclic stages of *Leishmania* which would inform the modifications in gene expression takes place at parasitic life differentiation. Differentiation of metacyclic stage of *L. major* and procyclic stage of *L. mexicana* from procyclic promastigotes have been studied and found out the sequential modifications in their gene expression (Holzer, McMaster, & Forney, 2006; Saxena et al., 2003). Previous studies have shown that around 8160 genes were used for DNA oligonucleotide genome microarrays to examine the mRNA expression profiles of *L. major* promastigotes and lesion derived amastigotes. It was also observed through DNA microarray assay that there are significant dissimilarities in gene expression behavior between *L. major* and *L. infantum* during their developmental stages (Rochette et al., 2008).

In VL, developmentally regulated genes were identified as a target by using promastigote and amastigote stage of *L. donovani* and *L. infantum* (Pandey, Pande, & Samant, 2020; Saxena et al., 2007, 2003; Srividya et al., 2007). In another study, gene expression for type 1 immune cytokine activation was reported in *L. chagasi* (Ettinger & Wilson, 2008; Samant, Sahu, Pandey, & Khare, 2021). Likewise, DNA microarray study has shown the expression in RNAs from BALB/c bone marrow macrophages with *L. chagasi* infection (Rodriguez et al., 2004). DNA microarray analysis has been done to examine the resistance mechanism of sodium antimony gluconate against *L. donovani* (El Fadili et al., 2008). Complementary DNA microarray analysis of bone marrow-derived macrophages has revealed the pathogenesis mechanism of *L. donovani* or *L. major* promastigotes through gene expression profiling (Gregory, Sladek, Olivier, & Matlashewski, 2008).

To control the VL, new target identification for novel drug discovery is a need of the hour. With the advances of global technology in the field of genomics which has great potential to discover new targets that can contribute to diagnosis, treatment, and prevention of leishmaniasis. In the last few years, many genes were identified for VL by using microarray technique and classified based on their ontology. Functions of these genes in drug or vaccine targeting were authenticated. By using the microarray technique out of verified genes *Enolase* and MAP kinase was found to be potential vaccine candidate (Gupta et al., 2007; Wei et al., 2002). In another report, gp63 surface gene was used as vaccine development in *L. donovani* (Jaffe, Rachamim, & Sarfstein, 1990). Gonzales Aseguinolaza, Taladriz, Marquet, & Larraga (1999) and Gurunathan et al. (1997) advocated LACK as strong vaccine candidate in *L. infantum* and *L. major*, respectively (Gonzales Aseguinolaza et al., 1999; Gurunathan et al., 1997). Promastigote surface antigen (PSA) a leucine rich repeats are the main epitopes in *L. infantum* (Boceta, Alonso, & Jiménez-Ruiz, 2000). Protective vaccination with PSA 2 from *L. major* is mediated by a Th1-type of immune response and acts as a potential vaccine candidate (Handman, Symons, Baldwin, Curtis, & Scheerlinck, 1995).

Together, these results provide a framework and emphasize for more microarray-based studies of *Leishmania* species to demonstrate that this high-throughput tools are valuable for identification of potential drug/vaccine targets and also to enhance our understanding in drug resistance mechanisms and factors involved.

5.6   Insight and issues with the use of DNA microarray

Leishmaniasis is a well-recognized infectious disease in tropical and subtropical countries. To date, Leishmaniasis treatments are unsatisfactory and have a serious problem with drug resistance. DNA microarray is an advanced technology that can contribute in discovering the new vaccine against Leishmaniasis. Microarray technologies already have been used for genome sequencing and gene expression of *Leishmania*. This technology aid the understanding of pathogenicity and drug resistance mechanism which characterize the respective gene expression. With the help of microarray we can study the differential expression of *Leishmania* genes as biomarkers for early diagnosis in the future. However, the microarray technology has not yet advanced substantially for validation and new gene discovery in parasites like *Trypanosoma* and *Leishmania* (Kumar, Sen, & Das, 2010).

DNA microarray was introduced for the first time in 1995 and is considered a massive achievement for field applications and technology (Schena et al., 1995). Schena et al. created the first microarray and with the use of robotic printer, printed a number of cDNAs on a glass microscope slide, thereby monitoring differential expression of multiple genes in parallel using that microarray. First, most of the microarray platforms developed so far have been used to obtain expression profiles of genes (Alizadeh et al., 2000). Second, development of genotyping array has made it quite easier to characterize the DNA (and sometimes RNA) so as to be able to characterize viral pathogens and also to detect mutations occurring in human genes. Third, array-based comparative genomic hybridization (array-CGH) has multiple advantages over classical karyotyping techniques such as it provides a high-resolution device to screen the copy number variations in whole genome (Shaw-Smith et al., 2004). Numerous studies have been elucidated that the gene expression of host cell in response to *Leishmania* infection using microarray analysis (Shadab et al., 2019).

While growing extremely fast, especially in the field of research, the microarray technology still lags behind in terms of development of its clinical applications. Much more problems rely in biostatistics than the technical issues. One challenge that microarray data faces is being considered as "noisy" (Dupuy & Simon, 2007). Several articles report that microarray studies have been highly criticized for reproducibility of the data and the validity of the data interpretation as inappropriate in terms of standardization, having inadequate quality control measures, and being unreliable in the context of data processing (Simon, Radmacher, Dobbin, & McShane, 2003). The concerns relating to the validity of clinical interpretation are grave in applications like expression profiling during introduction of new biomarkers as compared to other applications such as genotyping arrays, which deal with preexisting known biomarkers. Cut throat competition between microarray-based tests, PCR-based and tests based on sequencing is yet another challenge. Next-generation sequencing (NGS) techniques, a newly emerged field can provide with comprehensive information of whole genome in comparatively very low prices than the microarray tests (Jordan, 2010).

Besides, use of microarray technology for point-of-care (POC) diagnostics also meets numerous hurdles. For instance, the conventional format requires the sample solution to undergo various steps of sample preparation, typically on bulky bench-top instruments, before it can be introduced to DNA microarray slide (Wang & Li, 2011).

5.6.1   Toward microarray POC devices

On its way to become a POC device, microarray technology has to face multiple challenges. The first foremost being integration of whole assay into an individual, portable device. Currently microarray technologies make use of separate instruments for every step including sample preparation, DNA hybridization, signal visualization, and data interpretation. Furthermore, these include some very heavy and bulky components like the fluorescent scanners used for signal visualization, which are selectively available only in well-equipped laboratories. Another major challenge faced is that the time required for reaction in DNA hybridizations is very long, taking 12−17 hours (Bynum & Gordon, 2004).

5.6.2   Microfluidic microarrays

Microfluidics remain at the core of LOC devices (Stone, Stroock, & Ajdari, 2004). Integrating liquid handling operations and microarray assays adds following advantages to them:

1. Reduction in consumption of sample and reagent because of minute micrometer-sized channels.
2. Liquid being extremely efficient and controllable owing to small size of channels. Besides, delivery among these channels allows integration of several steps of microarray assays that are vital to implement the LOC devices (Hong et al., 2009).
3. Conventional microarrays allow delivery of target molecules to the probe spots by convective along with diffusion hence, reducing the time taken for hybridization from hours to minutes.
4. Last but not the least, microfluidic microarray provides the benefit of its potentially high sample throughput, apart from its adequate probe density.

Conventional microarray experiments in general allow applications only one sample per glass chip; however, a greater challenge of DNA microarrays is the inevitable variation amongst the samples, which might direct fake positive recognition of biomarkers in the early studies on microarrays (Simon et al., 2003). These variations generate replicate analysis of various crucial samples, which makes the multisample analysis ability of microfluidic microarray chips highly valuable. Delivering sample solutions over the probe spots in DNA hybridization requires the microfluidic flow. This can be achieved in two ways, use of either microfluidic chambers or the microfluidic channels in order to enhance DNA hybridization of target solutions (Liu, Williams, Gwirtz, Wold, & Quake, 2006; Peytavi et al., 2005; Wang & Cheng, 2006). First, the area with arrayed probes, where hybridization between sample DNA solutions and probe molecules occurs is covered with large microfluidic chambers (Liu et al., 2006). These chambers are attuned to both low-density and high-density microarrays. But, it is a huge challenge to design a liquid flow that is even and gets distributed equally over the large chamber. Second, microfluidic channels provide a better flow control of target solutions as compared to probe arrays (Peytavi et al., 2005). Numerous microfluidic chips have been designed so far that have straight and serpentine microchannels, mainly to conduct low-density microarray experiments (Wang & Li, 2011).

The microfluidic flow is also used to print probe solutions on the surface along with delivery of the sample solutions for hybridization. The quality of printed probe-spot morphology greatly influences the performance of hybridization assay. Being exposed to the air in pin-spotting method, spotting solutions are subjected to problems of splashing, not evaporating evenly, and cross contamination (Campas & Katakis, 2004). Moreover, unreacted probes formed from blocking and washing procedures after the process of probe spotting on glass surface could diffuse away and smear the chip leading to formation of comet-like spots (Sedighi & Li, 2014). In addition, during the further use of microchannel to enclose the spotted bioarray, use of steel clamps must be done so as to ensure proper alignment of entire hybridization microchannel to the probe rows (Sedighi & Li, 2014). The use of microchannel network as a microprinting technique can help obtain the probe spots with high homogeneity (Lee, Goodrich, & Corn, 2001; Sedighi & Li, 2014).

5.6.3 Label-free detection

Current DNA microarrays make use of fluorescent dyes to label target molecules in order to detect them. However, to achieve a high resolution in fluorescent detection, bulky fluorescent scanners are required. This is a major hurdle that limits the miniaturization required for the development of POC device. Besides, labeling the target molecules makes the process much complicated and costly. The results are also influenced to a great extent by the efficiency of labeling process and fluorescence quenching of the dye (Sassolas, Leca-Bouvier, & Blum, 2008). Development of numerous approaches in the past decade has taken to enhance efficiency of target labeling (Sassolas et al., 2008). Molecular beacon (MB) is a novel approach exploiting both the features of fluorescence, that is, sensitivity and convenience in label-free target detection (Fang, Liu, Schuster, & Tan, 1999). MB probes are some single-stranded nucleic acids that maintain a stem-and-loop structure and retain a pair of fluorophore-quencher at both the ends of their strands closely, thereby quenching the fluorescence emission in absence of target molecules. This loop region of MB strands gets hybridized to the target in presence of nonlabeled target molecules and as a result opens the MB structures up, thereby enhancing the fluorescence by removing the quenching (Fang et al., 1999).

5.6.4 Miniaturized nanoarray platforms

Fluorescence detectors make utilization of objectives having high numerical-aperture and great magnifications to detect even fairly weak fluorescence signals that are emitted from the microarray spots. Large magnification causes the detection of fewer microarray spots by the detector, which in turn makes the scanning of the whole area of array quite necessary. Therefore, an urgent need for development of large-format scanning fluorescent detectors is a major hindrance in development of portable microarray devices. Miniaturization of the microarray features in a way so as to make the whole array visible in the field of view of the objectives would make the scanning unnecessary. Miniaturized microarrays favor rapid mass and heat transport along with removing the need for bulky scanning therefore, reducing the assay time (Tsarfati-BarAd, Sauer, Preininger, & Gheber, 2011). Developing arrays with submicrometer features requires development of very accurate printing techniques with extremely high resolutions.

5.6.5 Integrated LOC devices

Not much time after microarray was introduced, it was noticed that it is highly beneficial to integrate all steps of the DNA microarray into a single device. However, integration is not as simple as attaching these subsystems together. All aspects of the integrated system like liquid handling techniques, thermal and pressure control, material of substrate, and units of signal transduction need to be compatible with every subsystem. Despite these challenges, great efforts have been put by researchers to develop LOC devices to be able to perform as many steps of the microarray assay as possible (Anderson, Su, Bogdan, & Fenton, 2000; Choi et al., 2012).

Use of integrated electrochemical micropumps was done to transfer liquids from reagent chambers to DNA microarray silicon chips. Microarray hybridization and further steps of washing and labeling were all performed in a self-contained device. The step including detection however was conducted on an external fluorescent scanner (Liu et al., 2006). In a recent study, a miniature fluorescent scanner, in place of a conventional bulky one, was used for the purpose of detection (Choi et al., 2012). Choi et al. used an integration of allele-specific PCR system and a disposable DNA microarray chip to achieve multiplex SNP detection. The hybridization process was accelerated using convective flows created by pneumatic micropumps, resulting in completion of whole on-site assay in 100 minutes (Choi et al., 2012). Even though significant progress has been made so far in developing the LOC devices, they are still not standalone devices, meeting requirements of POC diagnostics.

5.7 Conclusion

Recent advancements in various molecular biology and genome sequencing techniques hold great promise for fresh results and observations that would be helpful in leishmaniasis prevention, diagnosis, and treatment. Thorough knowledge of basic biology and the identification of new genes will lead to the discovery of possible candidates for vaccines and targets for drugs. One of the major steps in genome-wide technology is the DNA microarray. Microarray technology has an important influence on the study of parasite genomics. It also offers advantages, including antimicrobial discovery and toxicological testing, to other fields. In the design and implementation of DNA microarray experiments for gene expression analysis of the parasite, this review covers different strategies. Exciting drug targets, vaccine candidates, and biomarkers have been identified in these DNA microarray studies that can be tested as putative diagnostics, prognostics, and therapeutic targets.

Recent years have seen the development of some powerful LOC devices having integrated steps of the assay on their miniaturized platform. Nevertheless, they are still not capable of performing an assay without requirements of some external instrument. Particularly, for signal detection, they rely on the use the conventional methods (Anderson et al., 2000). Development of novel and compatible supporting technologies that shall allow their miniaturization is the major aspect in creation of LOC devices for POC. Another feature that can simplify future of LOC devices is developing the label-free detection techniques, other than fluorescent techniques. Microarray assays involve integration of several steps in standalone LOC devices in a more systematic way, which makes them capable of performing sample-in—answer-out assays efficiently and rapidly. These LOC devices exploit microfluidic networks both to connect their different compartments and help the device to become faster to use, smaller in size, and conveniently controlled. These LOC devices will be suitable candidates for POC diagnostics and shall play a vital role in personalized medicine in the future. With the passage of time, microarray technology approaches have reached their maturity, overcoming many of the issues they had at the start. Consequently, the microarrays of present day are sufficiently robust and reliable. While DNA microarray face fierce competition from NGS at the high end of throughput and from PCR-based techniques, hindering their progress in molecular diagnostic market, microarrays still have some advantages over these techniques. NGs techniques though sufficiently cheap, are still more expensive as compared the ones offered by microarray competitors. Some other unsettled difficulties in sequencing techniques, such as extensive sample preparation and data interpretation and the necessity of multiplexing in RNA sequencing (Morozova, Hirst, & Marra, 2009) will be go in favor of microarrays. On the other hand, with gaining familiarity among clinicians and getting more flexible in sample matrix, microarray techniques are moving to a better situation in their competition with PCR-based techniques. DNA microarrays have continued to exist, DNA microarrays have continued to exist in the fast-growing molecular diagnostic market even in the presence of NGS. Besides, more microarray-based diagnostic tests are gaining regulatory approval and entering the market at present. As per a recent report, microarray-based tests share the major portion of molecular diagnostics market with PCR-based tests and according to another report, their market is expected to grow by 15% in the coming years (Sedighi & Li, 2014). Overall, microarray technology seems to be progressively reviving in the clinical market, even though it does not dominate it as was expected in the days of its introduction.

References

Akopyants, N. S., Matlib, R. S., Bukanova, E. N., Smeds, M. R., Brownstein, B. H., Stormo, G. D., et al. (2004). Expression profiling using random genomic DNA microarrays identifies differentially expressed genes associated with three major developmental stages of the protozoan parasite Leishmania major. *Molecular and Biochemical Parasitology, 136*(1), 71−86.

Alizadeh, A. A., Eisen, M. B., Davis, R. E., Ma, C., Lossos, I. S., Rosenwald, A., et al. (2000). Distinct types of diffuse large B-cell lymphoma identified by gene expression profiling. *Nature, 403*(6769), 503−511.

Alonso, A., Larraga, V., & Alcolea, P. J. (2018). The contribution of DNA microarray technology to gene expression profiling in *Leishmania* spp.: A retrospective view. *Acta Tropica, 187*, 129−139.

Anderson, R. C., Su, X., Bogdan, G. J., & Fenton, J. (2000). A miniature integrated device for automated multistep genetic assays. *Nucleic Acids Research, 28*(12), e60.

Boceta, C., Alonso, C., & Jiménez-Ruiz, A. (2000). Leucine rich repeats are the main epitopes in Leishmania infantum PSA during canine and human visceral leishmaniasis. *Parasite Immunology, 22*(2), 55−62.

Brazas, M. D., & Hancock, R. E. W. (2005). Using microarray gene signatures to elucidate mechanisms of antibiotic action and resistance. *Drug Discovery Today, 10*(18), 1245−1252.

Bumgarner, R. (2013). Chapter 22: Overview of DNA microarrays: Types, applications, and their future. In Ausubel, F. M., et al., Current protocols in molecular biology, Unit 22 21.

Bynum, M. A., & Gordon, G. B. (2004). Hybridization enhancement using microfluidic planetary centrifugal mixing. *Analytical Chemistry, 76*(23), 7039−7044.

Campas, M., & Katakis, I. (2004). DNA biochip arraying, detection and amplification strategies. *Trends in Analytical Chemistry, 23*(1), 49−62.

Chen, M.-X., Ai, L., Chen, J.-H., Feng, X.-Y., Chen, S.-H., Cai, Y.-C., et al. (2016). DNA microarray detection of 18 important human blood protozoan species. *PLoS Neglected Tropical Diseases, 10*(12), e0005160.

Choi, J. Y., Kim, Y. T., Byun, J.-Y., Ahn, J., Chung, S., Gweon, D.-G., et al. (2012). An integrated allele-specific polymerase chain reaction-microarray chip for multiplex single nucleotide polymorphism typing. *Lab on a Chip, 12*(24), 5146−5154.

Clarke, P. A., te Poele, R., & Workman, P. (2004). Gene expression microarray technologies in the development of new therapeutic agents. *European Journal of Cancer, 40*(17), 2560−2591.

Dhami, D. S., Pandey, S. C., Shah, G. C., Bisht, M., & Samant, M. (2020). In vitro antileishmanial activity of the essential oil from *Agrimonia pilosa*. *National Academy Science Letters*, 1−4.

Duncan, R. C., Salotra, P., Goyal, N., Akopyants, N. S., Beverley, S. M., & Nakhasi, H. L. (2004). The application of gene expression microarray technology to kinetoplastid research. *Current Molecular Medicine, 4*(6), 611−621.

Dupuy, A., & Simon, R. M. (2007). Critical review of published microarray studies for cancer outcome and guidelines on statistical analysis and reporting. *Journal of the National Cancer Institute, 99*(2), 147−157.

El Deen, A. I. N., Zaki, M. S., & Fawzi, O. M. (2018). New diagnostic methods of parasitic infections in freshwater fishes. *Journal of Advanced Pharmacy Education & Research, 8*(1), 96−102.

El Fadili, K., Imbeault, Ml, Messier, N., Roy, Gt, Gourbal, B., Bergeron, M., et al. (2008). Modulation of gene expression in human macrophages treated with the anti-leishmania pentavalent antimonial drug sodium stibogluconate. *Antimicrobial Agents and Chemotherapy, 52*(2), 526−533.

El Fadili, K., Messier, N., Leprohon, P., Roy, G. t, Guimond, C., Trudel, N., et al. (2005). Role of the ABC transporter MRPA (PGPA) in antimony resistance in Leishmania infantum axenic and intracellular amastigotes. *Antimicrobial Agents and Chemotherapy, 49*(5), 1988−1993.

Ettinger, N. A., & Wilson, M. E. (2008). Macrophage and T-cell gene expression in a model of early infection with the protozoan Leishmania chagasi. *PLoS Neglected Tropical Diseases, 2* (6), e252.

Fang, X., Liu, X., Schuster, S., & Tan, W. (1999). Designing a novel molecular beacon for surface-immobilized DNA hybridization studies. *Journal of the American Chemical Society, 121*(12), 2921−2922.

Gonzales Aseguinolaza, G., Taladriz, S., Marquet, A., & Larraga, V. (1999). Molecular cloning, cell localization and binding affinity to DNA replication proteins of the p36/LACK protective antigen from *Leishmania infantum*. *European Journal of Biochemistry, 259*(3), 909−917.

Gregory, D. J., Sladek, R., Olivier, M., & Matlashewski, G. (2008). Comparison of the effects of *Leishmania major* or *Leishmania donovani* infection on macrophage gene expression. *Infection and Immunity, 76*(3), 1186−1192.

Guimond, C., Trudel, N., Brochu, C., Marquis, N., Fadili, A. E., Peytavi, R. g, et al. (2003). Modulation of gene expression in Leishmania drug resistant mutants as determined by targeted DNA microarrays. *Nucleic Acids Research, 31*(20), 5886−5896.

Gupta, S. K., Sisodia, B. S., Sinha, S., Hajela, K., Naik, S., Shasany, A. K., et al. (2007). Proteomic approach for identification and characterization of novel immunostimulatory proteins from soluble antigens of *Leishmania donovani* promastigotes. *Proteomics, 7*(5), 816−823.

Gurunathan, S., Sacks, D. L., Brown, D. R., Reiner, S. L., Charest, H., Glaichenhaus, N., et al. (1997). Vaccination with DNA encoding the immunodominant LACK parasite antigen confers protective immunity to mice infected with *Leishmania major*. *The Journal of Experimental Medicine, 186*(7), 1137−1147.

Handman, E., Symons, F. M., Baldwin, T. M., Curtis, J. M., & Scheerlinck, J. P. (1995). Protective vaccination with promastigote surface antigen 2 from *Leishmania major* is mediated by a TH1 type of immune response. *Infection and Immunity, 63*(11), 4261−4267.

Holzer, T. R., McMaster, W. R., & Forney, J. D. (2006). Expression profiling by whole-genome interspecies microarray hybridization reveals differential gene expression in procyclic promastigotes, lesion-derived amastigotes, and axenic amastigotes in *Leishmania mexicana*. *Molecular and Biochemical Parasitology, 146*(2), 198−218.

Hong, J., Edel, J. B., & Demello, A. J. (2009). Micro- and nanofluidic systems for high-throughput biological screening. *Drug Discovery Today, 14*(3-4), 134−146.

Hughes, T. R., & Shoemaker, D. D. (2001). DNA microarrays for expression profiling. *Current Opinion in Chemical Biology, 5*(1), 21−25.

Jaffe, C. L., Rachamim, N., & Sarfstein, R. (1990). Characterization of two proteins from *Leishmania donovani* and their use for vaccination against visceral leishmaniasis. *The Journal of Immunology, 144*(2), 699−706.

Jordan, B. R. (2010). Is there a niche for DNA microarrays in molecular diagnostics? *Expert Review of Molecular Diagnostics, 10*(7), 875−882.

Kumar, A., Pandey, S. C., & Samant, M. (2018). Slow pace of antileishmanial drug development. *Parasitology Open, 4*(e4), 1−11.

Kumar, A., Pandey, S. C., & Samant, M. (2020a). A spotlight on the diagnostic methods of a fatal disease Visceral Leishmaniasis. *Parasite Immunology, 42*, e12727.

Kumar, A., Pandey, S. C., & Samant, M. (2020b). DNA-based microarray studies in visceral leishmaniasis: Identification of biomarkers for diagnostic, prognostic and drug target for treatment. *Acta Tropica, 208*, 105512.

Kumar, A., Sen, A., & Das, P. (2010). Microarray based gene expression: A novel approach for identification and development of potential drug and effective vaccine against visceral Leishmaniasis. *International Journal of Advances in Pharmaceutical Sciences, 1*(1).

Lee, H. J., Goodrich, T. T., & Corn, R. M. (2001). SPR imaging measurements of 1-D and 2-D DNA microarrays created from microfluidic channels on gold thin films. *Analytical Chemistry, 73*(22), 5525−5531.

Leprohon, P., Légaré, D., Girard, I., Papadopoulou, B., & Ouellette, M. (2006). Modulation of Leishmania ABC protein gene expression through life stages and among drug-resistant parasites. *Eukaryotic Cell, 5*(10), 1713−1725.

Liu, J., Williams, B. A., Gwirtz, R. M., Wold, B. J., & Quake, S. (2006). Enhanced signals and fast nucleic acid hybridization by microfluidic chaotic mixing. *Angewandte Chemie International Edition, 45*(22), 3618−3623.

Liu, R. H., Nguyen, T., Schwarzkopf, K., Fuji, H. S., Petrova, A., Siuda, T., et al. (2006). Fully integrated miniature device for automated gene expression DNA microarray processing. *Analytical Chemistry, 78*(6), 1980−1986.

Martinez, M. A., de los Dolores Soto-del, M., Gutierrez, R. M., Chiu, C. Y., Greninger, A. L., Contreras, J. F., et al. (2015). DNA microarray for detection of gastrointestinal viruses. *Journal of Clinical Microbiology, 53*(1), 136−145.

Miller, M. B., & Tang, Y.-W. (2009). Basic concepts of microarrays and potential applications in clinical microbiology. *Clinical Microbiology Reviews, 22*(4), 611−633.

Mohammed, A. S. A., Tian, W., Zhang, Y., Peng, P., Wang, F., & Li, T. (2020). Leishmania lipophosphoglycan components: A potent target for synthetic neoglycoproteins as a vaccine candidate for Leishmaniasis (a review article). *Carbohydrate Polymers*, 116120.

Monzote, L. (2009). Current treatment of leishmaniasis: A review. *The Open Antimicrobial Agents Journal, 1*(1), 9−19.

Morozova, O., Hirst, M., & Marra, M. A. (2009). Applications of new sequencing technologies for transcriptome analysis. *Annual Review of Genomics and Human Genetics, 10*, 135−151.

Niemitz, E. (2007). The microarray revolution. *Nature Reviews Genetics, 8*, S15.

Pandey, S. C., Dhami, D. S., Jha, A., Shah, G. C., Kumar, A., & Samant, M. (2019). Identification of *trans-2-cis-8*-Matricaria-ester from the essential oil of *Erigeron multiradiatus* and evaluation of its antileishmanial potential by in vitro and in silico approaches. *ACS Omega, 4*(11), 14640.

Pandey, S. C., Jha, A., Kumar, A., & Samant, M. (2019). Evaluation of antileishmanial potential of computationally screened compounds targeting DEAD-box RNA helicase of *Leishmania donovani*. *International Journal of Biological Macromolecules, 121*, 480−487.

Pandey, S. C., Kumar, A., & Samant, M. (2020). Genetically modified live attenuated vaccine: A potential strategy to combat visceral leishmaniasis. *Parasite Immunology*, e12732.

Pandey, S. C., Pande, V., & Samant, M. (2020). DDX3 DEAD-box RNA helicase (Hel67) gene disruption impairs infectivity of *Leishmania donovani* and induces protective immunity against visceral leishmaniasis. *Scientific Reports, 10*(1), 1−10.

Patino, L. H., & Ramirez, J. D. (2017). RNA-seq in kinetoplastids: A powerful tool for the understanding of the biology and host-pathogen interactions. *Infection, Genetics and Evolution, 49*, 273−282.

Peytavi, R. g, Raymond, FdrR., GagnÃ©, D., Picard, F. J., Jia, G., Zoval, J., et al. (2005). Microfluidic device for rapid (<15 min) automated microarray hybridization. *Clinical Chemistry, 51*(10), 1836−1844.

Prasad, A., Hasan, S. M. A., Grouchy, S., & Gartia, M. R. (2019). DNA microarray analysis using a smartphone to detect the BRCA-1 gene. *Analyst, 144*(1), 197−205.

Pritchard, J. F., Jurima-Romet, M., Reimer, M. L. J., Mortimer, E., Rolfe, B., & Cayen, M. N. (2003). Making better drugs: Decision gates in non-clinical drug development. *Nature Reviews Drug Discovery, 2*(7), 542−553.

Rochette, A., Raymond, Fdr, Ubeda, J.-M., Smith, M., Messier, N., Boisvert, S. b, et al. (2008). Genome-wide gene expression profiling analysis of *Leishmania major* and *Leishmania infantum* developmental stages reveals substantial differences between the two species. *BMC Genomics, 9*(1), 255.

Rodriguez, A., Martinez, N., Camacho, F. I., Ruiz-Ballesteros, E., Algara, P., Garcia, J.-F., et al. (2004). Variability in the degree of expression of phosphorylated IκBα in chronic lymphocytic leukemia cases with nodal involvement. *Clinical Cancer Research, 10*(20), 6796−6806.

Samant, M., Sahu, U., Pandey, S. C., & Khare, P. (2021). Role of cytokines in experimental and human visceral leishmaniasis. *Frontiers in Cellular and Infection Microbiology, 11*, 624009. https://doi.org/10.3389/fcimb.2021.624009.

Sassolas, A., Leca-Bouvier, Ba. D., & Blum, Lc. J. (2008). DNA biosensors and microarrays. *Chemical Reviews, 108*(1), 109−139.

Saxena, A., Lahav, T., Holland, N., Aggarwal, G., Anupama, A., Huang, Y., et al. (2007). Analysis of the *Leishmania donovani* transcriptome reveals an ordered progression of transient and permanent changes in gene expression during differentiation. *Molecular and Biochemical Parasitology, 152*(1), 53−65.

Saxena, A., Worthey, E. A., Yan, S., Leland, A., Stuart, K. D., & Myler, P. J. (2003). Evaluation of differential gene expression in *Leishmania major* Friedlin procyclics and metacyclics using DNA microarray analysis. *Molecular and Biochemical Parasitology, 129*(1), 103−114.

Schena, M., Shalon, D., Davis, R. W., & Brown, P. O. (1995). Quantitative monitoring of gene expression patterns with a complementary DNA microarray. *Science, 270*(5235), 467–470.

Sedighi, A., & Li, P. C. H. (2014). *Challenges and future trends in DNA microarray analysis,. Comprehensive Analytical Chemistry* (Vol. 63, pp. 25–46). Elsevier.

Shadab, M., Das, S., Banerjee, A., Sinha, R., Asad, M., Kamran, M., et al. (2019). RNA-Seq revealed expression of many novel genes associated with *Leishmania donovani* persistence and clearance in the host macrophage. *Frontiers in Cellular and Infection Microbiology, 9*, 17.

Shaw-Smith, C., Redon, R., Rickman, L., Rio, M., Willatt, L., Fiegler, H., et al. (2004). Microarray based comparative genomic hybridisation (array-CGH) detects submicroscopic chromosomal deletions and duplications in patients with learning disability/mental retardation and dysmorphic features. *Journal of Medical Genetics, 41*(4), 241–248.

Simon, R., Radmacher, M. D., Dobbin, K., & McShane, L. M. (2003). Pitfalls in the use of DNA microarray data for diagnostic and prognostic classification. *Journal of the National Cancer Institute, 95*(1), 14–18.

Singh, N., Almeida, R., Kothari, H., Kumar, P., Mandal, G., Chatterjee, M., et al. (2007). Differential gene expression analysis in antimony-unresponsive Indian kala azar (visceral leishmaniasis) clinical isolates by DNA microarray. *Parasitology, 134*(6), 777.

Srividya, G., Duncan, R., Sharma, P., Raju, B. V. S., Nakhasi, H. L., & Salotra, P. (2007). Transcriptome analysis during the process of in vitro differentiation of *Leishmania donovani* using genomic microarrays. *Parasitology, 134*(11), 1527.

Stone, H. A., Stroock, A. D., & Ajdari, A. (2004). Engineering flows in small devices: Microfluidics toward a lab-on-a-chip. *Annual Review of Fluid Mechanics, 36*, 381–411.

Torres-Guerrero, E., Quintanilla-Cedillo, M. R., Ruiz-Esmenjaud, J., & Arenas, R. (2017). Leishmaniasis: A review. *F1000Research, 6*, 750.

Tsarfati-BarAd, I., Sauer, U., Preininger, C., & Gheber, L. A. (2011). Miniaturized protein arrays: Model and experiment. *Biosensors and Bioelectronics, 26*(9), 3774–3781.

Van den Kerkhof, M., Sterckx, Y. G. J., Leprohon, P., Maes, L., & Caljon, G. (2020). Experimental strategies to explore drug action and resistance in kinetoplastid parasites. *Microorganisms, 8*(6), 950.

Wang, L., & Li, P. C. H. (2011). Microfluidic DNA microarray analysis: A review. *Analytica Chimica Acta, 687*(1), 12–27.

Wang, S., & Cheng, Q. (2006). *Microarray analysis in drug discovery and clinical applications. Bioinformatics and Drug Discovery* (pp. 49–65). Springer.

Wei, S., Marches, F., Daniel, B., Sonda, S., Heidenreich, K., & Curiel, T. (2002). Pyridinylimidazole p38 mitogen-activated protein kinase inhibitors block intracellular *Toxoplasma gondii* replication. *International Journal for Parasitology, 32*(8), 969–977.

Wilson, M., DeRisi, J., Kristensen, H.-H., Imboden, P., Rane, S., Brown, P. O., & Schoolnik, G. K. (1999). Exploring drug-induced alterations in gene expression in *Mycobacterium tuberculosis* by microarray hybridization. *Proceedings of the National Academy of Sciences, USA, 96*(22), 12833–12838.

Yadav, A., Chandra, U., & Saha, S. (2016). Histone acetyltransferase HAT4 modulates navigation across G2/M and re-entry into G1 in *Leishmania donovani. Scientific Reports, 6*, 27510.

Chapter 6

Drug resistance and repurposing of existing drugs in Leishmaniasis

Ashutosh Paliwal, Rekha Gahtori, Amrita Kumari and Pooja Pandey
Department of Biotechnology, Kumaun University, Sir J C Bose Technical Campus, Bhimtal, India

6.1 Introduction

Leishmaniasis is commonly known as black fever or kala-azar, a parasitic infection transmitted by diphasic protozoans of the genus *Leishmania* (Oryan, Mehrabani, Owji, Motazedian, & Asgari, 2007; Shirian, Oryan, Hatam, Panahi, & Daneshbod, 2014). Worldwide, Leishmaniasis is spread by different species of protozoan parasite *Leishmania*, in several forms such as visceral leishmaniasis (VL) or kala-azar, mucocutaneous leishmaniasis (MCL), and cutaneous leishmaniasis (CL). Various strains of *Leishmania* thought to be accountable for the transmission of leishmaniasis into mammals by the bites of female sand-flies from the *Phlebotomus* and *Lutzomyia* genera via anthroponotic or zoonotic cycles (Murray, Berman, Davies, & Saravia, 2005; Oryan, 2015; Kumar, Pandey, & Samant, 2020a,b). Leishmaniasis is considered a complex vector-borne disease that has had a noteworthy impact on the world's population and is also reasoned to be among the top six tropical diseases by the World Health Organization. Report of Alvar, Yactayo, and Bern (2006) documented leishmaniasis under noncontagious infection which has pervasive morbidity and mortality rate around the globe. On the other hand, Shafiei et al. (2014) positioned leishmaniasis as third utmost common parasitic infection after toxoplasmosis and cryptosporidiosis. Infection of *Leishmania* has become convoluted with the coinfection of AIDS and it has acquired significant importance in HIV-infected people as an opportunistic infection in provinces where both infections are endemic (Alvar et al., 2008). There are several reports which claimed that generally human, wild, and domestic animals are mainly stricken with leishmaniasis. *Leishmania* is endemic in Europe and the name of that endemic species is *Leishmania infantum* and its most common

Pathogenesis, Treatment and Prevention of Leishmaniasis. DOI: https://doi.org/10.1016/B978-0-12-822800-5.00013-5
103

zymodeme is MON-1. The domestic dog is reported as the only reservoir host of major veterinary and human importance in Europe (Solano-Gallego et al., 2009). A report by Oryan et al. (2008) proclaimed the risk of parasitic infection for approximately 350 million people worldwide.

6.2 Treatment of leishmaniasis (available chemotherapy)

In India, visceral leishmania or kala-azar is the mutual type of disease spread by *Leishmania donovani* (Chakravarty & Sundar, 2019). Rather in India, Bangladesh, and Nepal are also affected by *L. donovani* in the visceral form of the infection. Therefore in 2005, these countries started a collaborative association for the elimination of *Leishmania* (Bhattacharya, Sur, Sinha, & Karbwang, 2006). This program was renewed in 2014 and extended up-to 2020 with several challenges such as drug resistance, toxicity issues, vaccine-related issues, and others (World Health Organization). Presently, in clinical research, advanced technologies provide evidences for the discovery of new drugs and therapies (Kumar, Pandey, & Samant, 2018; Kumar et al., 2020a,b). There are approximately 25 medications accessible for the treatment of leishmaniasis which is in the broad range and not species-specific (Uliana, Trinconi, & Coelho, 2018). The species-specific drug discovery is still a big challenge for the researchers while the coexistence of the diverse strains in same geographical region is very common. Some available antileishmanial agents are as follows:

6.2.1 Urea-stibamine

It is the first effective drug discovered in 1912 and proved as an antileishmanial drug in India by Prof. Bhrahmchari in 1922 and also selected for Nobel Prize in 1929 for saving the lives of millions of poor people of India (Singh & Sivakumar, 2004). Later on, other antileishmanial drugs were developed.

6.2.2 Pentavalent antimonials (Sb^V)

It is the second class drug used for the treatment of leishmaniasis. The compounds present in Sb^V are meglumine antimoniate (MA) and sodium stibogluconate (SSG) synthesized by Albert- David and Rhone−Poulenc. The dose of Sb^V 20 mg/kg body weight for 28−30 days, had been standardized for the treatment of the VL form of the disease (Chakravarty & Sundar, 2019). The complete mechanism of Sb^V is not well known but it inhibits the fatty acid oxidation pathways and glycolytic enzymatic pathways in *Leishmania* in a dose-dependent manner (Thakur, 1999; Thakur, Kumar, & Pandey, 1991). This drug was treatable since the 1970s, but in the 1980s, the epidemic war of *L. donovani* led to resistance against Sb^V in India (Berman, 1997). The higher dose of the Sb^V also drives certain adverse effects like abdominal pain, nausea, and pancreatic inflammations, and cardio-toxicity which cause sudden death. In India, the death rate was higher due to cardio-toxicity (Brummitt, Porter, & Herwaldt, 1996). Thus, till it was ineffective for *Leishmania*, due to drug resistance, the cure rate was also decreased (Chakravarty & Sundar, 2019).

6.2.3   Amphotericin B (AmB)

Amphotericin (deoxycholate) is a polyene, lipid-associated drug discovered in 1956 from the *Streptomyces* bacterium genus (Singh & Sivakumar, 2004). It is a well-known antifungal antibiotic agent. In India, for the treatment of *Leishmania*, it is used for the visceral infection at 0.75−1.0 mg/kg dose (Thakur et al., 1999; Mishra, Biswas, Jha, & Khan, 1992). It is also used for treatment of the post-kala-azar dermal *Leishmania*. The mechanism of action of AmB is, it binds to the cell wall of *Leishmania* especially in sterol and ergosterol, and obstructs the synthesis of the cell wall and create the holes in the membrane. It does not affect the mammalian cell wall but in human, it binds to the cholesterol and cause some side effect like fever, bone pains, and cardio-toxicity (Sundar, 2001). In this drug, deoxycholate was replaced with other lipids and prepared the lipid formulation which is easily taken by the body organs and is less toxic than amphotericin B. Three lipid formulations have been examined by the researchers for leishmaniasis are:

- Liposomal amphotericin B (L-AmB),
- Amphotericin B lipid complex, and
- Amphotericin B cholesterol dispersion.

These three L-AmB was approved by US-FDA (Sundar, Chakravarty, Agarwal, Rai, & Murray, 2010). The disadvantage of this drug is to maintain the proper cold chain for the long term use (Maintz et al., 2014). Frequently, this drug is effective for the VL form of *Leishmania* but only a few studies in CL and MCL forms are available which showed the less cure rate (Guery et al., 2017). Amphotericin B was in higher demand after antimonials resistance because the 100% success rate was observed in it. Amphotericin B is regularly directed as intravenous infusion daily or alternate days. It might be resistant due to the high regularity of its use (Akbari, Oryan, & Hatam, 2017).

6.2.4   Miltefosine

Miltefosine (MIL) is an alkyl phospholipid (hexadecyl phosphocholine) used as an antifungal, antibacterial, anticancer, and antileishmanial agents for a visceral and cutaneous form of diseases (Akbari et al., 2017). It is the first oral drug for *Leishmania* in India which is easy to use and has higher efficacy. Use of MIL is convenient than other drugs because oral treatment is also possible at home and hospitalization is not mandatory. Therefore it is cost-effective also (Das, Khan, Mohsin, & Kumar, 2011). Its 50−100 mg/day dose leads to a 94% cure rate (Sundar et al., 2002). MIL also showed a higher efficacy against the post-kala-azar dermal *Leishmania* (Ramesh, Katara, Verma, & Salotra, 2011). The extensive use of this drug developed resistance. The limitation of MIL is diarrhea, vomiting, gastrointestinal toxicity, nephrotoxicity, and hepatic toxicity (Sundar & Chatterjee, 2006). The failure of treatment leads to a relapse of the *Leishmania* which was also observed (Das et al., 2011).

6.2.5 Paromomycin (aminosidine)

Paromomycin (PM) is an aminoglycoside that has been used as an antibiotic and also as an antileishmanial, VL, and CL for both forms of *Leishmania*. PM was first discovered in the 1960s as a topical agent for CL (Uliana et al., 2018). It showed the synergistic effect with pentavalent antimonials (Sb^V) (Sundar & Chakravarty, 2008). A dose of PM at 16 and 20 mg/kg/day exhibited a cure rate of 93% and 97% (Jha et al., 1998), respectively. In 2006 the Indian government approved PM for curing of VL. PM is also used in amalgamation with stibogluconate, and pentostam. With pentostam, it showed 82% cure rate 20 days post treatment.

6.2.6 Pentamidine

It is an aromatic diamine synthesized in the 1930s and it is an analog of synthalin used for the *Trypanosoma*. Pentamidine was used for visceral diseases in India, in the 1940s (Bray, Barrett, Ward, & de Koning, 2003) and its treatment was effectively used in the 1970s to 1980s with a 98% cure rate (Jha, 1983). This drug is mainly used for the treatment of *Pneumocystis carinii* pneumonia. The administration of the pentamidine is intravenous in VL is much better than intramuscular (Christen et al., 2018). The mechanism of this pentamidine isothiocyanate is not well known but it inhibits the function of the kinetoplast DNA. The higher toxicity rate in pentamidine in comparison to SbV, is hardly used for visceral diseases in India and supplied only on the recommendation of government hospitals of India (Berman, 1997).

6.2.7 Nitroimidazole

The imidazole derivatives are also reported as antileishmanial agents. Fexinidazole is a nitroimidazole synthesized by Hoechst AG in the 1970s. It is a safe oral drug made up of two metabolites, Fexinidazole sulfoxide and sulfone (Wyllie et al., 2012). The combination of Fexinidazole with MIL showed significant antileishmanial activity against the VL form of diseases (Chakravarty & Sundar, 2019). Similarly, Pa-824 is another nitroimidazole compound reported as an antileishmanial compound and showed an additive effect in combination with fexinidazole (Patterson et al., 2013). Delamanid is another nitroimidazole, approved as an antitubercular drug, shown a potent inhibitory effect of *L. Donovani* (Chakravarty & Sundar, 2019). Some other azole derivatives such as metronidazole, ketoconazole, Itraconazole, and fluconazole also showed the antileishmanial activity by blocking the cell wall synthesis in *L. donovani* (Chakravarty & Sundar, 2019). All derivatives were used for CL in numerous studies.

6.2.8   Sitamaquine

It is an orally used 8-aminoquinoline and derivative of primaquine (Chakravarty & Sundar, 2019). This drug was first synthesized in the Walter Reed Army Institute of Research (United States). It was normally used for malaria but also showed strong activity against visceral *Leishmania* (Singh & Sivakumar, 2004). Other than these drugs, Allopurinol, a derivative of hypoxanthine also used as an oral drug. It inhibits purine catabolism and anabolism in mammalian and leishmanial cells, respectively. From decades allopurinol used for the treatment of *Leishmania* (Singh & Sivakumar, 2004). The alkyl phosphocholine analogs such as alkyl phosphocholine group, hexadecyl-phosphocholine, and Octadecyl-phosphocholine also used as an antileishmanial drug (Singh, 1996).

Some other synthetic compounds such as 9,9-dimethylxanthene tricyclics, Azasterols, edelfosine, Ilmofosine, *N*-acetyl-L-cysteine, Nicotinamide, Triazole SCH 56592, Perifosine, and 3-substituted quinolones also reported as an antileishmanial compound and proved as in vitro and in vivo studies. Some natural products also used for the treatment of the *leishmania* such as Plumbagin (*Pera benensis*), Trichothecenes (*Holarrhena floribunda*), Parthenolide (*Tanacetum parthenium*), Maesabalide III (*Maesa balansae*), Coronaridine (*Peschiera australis*), Licochalcone A (*Chinese licorice*), Canthin-6-one alkaloids (*Zanthoxylum chiloperone*), 2′,6′-dihydroxy-4′ methoxychalcone (*Piper aduncum*) also used as an antileishmanial agent (Monzote, 2009). Some phytoextracts like plumbagin, naphthoquinone (Awasthi, Kathuria, Pant, Kumari, & Mitra, 2016), essential oil and their derived compounds like *trans-2-cis-8-*Matricaria-ester from *Erigeron multiradiatus* and *Agrimonia pilosa* have also been reported as an antileishmanial agent by inhibiting various proteins of *L. donovani* (Dhami, Pandey, Shah, Bisht, & Samant, 2020; Pandey, Dhami, et al., 2019; Pandey, Jha, Kumar, & Samant, 2019).

6.3   Other approaches to the treatment of leishmaniasis

6.3.1   Local therapies

There are some local therapies also available for the treatment of leishmaniasis. Thermotherapy is one of them. The advantage of this therapy is its cost-effective nature and no need for a proper laboratory. *Leishmania* parasite cannot multiply at >39°C temperature in laboratory conditions (Chakravarty & Sundar, 2019). Thermotherapy is used in various ways such as the radio-frequency, generator, battery operator, etc. especially used for the treatment of CL. Similarly, cryotherapy is another local therapy. In this therapy liquid nitrogen (−195°C) is used once or twice which damages cell of the parasite (Leibovici & Aram, 1986). In a similar way, the CO_2 laser technology is also used for the thermolysis of infected tissues. The opposing effect of these therapies is hypo or hyper-pigmentation, edema, redness, etc. (Chakravarty & Sundar, 2019).

6.3.2 Combination therapy

Increasing the drug resistance towards antileishmanial agents, and growing the success rate of combination studies of malaria, HIV, Cancer, and tuberculosis increased the interest of the scientific community towards combinatorial therapies/studies. It is a multidrug therapy used according to the synergistic and additive effect between the two or more drugs in a different dose which enhanced the cure rate with fewer side effects and decreases the possibilities of drug resistance. Some experimental studies reported the combination of pentamidine with pentavalent antimonials (Sb^V) after growing resistance against Sb^V (Chunge, Owate, Pamba, & Donno, 1990). Similarly, MIL with Amphotericin B and pentamidine has been reported as the highest potential of antileishmanial (Seifert & Croft, 2006). Similarly, a combination of sodium antimony gluconate and indolylquinoline derivative A [2-2(2″-dichloroacetamidobenzyle)-3-(39-indolylquinoline)] reported for 100% elimination of parasite *Leishmania* from the liver and spleen in comparison to monotherapies (Pal et al., 2002). The efficacy of combination therapies in VL, CL, and MCL has been studied by the researchers (Pan American Health Organization (PAHO), 2018). Present therapies of the treatment of *Leishmania* have several side effects like high-cost, high toxicity, development of drug resistance. Therefore, the improvement of drug discovery for cure of *Leishmania* is more important. Today, the advanced science "nanoscience" is in high demand in the field of new drug discovery. Nanotechnology provided a new approach for the treatment of *Leishmania*. Nanotechnology functioned in different ways for many diseases, such as to develop a drug delivery system by using nanoparticle and polymers and development of the nano-drug formulation (Gershkovich et al., 2009). Thus, nanoparticles, liposomes, microspheres, and niosomes are new direct drug delivery approaches against parasitic infections. Some nanoparticles used as an antileishmanial agent are as follows:

6.3.2.1 Metal oxide and polymeric nanoparticles

The metal and metal oxide nanoparticles possess distinctive properties and also reported its strong potential for antimicrobial and anticancer activities.

Metal nanoparticle showed abundant chemical activities that showed the ability to produce reactive oxygen species and *Leishmania* parasites exhibit sensitivity towards reactive oxygen species, therefore these nanoparticles kill the parasite by its reactivity (Allahverdiyev, Abamor, Bagirova, & Rafailovich, 2011). Silver, zinc, and selenium nanoparticles demonstrated strong antimicrobial properties. Similarly, silver doped titanium dioxide alone showed the antileishmanial activity for VL and in combination with visible light used in the treatment of CL (Akbari et al., 2017). Similarly, selenium nanoparticles are also considered as antimicrobial and antioxidants and also play a role in the inhibition of production of amastigote and pro-mastigote forms of different species of *Leishmania.* They are also used as a unique therapeutic agent for the curing of CL (Beheshti et al., 2013). Zinc sulfate is also revealed as an antileishmanial agent with a high cure rate against CL (> 96%) (Minodier & Parola, 2007). Similarly, gold, platinum, and rhenium nanoparticles are also reported having a higher potential for antileishmanial properties (Fricker et al., 2008).

For reducing the dose requirement and increasing the mechanism of action of the drug, polymeric nanoparticle like nanospheres, and polymer-tagged nanoparticles are used as drug delivery systems (Kreuter, 1991). In some experimental studies, they used primaquine loaded poly-alkyl cyanoac-rylate nanoparticles as antileishmania and showed higher efficiency (21 times more) than primaquine alone. Similarly, polylactic-co-glycolic acid (PLGA), saponin β-aescin loaded nanoparticles demonstrated a higher efficiency of the killing parasite of *Leishmania* (Manoochehri et al., 2013; Van de Ven et al., 2011). Sitamaquine also had antileishmanial properties but Kumara et al. (2014) encapsulated Sitamaquine with PLGA-PEG involved with antibody to CD-14 and target the macrophage infested with the parasite and showed that polymeric nanoparticle tagged Sitamaquine has high efficacy compared to alone. The biological activity of natural compounds increased after tagging with polymeric nanoparticles (Akbari et al., 2017).

6.3.3 Other drug delivery systems

Biologically, there are lots of other drug delivery approaches perceived by the researchers, including nanodisks. The researchers used nanodisks loaded by amphotericin B and studied in vitro in BALB/c mice infected with the parasite *L. donovani*, which eliminated the infection (Yardley & Croft, 2000). Similarly, nanospheres and nanoparticles like nanochitosan, micro, and nano-immunostimulatory adjuvants are also used by researchers nowadays for the treatment of leishmaniasis (Badiee, Shargh, Khamesipour, & Jaafari, 2013).

Some emerging therapeutic targets using drugs are metabolic pathways, antimicrobial peptides, proteasome and cell cycle, secretory protein, and secretion pathways (Sundar & Singh, 2018). Thus, in growing, advanced nanotechnology and technical bioscience contributed an imperative part in the field of new drug discovery and delivery systems in the target region by using different models.

6.4 The problem of drug resistance

Statics of mortality and morbidity in leishmaniasis make it the most unattended tropical infectious disease in the world (Houweling et al., 2016). Among all forms of leishmaniasis, VL increase the number of infection upto 0.2−0.4 million cases worldwide. Additionally VL accounts for 30,000 deaths worldwide per annum (Alvar et al., 2012). A report by Gurunath, Joshi, Agrawal, and Shah (2014) claimed that the actual number of infected individuals by VL could be higher due to under-reporting and delayed diagnosis. Statics claimed the Indian subcontinent, as it accounts for approximately 60% VL burden on the globe, on the other hand, 50% visceral *Leishmania* infection cases come from Bihar (India), which makes it a hotspot for VL in India (Bhunia, Kesari, Chatterjee, Kumar, & Das, 2013; Muniaraj, 2014). The condition of ineffectiveness/inactiveness of drugs, which counters the disease-causing organism, is generally termed as drug resistance. It specifically refers to a particular lessening of the susceptibility of a certain *Leishmania* strain or species to a standard drug under the same predefined in vitro conditions and falsely anticipates that the initial susceptibility of the parasite population before treatment is always known (Croft, Sundar, & Fairlamb, 2006). Many drugs used in the treatment of leishmaniasis exhibit resistant property. Some of them and their mechanisms of resistance are enlisted in Table 6.1.

6.5 Repurposing of drugs used in the treatment of leishmaniasis

The de novo discovery of a new drug for a particular disease takes an extended period of time of an average about 10−12 years and goes through different stages to ensure its safety for human consumption (Neto, V. V, 2018). The process of de novo drug discovery or synthesis is quite hectic, time-consuming, and expensive. It takes screening of hundreds of potential candidate compounds and only a couple of them to fulfill all the criteria for the discovery of the drug. Another considerable challenge for the frequent discovery of a new target drug is that the patentability of a successful drug candidate for marketability is only 20 years to recover their manufacturing cost. Due to these shortcomings, the repurposing of an already existing drug for a particular clinical disease to another disease is gaining the attention of pharmaceutical industry as an alternative to de novo drug discovery.

A new and alternative strategy or approach in which identification of new chemical entities is called drug repurposing. Drug repurposing, a strategy where

TABLE 6.1 Different drugs used in leishmaniasis treatment and their mechanism of resistance.

S No.	Drug	Target(s)	Mechanism of resistance	Reference(s)
1.	Amphotericin B	Selective activity against fungi as well as *Leishmania* and *Trypanosoma cruzi*	1. In *L. donovani* promastigotes two transcripts of the enzyme, one of which was absent in the amphotericin B-resistant clone, the other over-expressed but without a splice leader sequence which would prevent translation 2. lizard parasite *L. tarentolae*, DNA amplification was observed with two extrachromosomal circles	Singh, Papadopoulou, and Ouellette (2001), Pourshafie et al. (2004)
2.	Miltefosine	Antileishmaniasis, anticancer	Due to a >95% reduced accumulation of 14C-labeled miltefosine	Pérez-Victoria, Castanys, and Gamarro (2003)
3.	Pentamidine	Second-line treatment for VL, CL, and DCL	Specific transporters for pentamidine uptake have been characterized and might have a role in resistance, accumulation of pentamidine in the *Leishmania* mitochondrion	Bray et al. (2003), Coelho, Beverley, and Cotrim (2003)
4.	Paromomycin (Aminosidine)	For the treatment of VL in a parenteral formulation	Remain unclear	Genest et al. (2008)
5.	Azoles	Inhibit C14-demethylase	–	Cauchetier et al. (2002)
6.	Sitamaquine	Treatment of VL, antiprotozoal activity	NO reported resistance	Neto, V. V, 2018
7.	Antimonials	Treatment of leishmaniasis	A novel resistance protein (LinJ34.0570) belongs to the superfamily of leucine-rich repeat (LRR) proteins involved in antimonial resistance in *L. infantum*	Genest et al. (2008), Nagle et al. (2014)

(Continued)

TABLE 6.1 (Continued)

S No.	Drug	Target(s)	Mechanism of resistance	Reference(s)
8.	Allopurinol	Allopurinol in combination with antimonials has been used with some efficacy against VL	Clinical resistance has not been reported; since this drug has not been used widely	Jin and Wong (2014)
9.	Atovaquone	Antileishmanial effects in murine models	Blocking the passage of atovaquone through	Cauchetier et al. (2002), Van Griensven et al. (2010)

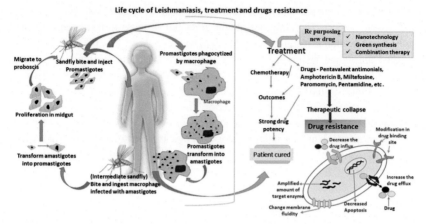

FIGURE 6.1 Schematic diagram represents the mode of infection, treatment, and mechanism of drug resistance in leishmaniasis.

a known compound or drug is already in use for the treatment of another disease could effectively be used in the treatment of other diseases. Drug repurposing exhibits less time and is a cost-effective treatment over de novo drug discovery, which are some prominent benefits of drug repurposing. Notable examples of drug repurposing for leishmaniasis include the use of MIL, amphotericin B, and pentamidine (Fig. 6.1), which were already considered or approved for other indications (Nagle et al., 2014). Due to the prolonged use of a functional antileishmanial drug, these parasites are evolving the coping mechanisms by utilizing the stimulus of natural selection.

Drug repurposing is a cost-effective and relatively less time-consuming process. In recent years, nearly 30% of USFDA approved new drugs are results of drug re-positioning (Jin & Wong, 2014). Drug resistance in the patients made popular drugs to be replaced with other alternative drugs. Pentavalent antimonial drugs have been the drug of choice for the treatment of Leishmaniasis around the world but it is embodied by associated the side effects in patients. Drugs like amphotericin B and pentamidine has also severe side effects. First oral medicine for VL in India, MIL is found to be teratogenic and resistant in affected areas (Van Griensven et al., 2010). The search for safer, cheaper, and effective drugs has been mitigated by repurposing drugs that have been already used in other diseases. Examples of such drugs include antifungal agents, antibiotics, anticancer agents, antidepressants, antiparasitic, antihypertensive, and other drugs (Andrade Neto et al., 2018).

6.5.1   Antifungal agents repurposed for leishmaniasis

Polyene antifungal drugs such as amphotericin B and nystatin have been repurposed for the treatment of Leishmaniasis. Liposome-infused Amphotericin B is also a drug of choice when the antimonial drug response fails the treatment (Hammond, 1977). The antipromastigote potential of nystatin has been evaluated having EC_{50} value 9.76 μg/mL against *Leishmania major* (Ali et al., 1997). These polyene antifungal agents exhibit their fungicidal effect by inhibiting the ergosterol biosynthesis pathway in fungal cells. The mode of action of these drugs as antileishmania is similar to the fungicidal action as here it targets the sterol biosynthesis pathway in the parasite making the pore in parasitic cell membrane thereby leaking the ions content and subsequent death (Ali et al., 1997). Another class of antifungal agents namely, Azole drugs have also been repurposed for their leishmanicidal potential. Itraconazole and posaconazole are examples of azole antifungal drugs and have been studied for their potential towards the treatment of this disease. These azoles have a similar modus operandi as polyene drugs and target C14α-demethylase (CYP51) enzyme which is essential for ergosterol biosynthesis (De Souza & Rodrigues, 2009). Ergosterol is thought to be a pathogen exclusive target for leishmaniasis and trypanosomiasis as it is not found in a human host. In vitro study of the antiproliferative effect of Itraconazole and posaconazole against *L. amazonensis* growth has shown their inhibitory potential towards both promastigote and amastigote stages by targeting mitochondrial malfunction and cellular disruption (De Macedo-Silva, Urbina, De Souza, & Rodrigues, 2013). Butenafine, another antifungal agent was evaluated for antipromastigote potential in vivo in mice model against *L. amazonensis* and *L. braziliensis*. The results showed that Butenafine is more effective than MIL in the case of *L. amazonensis* but similar to MIL against *L. braziliensis*, and the antipromastigote effect was found due to mitochondrial disruption by programmed cell death (Bezerra-Souza, Yamamoto, Laurenti, Ribeiro, & Passero, 2016).

6.5.2 Antihypertensive as antileishmaniasis

Ketanserin, an antidepressant, and the antihypertensive drug are effective against the growth of the promastigote and intracellular amastigote stages of *L. donovani* without any visible toxicity. This drug acts by obstructing a rate-limiting enzyme HMG-CoA reductase intricate in ergosterol biosynthesis (Singh, Dinesh, Kaur, & Shamiulla, 2014). Sodium nitroprusside, another antihypertensive drug was evaluated for its leishmanicidal effect against promastigotes and amastigote of *L. amazonensis* and elucidated to be more effective against promastigotes stage by oxidative damage to the parasite (Genestra et al., 2008). Dihydropyridine derivatives Amlodipine and Lacidipine have been studied in this regard. When amastigote-infected BALB/c mice were treated with these hypertensive drugs, it considerably condensed the parasitic load from the liver and spleen in 30 days in comparison to the control. Upon assessment of parasitic cell death, decreased oxygen consumption was observed. Additionally, apoptotic proteases (caspase-3 like) were also found active in apoptotic cells (Palit & Ali, 2008a,b).

An antianginal agent, Bepridil, is operative against *L. major*, *L. braziliensis*, *L. chagasi*, and *L. amazonensis* (Reimão, Colombo, Pereira-Chioccola, &

Tempone, 2011). Nimodipine, a Ca^+ channel blocker agent was found very effective against both the stages of *L. chagasi.* However, *L. major* and *L. amazonensis* promastigote were found susceptible too (Tempone, Taniwaki, & Reimão, 2009). Another Ca^+ channel inhibitor such as Amlodipine, Azelnidipine, Cilnidipine, Lercanidipine, Nicardipine, Nifedipine, Nitrendipine, and Nimodipine has also been studied for repurposing as antileishmania agents and showed their positive outcomes (Reimão & Tempone, 2011).

6.5.3 Antidepressant as antileishmaniasis

An antidepressant drug, the tetracyclic Mianserin has been examined for its effect against leishmaniasis agent and found out to be effective against *L. donovani* promastigotes as well as amastigote stages by inhibiting the HMG-CoA reductase enzyme essential for ergosterol biosynthesis (Dinesh, Kaur, Swamy, & Singh, 2014). Another important antidepressant drug used in many psychological disorders, a selective serotonin reuptake inhibitor, namely, Sertraline, was also evaluated for its re-positioning and was effectively able to kill *L. donovani* by causing a decrease in oxygen consumption in the parasite (Palit & Ali, 2008a,b). Monoamine oxidase inhibitors Nialamide and Phenelzine were found out to be promising against cutaneous and VL (Evans, Croft, Peters, & Neal, 1989).

6.5.4 Anticancer agents as antileishmaniasis

Hydroxyurea, an anticancer agent was demonstrated to arrest the cell cycle progression in vitro in *L. major* and *L. mexicana* promastigotes during the G2/M phase. Hydroxyurea at 10 or 100 µg/mL concentration, it destroyed the parasite of *Leishmania* in 9 or 3 days, respectively (Martinez-Rojano, Mancilla-Ramirez, Quiñonez-Diaz, & Galindo-Sevilla, 2008). In vitro and in vivo leishmanicidal effect of testicular and ovarian anticancer drug cisplatin was found to be significant in treating leishmaniasis by inducing cell cycle damages and arrest (Tavares, Ouaissi, Ouaissi, & Cordeiro-da-Silva, 2007). Tetracyclic diterpene, Paclitaxel is also functioning similarly and promotes tubulin damage, cell cycle alteration, and arrest in promastigotes and intracellular amastigotes of *Leishmania* (Doherty, Sher, & Vogel, 1998). Other anticancer drugs such as Sunitinib, Lapatinib, and Doxorubicin-based nanoparticles have been evaluated for their potential and found very effective against VL under experimental conditions (Kansal, Tandon, Verma, Dube, & Mishra, 2013; Sanderson, Yardley, & Croft, 2014).

6.5.5 Antibiotics as antileishmaniasis

DNA topoisomerases (I & II) of the *Leishmania* parasite is a potent target for drug treatment. This enzyme plays a central role in maintaining DNA topology in cells. Studies have suggested that many of the antibiotics and other drugs specifically target this enzyme due to structural and biochemical variations with the human counterpart of this enzyme (Cheesman, 2000; Cortázar, Coombs, & Walker, 2007). The parasite DNA topoisomerases are crucial for the maintenance of kinetoplast DNA, which is exclusive to the parasite. Antibiotics like enoxacin, ciprofloxacin, norfloxacin, ofloxacin, pentamidine, and lomefloxacin had been demonstrated to show significant target selectivity towards DNA topoisomerase II enzyme of *L. panamensis* (Cortázar et al., 2007). Aminoglycoside antibiotics streptomycin and tobramycin was found to inhibit the growth of Amastigote as well as promastigote stages of *L. donovani* at a concentration of $\geq 50 \, \mu g/mL$ (Navin & Pearson, 1987). Another common antibiotic has exhibited its antipromastigote and amastigote activity against *L. tropica, L. major, L. infantum chagasi, L. amazonensis*, and *L. braziliensis* (De Oliveira-Silva, de Morais-Teixeira, & Rabello, 2008). Combination therapy with multiple sets of drugs such as Clofazimine, rifampicin, and dapsone (Neal & Croft, 1984); sulfadiazine, trimethoprim, and metronidazole or tinidazole (Bano & Shahab, 1994) as well as Rifampicin and amphotericin B (El-On, Messer, & Greenblatt, 1984) had shown their promising antileishmanial potential.

6.6 Conclusion

Parasitic zoonoses comprise some types of life-threatening infectious diseases in the human population around the globe. Leishmaniasis remains a serious public health burden in various parts of the world. In this section, it can be concluded that visceral, cutaneous, and MCL is reported as the most destructive and neglected tropical disease with less medical treatment. The worst part is that during the previous century only slightly upgraded treatment alternatives are available for it. Different hosts of *Leishmania* transmission including diverse mammalian hosts, and reservoir hosts also increased its complexity. Thus, the control and treatment of leishmaniasis mostly depend on the understanding of how leishmaniasis involves various mammalian reservoir hosts, whose epidemiological role is yet to be elucidated. Available treatment options generally face severe challenges such as development of resistance, and toxicity of drugs as well. Therapeutic efficacy varies depending upon the species, symptoms, and geographical regions of the *Leishmania* parasite. Great scientific knowledge/literature available on the epidemiology of leishmaniasis, the rate of spreading of this infection and its control remains inadequate. The main reason behind the high rate of spreading of leishmaniasis could be the unavailability of an effective vaccine (Pandey, Kumar, & Samant, 2020; Pandey, Pande, & Samant, 2020). The development of novel drug for intracellular pathogens is a complex practice that generally had a low success rate.

To give it the best chance, the evidence needed to support the process must be of a high standard. Still, many drugs could be used against leishmaniasis, but most drugs have their limitations. The main issue of using drugs is drug toxicity and drug resistance. Broadly speaking, the discovery of a drug for a disease, which includes identification, characterization, and development for clinical application is very expensive and it's a time-consuming process with an average of 10−20 years. Therefore, the development of such drugs which are mainly targeting *Leishmania* could be quite difficult. So we should go with some alternative approaches which not only be less time taking but also be active in the treatment of *Leishmania*. In last few years, the use of nanotechnology exhibited a great impact on drug delivery and other medical aspects also. For effective and safe control overspreading of leishmaniasis is different delivery techniques could play an important role. New drug delivery applications such as nanoparticles, microparticles, liposomes, and niosomes transport drugs to the target cell specifically with less toxicity on normal cells. The recent advances, techniques, and nanostructured carriers improved efficiency, bioavailability, solubility, and tolerance level of many potent antileishmanial agents that faces challenges in oral delivery and have narrow therapeutic indices.

Drug repurposing could be an alternative and better option to overcome this issue. In this arena, repurposing or re-positioning of existing drugs could exhibit beneficial activities like reduced costs during discovery, development, and clinical phases; an accelerated drug development process; possible extension of patent life; the potential to recover and repurpose previously failed compounds; and minimize the overall risk. With the development of new scientific protocols and approaches different methods and assays are being developed for the screening of antileishmanial compounds that are cost-effective, robust, and precise, automated to minimize the risk related with human error and escalate throughput, empowering large numbers of molecules to be rapidly evaluated. More combinatorial therapies of these potential antileishmanial agents should be studied in vitro and in vivo models. This could greatly enhance our understanding of the effects of different drug combinations for the disease.

References

Akbari, M., Oryan, A., & Hatam, G. (2017). Application of nanotechnology in treatment of leishmaniasis: A review. *Acta Tropica, 172,* 86−90.

Ali, S. A., Iqbal, J., Khalil, N. Y., Manzoor, A., Bukhari, I., Ahmad, B., & Yasinzai, M. M. (1997). Leishmanicidal activity of Nystatin (mycostatin): A potent polyene compound. *Journal-Pakistan Medical Association, 47,* 246−247.

Allahverdiyev, A. M., Abamor, E. S., Bagirova, M., & Rafailovich, M. (2011). Antimicrobial effects of TiO_2 and Ag_2O nanoparticles against drug-resistant bacteria and *leishmania* parasites. *Future Microbiology, 6*(8), 933−940.

Alvar, J., Aparicio, P., Aseffa, A., Den Boer, M., Canavate, C., Dedet, J. P., & Moreno, J. (2008). The relationship between leishmaniasis and AIDS: The second 10 years. *Clinical Microbiology Reviews, 21*(2), 334−359.

Alvar, J., Vélez, I. D., Bern, C., Herrero, M., Desjeux, P., & Cano, J.WHO Leishmaniasis Control Team. (2012). Leishmaniasis worldwide and global estimates of its incidence. *PLoS One, 7*(5), e35671.

Alvar, J., Yactayo, S., & Bern, C. (2006). Leishmaniasis and poverty. *Trends in Parasitology, 22* (12), 552−557.

Andrade Neto, V. V., Cunha Junior, E. F., Faioes, V. D. S., Martins, T. P., Silva, R. L., Leon, L. L., & Santos, E. C. T. (2018). Leishmaniasis treatment: update of possibilities for drug repurposing. *Frontiers in Bioscience, 23*, 967−996. https://www.arca.fiocruz.br/handle/icict/28846.

Awasthi, B. P., Kathuria, M., Pant, G., Kumari, N., & Mitra, K. (2016). Plumbagin, a plant-derived naphthoquinone metabolite induces mitochondria mediated apoptosis-like cell death in *Leishmania donovani*: An ultrastructural and physiological study. *Apoptosis, 21*(8), 941−953.

Badiee, A., Shargh, V. H., Khamesipour, A., & Jaafari, M. R. (2013). Micro/nanoparticle adjuvants for antileishmanial vaccines: Present and future trends. *Vaccine, 31*(5), 735−749.

Bano, P., & Shahab, S. M. (1994). A combination of sulphadiazine, trimethoprim and metronidazole or tinidazole in kala-azar. *The Journal of the Association of Physicians of India, 42*(7), 535−536.

Beheshti, N., Soflaei, S., Shakibaie, M., Yazdi, M. H., Ghaffarifar, F., Dalimi, A., & Shahverdi, A. R. (2013). Efficacy of biogenic selenium nanoparticles against *Leishmania major*: In vitro and in vivo studies. *Journal of Trace Elements in Medicine and Biology, 27*(3), 203−207.

Berman, J. D. (1997). Human leishmaniasis: Clinical, diagnostic, and chemotherapeutic developments in the last 10 years. *Clinical Infectious Diseases, 24*(4), 684−703.

Bezerra-Souza, A., Yamamoto, E. S., Laurenti, M. D., Ribeiro, S. P., & Passero, L. F. D. (2016). The antifungal compound butenafine eliminates promastigote and amastigote forms of *Leishmania (Leishmania) amazonensis* and *Leishmania (Viannia) braziliensis*. *Parasitology International, 65*(6), 702−707.

Bhattacharya, S. K., Sur, D., Sinha, P. K., & Karbwang, J. (2006). Elimination of leishmaniasis (kala-azar) from the Indian subcontinent is technically feasible & operationally achievable. *Indian Journal of Medical Research, 123*(3), 195.

Bhunia, G. S., Kesari, S., Chatterjee, N., Kumar, V., & Das, P. (2013). Spatial and temporal variation and hotspot detection of kala-azar disease in Vaishali district (Bihar), India. *BMC Infectious Diseases, 13*(1), 64.

Bray, P. G., Barrett, M. P., Ward, S. A., & de Koning, H. P. (2003). Pentamidine uptake and resistance in pathogenic protozoa: Past, present and future. *Trends in Parasitology, 19*(5), 232−239.

Brummitt, C. F., Porter, J. A., & Herwaldt, B. L. (1996). Reversible peripheral neuropathy associated with sodium stibogluconate therapy for American cutaneous leishmaniasis. *Clinical Infectious Diseases, 22*(5), 878−879.

Cauchetier, E., Loiseau, P. M., Lehman, J., Rivollet, D., Fleury, J., Astier, A., & Paul, M. (2002). Characterisation of atovaquone resistance in *Leishmania infantum promastigotes*. *International Journal for Parasitology, 32*(8), 1043−1051.

Chakravarty, J., & Sundar, S. (2019). Current and emerging medications for the treatment of leishmaniasis. *Expert Opinion on Pharmacotherapy, 20*(10), 1251−1265.

Cheesman, S. J. (2000). The topoisomerases of protozoan parasites. *Parasitology Today, 16*(7), 277−281.

Christen, J. R., Bourreau, E., Demar, M., Lightburn, E., Couppie, P., Ginouves, M., & de Santi, V. P. (2018). Use of the intramuscular route to administer pentamidine isethionate in *Leishmania guyanensis* cutaneous leishmaniasis increases the risk of treatment failure. *Travel Medicine and Infectious Disease, 24*, 31−36.

Chunge, C. N., Owate, J., Pamba, H. O., & Donno, L. (1990). Treatment of visceral leishmaniasis in Kenya by aminosidine alone or combined with sodium stibogluconate. *Transactions of the Royal Society of Tropical Medicine and Hygiene, 84*(2), 221−225.

Coelho, A. C., Beverley, S. M., & Cotrim, P. C. (2003). Functional genetic identification of PRP1, an ABC transporter superfamily member conferring pentamidine resistance in *Leishmania major. Molecular and Biochemical Parasitology, 130*(2), 83−90.

Cortázar, T. M., Coombs, G. H., & Walker, J. (2007). Leishmania panamensis: Comparative inhibition of nuclear DNA topoisomerase II enzymes from promastigotes and human macrophages reveals anti-parasite selectivity of fluoroquinolones, flavonoids and pentamidine. *Experimental Parasitology, 116*(4), 475−482.

Croft, S. L., Sundar, S., & Fairlamb, A. H. (2006). Drug resistance in leishmaniasis. *Clinical Microbiology Reviews, 19*(1), 111−126.

Das, S., Khan, W., Mohsin, S., & Kumar, N. (2011). Miltefosine loaded albumin microparticles for treatment of visceral leishmaniasis: Formulation development and *in vitro* evaluation. *Polymers for Advanced Technologies, 22*(1), 172−179.

De Macedo-Silva, S. T., Urbina, J. A., De Souza, W., & Rodrigues, J. C. F. (2013). In vitro activity of the antifungal azoles itraconazole and posaconazole against *Leishmania amazonensis. PLoS One, 8*(12), e83247.

De Oliveira-Silva, F., de Morais-Teixeira, E., & Rabello, A. (2008). Antileishmanial activity of azitahromycin against *Leishmania (Leishmania) amazonensis, Leishmania (Viannia) braziliensis*, and *Leishmania (Leishmania) chagasi. The American Journal of Tropical Medicine and Hygiene, 78*(5), 745−749.

De Souza, W., & Rodrigues, J. C. F. (2009). Sterol biosynthesis pathway as target for anti-trypanosomatid drugs. *Interdisciplinary Perspectives on Infectious Diseases, 2009*, 642502.

Dhami, D. S., Pandey, S. C., Shah, G. C., Bisht, M., & Samant, M. (2020). In vitro antileishmanial activity of the essential oil from *Agrimonia pilosa. National Academy Science Letters*, 1−4.

Dinesh, N., Kaur, P. K., Swamy, K. K., & Singh, S. (2014). Mianserin, an antidepressant kills *Leishmania donovani* by depleting ergosterol levels. *Experimental Parasitology, 144*, 84−90.

Doherty, T. M., Sher, A., & Vogel, S. N. (1998). Paclitaxel (Taxol)-induced killing of *Leishmania major* in murine macrophages. *Infection and Immunity, 66*(9), 4553−4556.

El-On, J., Messer, G., & Greenblatt, C. L. (1984). Growth inhibition of *Leishmania tropica* amastigotes *in vitro* by rifampicin combined with amphotericin B. *Annals of Tropical Medicine & Parasitology, 78*(2), 93−98.

Evans, A. T., Croft, S. L., Peters, W., & Neal, R. A. (1989). Hydrazide antidepressants possess novel antileishmanial activity *in vitro* and *in vivo. Annals of Tropical Medicine & Parasitology, 83*(1), 19−24.

Fricker, S. P., Mosi, R. M., Cameron, B. R., Baird, I., Zhu, Y., Anastassov, V., & Langille, J. (2008). Metal compounds for the treatment of parasitic diseases. *Journal of Inorganic Biochemistry, 102*(10), 1839−1845.

Genest, P. A., Haimeur, A., Légaré, D., Sereno, D., Roy, G., Messier, N., & Ouellette, M. (2008). A protein of the leucine-rich repeats (LRRs) superfamily is implicated in antimony resistance in *Leishmania infantum amastigotes*. *Molecular and Biochemical Parasitology*, *158*(1), 95–99.

Genestra, M., Soares-Bezerra, R. J., Gomes-Silva, L., Fabrino, D. L., Bellato-Santos, T., Castro-Pinto, D. B., & Leon, L. L. (2008). In vitro sodium nitroprusside-mediated toxicity towards *Leishmania amazonensis promastigotes* and axenic amastigotes. *Cell Biochemistry and Function*, *26*(6), 709–717.

Gershkovich, P., Wasan, E. K., Lin, M., Sivak, O., Leon, C. G., Clement, J. G., & Wasan, K. M. (2009). Pharmacokinetics and biodistribution of amphotericin B in rats following oral administration in a novel lipid-based formulation. *Journal of Antimicrobial Chemotherapy*, *64*(1), 101–108.

Guery, R., Henry, B., Martin-Blondel, G., Rouzaud, C., Cordoliani, F., Harms, G., & Morizot, G. (2017). Liposomal amphotericin B in travelers with cutaneous and muco-cutaneous leishmaniasis: Not a panacea. *PLoS Neglected Tropical Diseases*, *11*(11), e0006094.

Gurunath, U., Joshi, R., Agrawal, A., & Shah, V. (2014). An overview of visceral leishmaniasis elimination program in India: A picture imperfect. *Expert Review of Anti-infective Therapy*, *12*(8), 929–935.

Hammond, S. I. (1977). *3 Biological activity of polyene antibiotics, . Progress in medicinal chemistry* (14, pp. 105–179). Elsevier.

Houweling, T. A., Karim-Kos, H. E., Kulik, M. C., Stolk, W. A., Haagsma, J. A., Lenk, E. J., & de Vlas, S. J. (2016). Socioeconomic inequalities in neglected tropical diseases: A systematic review. *PLoS Neglected Tropical Diseases*, *10*(5), e0004546.

Jha, T. K. (1983). Evaluation of diamidine compound (pentamidine isethionate) in the treatment of resistant cases of kala-azar occurring in North Bihar, India. *Transactions of the Royal Society of Tropical Medicine and Hygiene*, *77*(2), 167–170.

Jha, T. K., Lockwood, D. N., Olliaro, P., Thakur, C. P. N., Kanyok, T. P., Singhania, B. L., & Jha, S. (1998). Randomised controlled trial of aminosidine (paromomycin) v sodium stibogluconate for treating visceral leishmaniasis in North Bihar, India Commentary: Some good news for treatment of visceral leishmaniasis in Bihar. *British Medical Journal*, *316*(7139), 1200–1205.

Jin, G., & Wong, S. T. (2014). Toward better drug repositioning: Prioritizing and integrating existing methods into efficient pipelines. *Drug Discovery Today*, *19*(5), 637–644.

Kansal, S., Tandon, R., Verma, P. R. P., Dube, A., & Mishra, P. R. (2013). Development of doxorubicin loaded novel core shell structured nanocapsules for the intervention of visceral leishmaniasis. *Journal of Microencapsulation*, *30*(5), 441–450.

Kreuter, J. (1991). Liposomes and nanoparticles as vehicles for antibiotics. *Infection*, *19*(4), S224–S228.

Kumar, A., Pandey, S. C., & Samant, M. (2018). Slow pace of antileishmanial drug development. *Parasitology Open*, *4*(4), 1–11.

Kumar, A., Pandey, S. C., & Samant, M. (2020a). A spotlight on the diagnostic methods of a fatal disease Visceral Leishmaniasis. *Parasite Immunology*, e12727.

Kumar, A., Pandey, S. C., & Samant, M. (2020b). DNA-based microarray studies in visceral leishmaniasis: Identification of biomarkers for diagnostic, prognostic and drug target for treatment. *Acta Tropica*, *208*, 105512.

Kumara, R., Sahoo, G. C., Pandeya, K., Dasa, V., Yousuf, M., Ansaria, S. R., & Dasa, P. (2014). PLGA-PEG encapsulated sitamaquine nanoparticles drug delivery system against *Leishmania donovani*. *Journal of Innovation Science and Research*, *3*(1), 85–90.

Leibovici, V., & Aram, H. (1986). Cryotherapy in acute cutaneous leishmaniasis. *International Journal of Dermatology, 25*(7), 473—475.

Maintz, E. M., Hassan, M., Huda, M. M., Ghosh, D., Hossain, M., Alim, A., & Mondal, D. (2014). Introducing single dose liposomal amphotericin B for the treatment of visceral leishmaniasis in rural bangladesh: Feasibility and acceptance to patients and health staff. *Journal of Tropical Medicine, 2014,* 676817.

Manoochehri, S., Darvishi, B., Kamalinia, G., Amini, M., Fallah, M., Ostad, S. N., & Dinarvand, R. (2013). Surface modification of PLGA nanoparticles via human serum albumin conjugation for controlled delivery of docetaxel. *DARU Journal of Pharmaceutical Sciences, 21*(1), 58.

Martinez-Rojano, H., Mancilla-Ramirez, J., Quiñonez-Diaz, L., & Galindo-Sevilla, N. (2008). Activity of hydroxyurea against *Leishmania mexicana. Antimicrobial Agents and Chemotherapy, 52*(10), 3642—3647.

Minodier, P., & Parola, P. (2007). Cutaneous leishmaniasis treatment. *Travel Medicine and Infectious Disease, 5*(3), 150—158.

Mishra, M., Biswas, U. K., Jha, D. N., & Khan, A. B. (1992). Amphotericin versus pentamidine in antimony-unresponsive kala-azar. *The Lancet, 340*(8830), 1256—1257.

Monzote, L. (2009). Current treatment of leishmaniasis: A review. *The Open Antimicrobial Agents Journal, 1*(1), 9—19.

Muniaraj, M. (2014). The lost hope of elimination of Kala-azar (visceral leishmaniasis) by 2010 and cyclic occurrence of its outbreak in India, blame falls on vector control practices or co-infection with human immunodeficiency virus or therapeutic modalities? *Tropical Parasitology, 4*(1), 10.

Murray, H. W., Berman, J. D., Davies, C. R., & Saravia, N. G. (2005). Advances in leishmaniasis. *The Lancet, 366*(9496), 1561—1577.

Nagle, A. S., Khare, S., Kumar, A. B., Supek, F., Buchynskyy, A., Mathison, C. J., & Molteni, V. (2014). Recent developments in drug discovery for leishmaniasis and human African trypanosomiasis. *Chemical Reviews, 114*(22), 11305—11347.

Navin, T. R., & Pearson, R. D. (1987). Inhibition of *Leishmania donovani* growth by streptomycin and tobramycin. *Annals of Tropical Medicine & Parasitology, 81*(6), 731—733.

Neal, R. A., & Croft, S. L. (1984). An in-vitro system for determining the activity of compounds against the intracellular amastigote form of *Leishmania donovani. Journal of Antimicrobial Chemotherapy, 14*(5), 463—475.

Oryan, A. (2015). Plant-derived compounds in treatment of leishmaniasis. *Iranian Journal of Veterinary Research, 16*(1), 1.

Oryan, A., Mehrabani, D., Owji, S. M., Motazedian, M. H., & Asgari, Q. (2007). Histopathologic and electron microscopic characterization of cutaneous leishmaniasis in *Tatera indica* and *Gerbillus* spp. infected with *Leishmania major. Comparative Clinical Pathology, 16*(4), 275—279.

Oryan, A., Mehrabani, D., Owji, S. M., Motazedian, M. H., Hatam, G. H., & Asgari, Q. (2008). Morphologic changes due to cutaneous leishmaniosis in BALB/c mice experimentally infected with *Leishmania major. Journal of Applied Animal Research, 34*(1), 87—92.

Pal, C., Raha, M., Basu, A., Roy, K. C., Gupta, A., Ghosh, M., & Bandyopadhyay, S. (2002). Combination therapy with indolylquinoline derivative and sodium antimony gluconate cures established visceral leishmaniasis in hamsters. *Antimicrobial Agents and Chemotherapy, 46* (1), 259—261.

Palit, P., & Ali, N. (2008a). Oral therapy with amlodipine and lacidipine, 1, 4-dihydropyridine derivatives showing activity against experimental visceral leishmaniasis. *Antimicrobial Agents and Chemotherapy, 52*(1), 374−377.

Palit, P., & Ali, N. (2008b). Oral therapy with sertraline, a selective serotonin reuptake inhibitor, shows activity against *Leishmania donovani*. *Journal of Antimicrobial Chemotherapy, 61*(5), 1120−1124.

Pan American Health Organization (PAHO). (2018). *Leishmaniasis in the Americas: Treatment recommendations*. Washington, DC: PAHO.

Pandey, S. C., Dhami, D. S., Jha, A., Shah, G. C., Kumar, A., & Samant, M. (2019). Identification of *trans-2-cis-8-Matricaria-ester* from the essential oil of *Erigeron multiradiatus* and evaluation of its antileishmanial potential by in vitro and in silico approaches. *ACS Omega, 4*(11), 14640.

Pandey, S. C., Jha, A., Kumar, A., & Samant, M. (2019). Evaluation of antileishmanial potential of computationally screened compounds targeting DEAD-box RNA helicase of *Leishmania donovani*. *International Journal of Biological Macromolecules, 121*, 480−487.

Pandey, S. C., Pande, V., & Samant, M. (2020). DDX3 DEAD-box RNA helicase (Hel67) gene disruption impairs infectivity of Leishmania donovani and induces protective immunity against visceral leishmaniasis. *Sci Rep, 10*(1), 18218. Available from https://doi.org/ 10.1038/s41598-020-75420-y.

Patterson, S., Wyllie, S., Stojanovski, L., Perry, M. R., Simeons, F. R., Norval, S., & Fairlamb, A. H. (2013). The R enantiomer of the antitubercular drug PA-824 as a potential oral treatment for visceral leishmaniasis. *Antimicrobial Agents and Chemotherapy, 57*(10), 4699−4706.

Pérez-Victoria, F. J., Castanys, S., & Gamarro, F. (2003). *Leishmania donovani* resistance to miltefosine involves a defective inward translocation of the drug. *Antimicrobial Agents and Chemotherapy, 47*(8), 2397−2403.

Pourshafie, M., Morand, S., Virion, A., Rakotomanga, M., Dupuy, C., & Loiseau, P. M. (2004). Cloning of S-adenosyl-l-methionine: C-24-Δ-sterol-methyltransferase (ERG6) from *Leishmania donovani* and characterization of mRNAs in wild-type and amphotericin B-resistant promastigotes. *Antimicrobial Agents and Chemotherapy, 48*(7), 2409−2414.

Ramesh, V., Katara, G. K., Verma, S., & Salotra, P. (2011). Miltefosine as an effective choice in the treatment of post-kala-azar dermal leishmaniasis. *British Journal of Dermatology, 165* (2), 411−414.

Reimão, J. Q., Colombo, F. A., Pereira-Chioccola, V. L., & Tempone, A. G. (2011). In vitro and experimental therapeutic studies of the calcium channel blocker bepridil: Detection of viable Leishmania (L.) chagasi by real-time PCR. *Experimental Parasitology, 128*(2), 111−115.

Reimão, J. Q., & Tempone, A. G. (2011). Investigation into in vitro anti-leishmanial combinations of calcium channel blockers and current anti-leishmanial drugs. *Memórias do Instituto Oswaldo Cruz, 106*(8), 1032−1038.

Sanderson, L., Yardley, V., & Croft, S. L. (2014). Activity of anti-cancer protein kinase inhibitors against *Leishmania* spp. *Journal of Antimicrobial Chemotherapy, 69*(7), 1888−1891.

Seifert, K., & Croft, S. L. (2006). In vitro and in vivo interactions between miltefosine and other antileishmanial drugs. *Antimicrobial Agents and Chemotherapy, 50*(1), 73−79.

Shafiei, R., Mohebali, M., Akhoundi, B., Galian, M. S., Kalantar, F., Ashkan, S., & Ghasemian, M. (2014). Emergence of co-infection of visceral leishmaniasis in HIV-positive patients in northeast Iran: A preliminary study. *Travel Medicine and Infectious Disease, 12*(2), 173−178.

Shirian, S., Oryan, A., Hatam, G. R., Panahi, S., & Daneshbod, Y. (2014). Comparison of conventional, molecular, and immunohistochemical methods in diagnosis of typical and atypical cutaneous leishmaniasis. *Archives of Pathology and Laboratory Medicine, 138*(2), 235−240.

Singh, A. K., Papadopoulou, B., & Ouellette, M. (2001). Gene amplification in amphotericin B-resistant *Leishmania tarentolae. Experimental Parasitology, 99*(3), 141−147.

Singh, S. (1996). Alkylphosphocholine in visceral leishmaniasis: *In-vitro* and *in-vivo* study. *Journal of Parasitic Diseases: Official Organ of the Indian Society for Parasitology, 20,* 185−188.

Singh, S., Dinesh, N., Kaur, P. K., & Shamiulla, B. (2014). Ketanserin, an antidepressant, exerts its antileishmanial action via inhibition of 3-hydroxy-3-methylglutaryl coenzyme A reductase (HMGR) enzyme of *Leishmania donovani. Parasitology Research, 113*(6), 2161−2168.

Singh, S., & Sivakumar, R. (2004). Challenges and new discoveries in the treatment of leishmaniasis. *Journal of Infection and Chemotherapy, 10*(6), 307−315.

Solano-Gallego, L., Koutinas, A., Miró, G., Cardoso, L., Pennisi, M. G., Ferrer, L., & Baneth, G. (2009). Directions for the diagnosis, clinical staging, treatment and prevention of canine leishmaniosis. *Veterinary Parasitology, 165*(1-2), 1−18.

Sundar, S. (2001). Treatment of visceral leishmaniasis. *Medical Microbiology and Immunology, 190*(1-2), 89−92.

Sundar, S., & Chakravarty, J. (2008). Paromomycin in the treatment of leishmaniasis. *Expert Opinion on Investigational Drugs, 17*(5), 787−794.

Sundar, S., Chakravarty, J., Agarwal, D., Rai, M., & Murray, H. W. (2010). Single-dose liposomal amphotericin B for visceral leishmaniasis in India. *New England Journal of Medicine, 362*(6), 504−512.

Sundar, S., & Chatterjee, M. (2006). Visceral leishmaniasis-current therapeutic modalities. *Indian Journal of Medical Research, 123*(3), 345.

Sundar, S., Jha, T. K., Thakur, C. P., Engel, J., Sindermann, H., Fischer, C., & Berman, J. (2002). Oral miltefosine for Indian visceral leishmaniasis. *New England Journal of Medicine, 347*(22), 1739−1746.

Sundar, S., & Singh, B. (2018). Emerging therapeutic targets for treatment of leishmaniasis. *Expert Opinion on Therapeutic Targets, 22*(6), 467−486.

Tavares, J., Ouaissi, M., Ouaissi, A., & Cordeiro-da-Silva, A. (2007). Characterization of the anti-Leishmania effect induced by cisplatin, an anticancer drug. *Acta Tropica, 103*(2), 133−141.

Tempone, A. G., Taniwaki, N. N., & Reimão, J. Q. (2009). Antileishmanial activity and ultrastructural alterations of *Leishmania* (L.) chagasi treated with the calcium channel blocker nimodipine. *Parasitology Research, 105*(2), 499−505.

Thakur, C. P. (1999). Drug resistance in kala-azar: An overviews. In *Proceedings of round table conference series, 1999.* Ranbaxy Science Foundation.

Thakur, C. P., Kumar, M., & Pandey, A. K. (1991). Comparison of regimes of treatment of antimony-resistant kala-azar patients: A randomized study. *The American Journal of Tropical Medicine and Hygiene, 45*(4), 435−441.

Thakur, C. P., Singh, R. K., Hassan, S. M., Kumar, R., Narain, S., & Kumar, A. (1999). Amphotericin B deoxycholate treatment of visceral leishmaniasis with newer modes of administration and precautions: A study of 938 cases. *Transactions of the Royal Society of Tropical Medicine and Hygiene, 93*(3), 319−323.

Uliana, S. R., Trinconi, C. T., & Coelho, A. C. (2018). Chemotherapy of leishmaniasis: Present challenges. *Parasitology, 145*(4), 464.

Van de Ven, H., Vermeersch, M., Matheeussen, A., Vandervoort, J., Weyenberg, W., Apers, S., & Ludwig, A. (2011). PLGA nanoparticles loaded with the antileishmanial saponin β-aescin: Factor influence study and in vitro efficacy evaluation. *International Journal of Pharmaceutics*, *420*(1), 122–132.

Van Griensven, J., Balasegaram, M., Meheus, F., Alvar, J., Lynen, L., & Boelaert, M. (2010). Combination therapy for visceral leishmaniasis. *The Lancet Infectious Diseases*, *10*(3), 184–194.

World Health Organization. (2015). Kala-Azar elimination programme: report of a WHO consultation of partners, Geneva, Switzerland. (Accessed 11 February 2015).

Wyllie, S., Patterson, S., Stojanovski, L., Simeons, F. R., Norval, S., Kime, R., & Fairlamb, A. H. (2012). The anti-trypanosome drug fexinidazole shows potential for treating visceral leishmaniasis. *Science Translational Medicine*, *4*(119), 119re1.

Yardley, V., & Croft, S. L. (2000). A comparison of the activities of three amphotericin B lipid formulations against experimental visceral and cutaneous leishmaniasis. *International Journal of Antimicrobial Agents*, *13*(4), 243–248.

Chapter 7

Novel nanotechnology-based approaches in the treatment of leishmaniasis

Khushboo Dasauni, Deepa Bisht and Tapan Kumar Nailwal

Department of Biotechnology, Kumaun University, Sir J C Bose Technical Campus, Bhimtal, India

7.1 Introduction

Leishmania is an obligate intracellular and unicellular kinetoplastid dimorphic protozoan alternating between the promastigotes (in insect vector) and amastigotes (in vertebrate hosts). A bite from a phlebotomine sandfly spreads the parasite to mammals, including humans, and it is also transmitted by sharing needles, blood transfusions, and innate transmissions (Kaye & Scott, 2011; Pinto et al., 2011). According to reports, leishmaniasis is the third most important vector-borne disease, endemic in 98 countries and there are about 12 million infected people with 350 million people at the risk of infection, in Asia, Africa, southern Europe, South and Central America with several reported epidemics of leishmaniasis such as in Sudan and Afghanistan. Leishmaniasis is a parasitic disease, mainly manifested in the following three clinical forms: visceral leishmaniasis (VL), cutaneous leishmaniasis (CL), and mucocutaneous leishmaniasis. Among them, VL is the most serious form of the disease which is fatal if left untreated. VL has become an important opportunistic infection associated with human immunodeficiency virus (HIV). In southern Europe, up to 70% of adult VL cases are related to HIV infection (Barrett & Croft, 2012; Van Griensven & Diro, 2012). According to the World Health Organization, the annual incidence of VL and CL is estimated at 0.3 million and 1 million, respectively. Here, we have reviewed current modern approaches for the diagnosis of leishmaniasis, primarily focusing on the detection of disease in humans (Kumar, Pandey, & Samant, 2020). The number of real cases of leishmaniasis is incorrect because out of 88 countries suffering from it, only 40 countries regularly and annually report the disease. Currently treatment of leishmaniasis includes using drugs to alleviate disease and vector

Pathogenesis, Treatment and Prevention of Leishmaniasis. DOI: https://doi.org/10.1016/B978-0-12-822800-5.00005-6

control to reduce its transmission. Pentavalent antimonials (namely, sodium stibogluconate and meglumine antimoniate) are the mainstay of antileishmanial therapy (Sundar & Chakravarty, 2010). Although glucantime is often used to treat leishmaniasis, it has some side effects, including increased liver enzymes and changes in the electrocardiogram. Besides, pentamidine isethionates, miltefosine, and paromomycin (PM), can also be used, but their use is limited due to toxicity and high cost of treatment. Furthermore, the drug is painful to inject, and research shows that resistance of the parasite to glucantime is increasing in different parts of the world (Sundar & Rai, 2002). Also, strains of most of the human-infective *Leishmania* species are reportedly to be resistant to standard chemotherapeutics. Therefore there is an urgent need to develop new treatments for leishmaniasis (Kumar, Pandey, & Samant, 2018).

Nowadays, there are two ways to develop new therapies; one is to find new drugs and the other is to optimize certain drug formulations. The discovery of a traditional drug takes 10−12 years and is costly; about 1 billion dollars on an average is required to develop a drug. One strategy to improve the treatment of leishmaniasis is to apply a drug delivery system that can enhance the effectiveness of the treatment by optimizing the absorption, distribution, metabolism, and excretion of existing drugs with reduced toxicity (Dorlo, Balasegaram, Beijnen, & de Vries, 2012). However, *Leishmania* poses a further challenge to drug delivery since the drug has to achieve therapeutic levels at multiple sites (bone marrow, liver, spleen, cutaneous lesions) and reach within phagolysosome of macrophages (Santos, Oyafuso, Kiill, Daflon-Gremiao, & Chorilli, 2013). Hence, the development of systems that are capable of delivering drugs and target parasites within host cells is crucial (Fig. 7.1). Novel advances in nanotechnology have proven beneficial in therapeutic fields such as drug, gene/protein delivery, and developing drug carriers for a range of different diseases caused by parasitic or bacterial pathogens such as leishmaniasis, malaria, Chagas disease, and tuberculosis (Romero & Morilla, 2010). In this context, researchers have demonstrated the benefits of nanotechnology to improve efficacy as well as a reduction in side effects/toxicity of drugs used for the treatment of these infectious diseases. Nanotechnology involves the engineering of macromolecular devices to nanometer range and has already been used in medicine extensively (Davis et al., 2010). Some nanotherapeutics have been approved by Food and Drug Administration and are presently accessible for clinical use for different diseases such as fungal infections and leishmaniasis, HIV-associated sarcoma, and several other conditions (Hrkach et al., 2012).

In today's technologically advanced world, the use of nanotechnology is constantly expanding. This form of technology has many advantages over existing technologies in many fields and medicine is one of them (Croft & Olliaro, 2011). With the help of nanotechnology, a variety of devices and mechanisms have been developed, which can help cure diseases/disorders in a better and more competent way. Usefulness of nanotechnology can

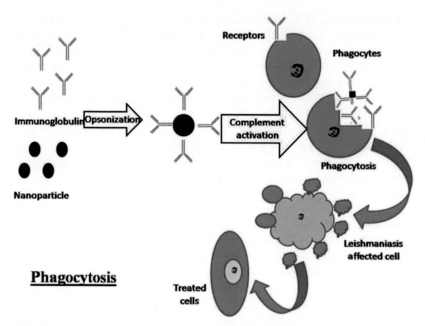

FIGURE 7.1   Process of phagocytosis for absorption of nanoparticle.

especially be seen in the treatment of infectious diseases. This chapter considers treatment of leishmaniasis by different nanotechnology-based techniques, namely nanodrugs, silver nano particles (SNPs), lipid nanocapsules, nanovaccines, nanotubes, etc.

7.2   Nanodrugs: A new horizon against leishmaniasis

Nanotechnology must be used to treat infectious diseases such as leishmaniasis. Many antiprotozoan drugs have been manufactured and are still being discovered (Pandey, Jha, Kumar, & Samant, 2019) (Pandey et al., 2019), but protozoans have re-emerged with resistance to these drugs. Nanotechnology has recently shown its promise in developing a liposomal formulation called amphotericin B (AmB) for leishmaniasis but it has shown side effects and is not cost-effective for developing countries (Laniado-Laborin & Cabrales-Vargas, 2009). Initial nanodelivery systems for delivering chemotherapeutics were nanodisks impregnated with AmB, polymeric-nanoparticle loaded with pentamidine, primaquine, and niosomes, and it still needs clinical level validation. There is an urgent need to undertake the task to use effective nanotechnology devices in combating this infectious disease (Zampa et al., 2009).

Before penicillin, colloidal silver was the treatment of choice for many diseases and infections. Many reports show colloidal silver is effective against approximately 650 different microorganisms. Therefore it seems that the size of nanosilver particles is very small and can penetrate skin lesions, thus has a good curative effect on *Leishmania* (Wagner, Dullaart, Bock, & Zweck, 2006). Silver has been used to treat various infections for many years, and with the development of nanotechnology, and the use of silver nanoparticles (AgNPs) has provided us new treatment to combat infectious diseases methods. Nanosilver compounds have effects on various microorganisms (including bacteria, viruses, fungi), and can even defend against protozoa. Nanosilver solution is a new drug, with good antibacterial, antifungal, and antiviral properties at low concentrations. Studies have shown that nanosilver cement has high antibacterial activity and high effectiveness against multidrug-resistant bacteria without cytotoxicity in vitro. Recently, researchers have shown that silver nanoparticles have antiinflammatory effects and can promote wound healing and wound dressings (Jebali & Kazemi, 2013). Nano-mediated drug delivery of plant-derived products is one of the most important strategies for the treatment of VL in the absence of sufficient antileishmanial drugs. According to reports, Artemisinin, which is traditionally used to treat malaria, has antileishmanial and antitumor activities (Srivastava, Shankar, Mishra, & Singh, 2016). Earlier, it has been demonstrated that nanoparticle preparations loaded with artemisinin can improve its in vitro activity against *Leishmania donovani* amastigotes ex vivo. Nanoparticles of AmB have greater efficacy than conventional AmB. This formulation may have a good safety profile, and with low cost of production, it may prove to be a feasible alternative to conventional AmB in the treatment of VL (Jebali & Kazemi, 2013). If nanoparticles are systemically administered, they will be agglomerated after exposure to plasma, and their efficacy will be decreased. Antileishmanial nanoparticles must be conjugated with biological compounds such as antibodies or lectin, which bind to specific targets, to exert more toxicity for parasites and less toxicity for normal cells (Gedda, Singh, Srivastava, & Sundar, 2019; Singh, Hasker, Boelaert, & Sundar, 2016; Singh, Mishra, Bajpai, Singh, & Tiwari, 2014).

Some nanoparticles are highly cytotoxic to macrophages and this must be considered. The use of nanoparticles to treat CL may have both positive and negative effects. Some reports indicate that gold nanoparticles (AuNPs), titanium dioxide nanoparticles (TiO_2NPs), zinc oxide nanoparticles (ZnONPs), magnesium oxide nanoparticles (MgONPs), etc., have antibacterial properties. *Leishmania* parasites are said to be sensitive to heat, and some nanoparticles have a photothermal effect after being exposed to near-infrared (NIR) light. These nanoparticles absorb NIR energy and convert it into heat. Then, as the temperature rises, cells are damaged. Leishmaniasis vaccine development is another major area where DNA nanotechnology may play an important role. So far, many efforts have been made to develop a successful leishmaniasis vaccine, but its realization into the clinics has been a bottleneck (Pandey, Kumar, & Samant, 2020; Singh et al., 2014, 2016).

7.2.1 Polymeric nanoparticles

Polymers are the most widely studied and researched form of carriers used in nanomedicine. Poly alkyl cyanoacrylate nanoparticles were used to adsorb anticancer drugs. It was first used in cancer treatment in 1979. These nanoparticles are made of various types of biocompatible and biodegradable colloidal particles. They have a size of 10–1000 nm. They carry drugs in different ways like adsorption, encapsulation, dissolution, entrapment, or by chemical binding of the drug on to the surface of polymeric nanoparticles (PNPs). Advanced physicochemical properties of PNPs can improve bioavailability, enhance cell dynamics, are biodegradable, and provide controlled drug delivery. PNPs include synthetic polymers, such as polylactic acid, polyglycolic acid, polylactide-co-glycolide (PLGA), polycaprolactone, polycyanoacrylate, and also natural polymers, such as gelatin, albumin, chitosan, and alginate. Among these polymers, PLGA has been mainly used in drug delivery and tissue engineering. PNPs exist in two different forms: nanospheres and nanocapsules. In the case of nanocapsules, the drug is encapsulated in a cavity surrounded by a polymer membrane, whereas the drug is not confined in a cavity, but is dispersed uniformly in the case of nanospheres. PNPs appear to be a great choice for the delivery of drugs and proteins to target cells because of their easy permeation due to their small size and these polymers can be designed in various molecular designs with many applications (Tiwari et al., 2012). PNPs deliver the drug to the targeted site through three mechanisms:

1. Degradation of the polymer at the target site through an enzymatic reaction, leading to drug release.
2. Drug is released by swelling of PNP, then hydrating and diffusing.
3. Separation of drug from polymer.

PNP is currently being investigated as a drug carrier and different types of PNPs are being studied on mouse models for treatment of leishmaniasis (Das, Roy, Mondal, Bera, & Mukherjee, 2013).

7.2.2 Lipid nanocapsules

Lipid nanocapsules (LNs) are nanocarriers between 20 and 100 nm in size that mimic lipoproteins. LNs consist of a lipid core and a surfactant film surrounding it (Omwoyo et al., 2014). It is a hybrid structure made using liposomes and polymer nanocapsules (Kozako, Arima, Yoshimitsu, Honda, & Soeda, 2012). LN is prepared by using a solvent-free method that provides stability and higher bioavailability. The main advantage of LN is that they can deliver drugs on-site, require highly reduced dosage with minimal toxic side effects, and reduce toxic side effects (Zhai & Zhai, 2014). In a study on the development of LNs, the core was made of hydrophobic olive oil, and the shell was made of hydrophilic component chitosan. Miltefosine is an alkyl phospholipid used to treat leishmaniasis by the destruction of its Ca^{2+} homeostasis (Verma & Dey, 2006). Formulation of nanoparticles containing miltefosine enhances efficacy against leishmaniasis, which can be proved by its damaged anterior flagella. LN also ensures stability and sustained release of the drug. LN oral medications have also been developed with advances in technology (Bhandari et al., 2012).

7.2.3 Solid lipid nanoparticles (SLNs) and nanostructured lipid carriers (NLCs)

SLNs are a relatively new class of nanocarriers and NLCs belonging to this class and differing from each other based on their matrix. SLN was first developed in 1996 and can be classified into three types of structures: SLN, NLCs, and lipid conjugates. These particles are solid at room and body temperatures and comprised of lipids such as glyceryl monostearate and stearic acid (Bawa, Melethil, Simmons, & Harris, 2008). Because SLN contains lipids, they retain a biocompatible and biodegradable profile, and since they are solid and rigid, they allow good protection of incorporated drug, even in inhospitable environments with a great variation of pH, humidity, and temperature. These have various advantages since they protect the drug against harsh environmental conditions; their large-scale production is easy using the high-pressure homogenization technique. However, they have some limitations as well, that is, SLNs have low drug loading efficacy due to their crystalline structure and there is a chance of drug expulsion during storage of crystalline structure and initial burst release can occur. NLCs are similar to SLN but have a greater ability to incorporate drugs, and do not usually crystallize during storage processes, and have liquid lipids inside them instead of solid (Peer et al., 2007). These particles are ideal for delivering hydrophobic drugs as they are composed entirely of lipids. A recent study associated SLN with PM, an antileishmanial drug, to improve its effectiveness (Souto et al., 2015). PM-loaded SLN (PM-SLN) was evaluated in vivo against infection of *Leishmania major* in BALB/c mice. PM-SLN had greater apparent safety compared to free drugs and are more efficient as they increased penetration of the drug into macrophages in addition to enhancing immune response (Souto et al., 2015). Furthermore, NLC systems can improve the efficacy of poorly water-soluble drugs against protozoan diseases. For instance, NLC carrying cedrol has shown improved antiparasitic activity against *L. donovani*, in vitro, and in vivo compared to treatment with free drug (Chawla & Madhubala, 2010).

In a study, chitosan-coated SLNs carrying AmB were synthesized for chemotherapy of *Leishmania* infections. Their antileishmanial activity showed that SLNs have a much better effect than formulations of AmBisome and Fungizone, available in the market. Additionally, this study showed SLNs are

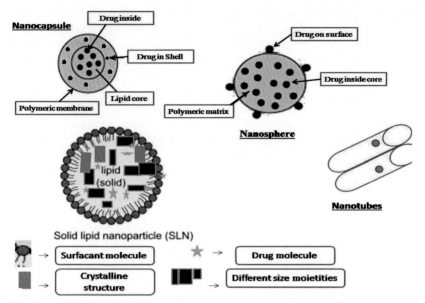

FIGURE 7.2   Graphical representations of the structure of various nanoparticle systems.

safer than market products, by evaluating acute toxicity studies in mice (Prajapati et al., 2011). NLCs are referred to as second-generation SLNs. They are the combination of both solids and lipids, unlike SLNs (Fig. 7.2).

7.2.4   Metallic nanoparticles

Since early history metals have been used in medications, these nanoparticles first came into existence in the 1850s (Ribeiro et al., 2004). There is a wide range of metallic nanoparticles that are being used for antileishmanial activity providing negligible toxicity and high efficiency (Allahverdiyev et al., 2011; Sazgarnia et al., 2013).

7.2.4.1   Iron

A study was conducted for the treatment of VL using iron oxide nanoparticles coated with glycine (peptide), and with encapsulated AmB drug. A 10−15 nm nanoparticle size was used, which reduced parasitic content in the spleen of treated subjects (Khatami et al., 2017). Glycine-coated nanoparticles could be employed further in leishmanial treatments.

7.2.4.2   Zinc

ZnONPs are massively produced and used. A study was conducted in which ZnONPs were employed in varying concentrations (0.18, 0.37, 0.75, and

1.5 g/mL) against the *L. donovani* amastigotes. Results were analyzed by colorimetric assay which suggested that ZnONPs exerted a cytotoxic effect on amastigote cells, causing hindrance in their proliferation and suppression of *L. donovani* activity. The study suggests that ZnONPs could be a cost-effective means for antileishmanial drug development. ZnONPs were prepared from *Verbena officinalis* and *Verbena tenuisecta* plant leaf extracts (Afridi, Hashmi, Ali, Zia, & Haider Abbasi, 2018; Delavari, Dalimi, Ghaffarifar, & Sadraei, 2014). Results suggested that *V. officinalis* had more phenolic content, and both plant ZnONPs were tested for antileishmanial activity, where the *V. officinalis* ZnONPs had better activity due to greater phenolic content and smaller size as compared to ZnONPs from *V. tenuisecta*.

7.2.4.3 Silver

Being very useful in medications and initially used for treating infections, around 650 different diseases and illnesses were reported to be treated by using it (Kalishwaralal, Barath Mani Kanth, Pandian, Deepak, & Gurunathan, 2010; Kim et al., 2008). Later, with further technological developments, improved nanosilver or silver nanoparticles have been developed. Various studies have been conducted on the biogenic synthesis of AgNPs and their mode of action in different biomedical applications (Baiocco et al., 2010; Mayelifar, Taheri, Rajabi, & Sazgarnia, 2015). Antileishmanial activity of AgNPs was checked, obtained from a fungal source, *Fusarium oxysporum*, and evaluated by a group of researchers (Allahverdiyev et al., 2011). Results were promising as AgNPs led to the death of promastigotes enabling its apoptosis. In further studies, it was found that AgNPs release reactive oxygen species (ROS) that cause damage to membranes of promastigotes. In the case of amastigotes, AgNPs led to a reduction of infected macrophages (Allahverdiyev et al., 2011). Another AgNP study suggested that the antibacterial activities of AgNPs helps fight leishmaniasis. In the study, the effects of AgNPs were checked against leishmanial parasite morphology, infectivity, metabolic activity, survival abilities, and proliferation rates. AgNPs led to the impairment of morphological characteristics and infectivity rates of the parasite. Additionally, metabolic activity and proliferation were reduced by 1.5-fold (Fanti et al., 2018). Overall, AgNPs could be a new therapeutic source for the treatment of leishmaniasis (Fanti et al., 2018; Rahul et al., 2015).

7.2.4.4 Others

Use of nanoparticles under ultraviolet (UV) and infrared (IR) light generates ROS, causes the death of parasites. In one study, antileishmanial effects of some nanoparticles, such as AgNPs, AuNPs, TiO$_2$NPs, ZnONPs, and MgONPs were evaluated on *L. major* parasite (Jebali & Kazemi, 2013; Kalangi et al., 2016). The increased antileishmanial activity was observed for AgNPs, followed by AuNPs, TiO$_2$NPs, ZnONPs, and MgONPs under UV and IR light conditions as compared to dark. Thus these light-improved antileishmanial properties of the abovementioned nanoparticles must be considered in forthcoming studies (Jebali & Kazemi, 2013). Similarly, in another study, chitosan-derived TiO$_2$NPs were used as an effective antileishmanial agent against amastigote and promastigote forms of the parasite. Chitosan-derived TiO$_2$NPs were loaded with meglumine antimoniate to enhance the activity of TiO$_2$NPs. The activity of nanoparticles was checked and formulations were found to be effective against amastigote as well as promastigote forms of the parasite (Varshosaz, Arbabi, Pestehchian, Saberi, & Delavari, 2018). Overall, metallic oxide nanoparticles provide an approach for the reduction and treatment of all types of leishmanial activity (Varshosaz et al., 2018) (Fig. 7.3).

7.2.5   Nanotubes

Nanotubes are cylindrical hollow molecules that are synthesized from inorganic and metallic materials. Many studies have been conducted that prove that nanotubes are excellent nanocarriers. The antileishmanial effect of AmB carbon nanotubes was examined. They used a formulation of linked AmB, an antileishmanial drug, with functionalized carbon nanotubes to reduce toxicity caused by the drug. This formulation was able to inhibit parasite growth more effectively than AmB alone. Thus the drug carrier improves the efficacy of the drug (Wu et al., 2005). Carbon nanotubes for drug delivery have not been considered for humans yet, and are in preclinical stage (Table 7.1).

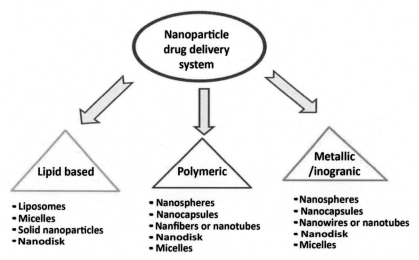

FIGURE 7.3   Overview of the relationship between nanoparticle drug delivery system.

TABLE 7.1 Advantages and disadvantages of current nanomedicines.

Nanotechnology-based system	Advantages	Disadvantages	Reference
Liposomes	Drug stability increased via encapsulation; nontoxic, flexible, biocompatible, biodegradable; increased efficacy and therapeutic index of drug; flexibility to couple with site-specific ligands to achieve active targeting; used preferentially for parenteral or cutaneous route	Leakage, fusion of encapsulated drugs; production costs can be high	Frezard and Demicheli (2010)
Polymeric nanoparticles	High level of biocompatibility with reduced cytotoxicity	Toxicity related to surfactant	Lembo and Cavalli (2010)
Lipid nanocapsules	Easy to scale-up; encapsulating lipophilic and hydrophilic drugs; evading of organic solvents		Zhai and Zhai (2014)
Solid lipid nanoparticles	Easy to scale-up and sterilized develop stability of drugs; encapsulating lipophilic and hydrophilic drugs; avoiding of organic solvents; used for oral, parenteral, or cutaneous routes	Low drug loading and expulsion of matrix; short half-life; toxicity related to surfactant	Zhai and Zhai (2014)
Carbon nanotubes	Exhibit biocompatibility, excretion, and less toxicity		Liu et al. (2008)

7.3   Nanovaccines: Emerging methods of nanotechnology to combat leishmaniasis

Drugs used for chemotherapy are the main treatment for leishmaniasis, including AmB, PM, fluconazole, antimony containing compounds, and pentamidine. However, these therapeutic drugs have their limitations, such as toxicity, low efficacy, and drug resistance (Gedda et al., 2019; Kumar et al., 2018). Other therapies, that may be effective in eradicating leishmaniasis, are vaccine based. Two types of leishmanial vaccines are under preparation: first generation and second generation. First-generation leishmanial vaccines consist of live vaccines (Pandey, Pande, & Samant, 2020) while second-generation vaccines are prepared using recombinant technology (Coler & Reed, 2005). To date, there is no licensed leishmaniasis vaccine. Three leishmanial vaccines, Leish-F1, F2, and F3, designed at the Infectious Disease Research Institute, United States, are in clinical trials (Handman, 2001). These are formulated based on the selective antigen epitope properties of *Leishmania*. Recombinant *Leishmania* vaccines are also being developed at the Sabin Vaccine Institute (Gillespie et al., 2016).

With the advent of nanotechnology, nanoparticles are now used as carriers for new antigen preparations. Nanoparticles can provide a safe, effective, and efficient vaccine delivery system. According to a study, SLNs can be used as an efficient tool to synthesize leishmanial vaccine (Saljoughian et al., 2013). The use of nanoparticles to deliver antigens and adjuvants has different purposes:

1. Increased uptake of antigen, loaded in nanoparticles, by antigen-presenting cells (APCs) (Heidari-Kharaji et al., 2016).
2. Activation of stronger immune response because different nanoparticles deliver to the same APC at the same time, activating immune response strongly as compared to free antigen and adjuvant (Pham, Loiseau, & Barratt, 2013).
3. Activation of Th1 (type 1 helper cell)-type immune response (Thakur, Sharma, Singh, & Katare, 2018).

In 2005 a team of researchers prepared a nanovaccine by loading recombinant *Leishmania* superoxide dismutase (SODB1) into chitosan nanoparticles in mice using the ionotropic gelation method. This study evaluated the loading efficacy and size of SODB1-loaded nanoparticles. Results showed that the use of stable chitosan nanoparticles can produce a higher cell-mediated immune response and have a higher IgG_2a level, which can be used as leishmaniasis nanovaccine (Tyagi et al., 2005). In another study, nanoliposomes were used as nanocarriers for soluble *Leishmania* antigens. Although there is no nanovaccine available for leishmaniasis, studies have been done on the use of nanoparticles as vaccine carriers and on adjuvants to form nanovaccines that have led to higher efficacy, which may reduce leishmaniasis cases (Sharma, Agrawal, Mody, & Vyas, 2015).

7.4 Conclusion

Nanotechnology for treatment of leishmaniasis is a relatively new research area. It can be applied to address all aspects of leishmaniasis, still a lot of research and development needs to be done. Although there are numerous treatment options, there is not even an effective option to effectively control the incidence of leishmaniasis. Drugs that can be used to treat leishmaniasis have many disadvantages, such as high cost, toxicity, and development of resistance in parasites. Various studies are underway to establish nanotechnology, namely designing nanomedicines and nanovaccines for treatment of leishmaniasis (Chen et al., 2014). Various nanomaterials are being researched to develop safe and cost-effective drugs for treatment of leishmaniasis. Many studies have shown that potentially effective drugs for treatment of leishmaniasis may be liposomes, PLGA nanoparticles, carbon nanotubes, and SLNs that enhance targeted drug delivery to parasites. Commercial viability of nanomedicine is a major concern for researchers. The most desirable feature of any drug delivery system is its commercial viability. The cost of drugs will affect resources and upscaling of drug production. AmB is currently the most cost-effective drug for treatment of leishmaniasis. Other drug delivery strategies based on nanoparticles are under developmental and experimental stages, and their production costs have not yet been analyzed. However, in-depth research is needed to develop low-cost drugs against leishmaniasis. Nanovaccines are quite a new concept for treating leishmaniasis. While, there is a lot of research being done to find effective nanotechnology-based leishmaniasis drugs, in addition to the liposomal drugs (AmB) that are commercially available, they are still in the preclinical stage (Casa, Scariot, Khalil, Nakamura, & Mainardes, 2018).

References

Afridi, M. S., Hashmi, S. S., Ali, G. S., Zia, M., & Haider Abbasi, B. (2018). Comparative anti-leishmanial efficacy of the biosynthesised ZnONPs from genus Verbena. *IET Nanobiotechnology, 12*, 1067−1073.

Allahverdiyev, A. M., Abamor, E. S., Bagirova, M., Ustundag, C. B., Kaya, C., Kaya, F., & Rafailovich, M. (2011). Antileishmanial effect of silver nanoparticles and their enhanced antiparasitic activity under ultraviolet light. *International Journal of Nanomedicine, 6*, 2705−2714.

Baiocco, P., Ilari, A., Ceci, P., Orsini, S., Gramiccia, M., Di Muccio, T., & Colotti, G. (2010). Inhibitory effect of silver nanoparticles on trypanothione reductase activity and Leishmania infantum proliferation. *ACS Medicinal Chemistry Letters, 2*, 230−233.

Barrett, M. P., & Croft, S. L. (2012). Management of trypanosomiasis and leishmaniasis. *British Medical Bulletin, 104*, 175.

Bawa, R., Melethil, S., Simmons, W. J., & Harris, D. (2008). Nano pharmaceuticals: patenting issues and FDA regulatory challenges. *SciTech Lawyer, 5*, 10−15.

Bhandari, V., Kulshrestha, A., Deep, D. K., Stark, O., Prajapati, V. K., Ramesh, V., . . . Salotra, P. (2012). Drug susceptibility in leishmania isolates following miltefosine treatment in cases of visceral leishmaniasis and post kala-azar dermal leishmaniasis. *PLoS Neglected Tropical Diseases*, *6*, 1657.

Casa, D., Scariot, D., Khalil, N., Nakamura, C., & Mainardes, R. (2018). Bovine serum albumin nanoparticles containing amphotericin B were effective in treating murine cutaneous leishmaniasis and reduced the drug toxicity. *Experimental Parasitology*, *192*, 12–18.

Chawla, B., & Madhubala, R. (2010). Drug targets in Leishmania. *Journal of Parasitic Diseases*, *34*, 1.

Chen, R., Chen, Q., Kim, H., Siu, K. H., Sun, Q., Tsai, S. L., & Chen, W. (2014). Biomolecular scaffolds for enhanced signaling and catalytic effciency. *Current Opinion in Biotechnology*, *28*, 59–68.

Coler, R. N., & Reed, S. G. (2005). Second-generation vaccines against leishmaniasis. *Trends in Parasitology*, *21*, 244–249.

Croft, S. L., & Olliaro, P. (2011). Leishmaniasis chemotherapy-challenges and opportunities. *Clinical Microbiology and Infection*, *17*, 1478.

Das, S., Roy, P., Mondal, S., Bera, T., & Mukherjee, A. (2013). One pot synthesis of gold nanoparticles and application in chemotherapy of wild and resistant type visceral leishmaniasis. *Colloids and Surfaces B: Biointerfaces*, *107*, 27.

Davis, M. E., Zuckerman, J. E., Choi, C. H. J., Seligson, D., Tolcher, A., Alabi, C. A., ... Ribas. (2010). Evidence of RNAi in humans from systemically administered siRNA via targeted nanoparticles. *Nature*, *464*(7291), 1067–1070.

Delavari, M., Dalimi, A., Ghaffarifar, F., & Sadraei, J. (2014). *In vitro* study on cytotoxic effects of ZnO nanoparticles on promastigote and amastigote forms of Leishmania major (MRHO/IR/75/ER). *Iran Journal of Parasitology*, *9*, 6–13.

Dorlo, T. P. C., Balasegaram, M., Beijnen, J. H., & de Vries, P. J. (2012). Miltefosine: a review of its pharmacology and therapeutic efficacy in the treatment of leishmaniasis. *The Journal of Antimicrobial Chemotherapy*, *67*, 2576.

Fanti, J. R., Tomiotto-Pellissier, F., Miranda-Sapla, M. M., Cataneo, A. H. D., Andrade, C., Panis, C., ... Costa, I. N. (2018). Biogenic silver nanoparticles inducing *Leishmania amazonensis* promastigote and amastigote death *in vitro*. *Acta Tropica*, *178*, 46–54.

Frezard, F., & Demicheli, C. (2010). New delivery strategies for the old pentavalent antimonial drugs. *Expert Opinion on Drug Delivery*, *7*, 1343–1358.

Gedda, M. R., Singh, O. P., Srivastava, O. N., & Sundar, S. (2019). Therapeutic leishmaniasis: recent advancement and developments in nanomedicines. *Nanotechnology in Modern Animal Biotechnology*, 195–220.

Gillespie, P. M., Beaumier, C. M., Strych, U., Hayward, T., Hotez, P. J., & Bottazzi, M. E. (2016). Status of vaccine research and development of vaccines for leishmaniasis. *Vaccine*, *34*, 2992–2995.

Handman, E. (2001). Leishmaniasis: current status of vaccine development. *Clinical Microbiology Reviews*, *14*, 229–243.

Heidari-Kharaji, M., Taheri, T., Doroud, D., Habibzadeh, S., Badirzadeh, A., & Rafati, S. (2016). Enhanced paromomycin efficacy by solid lipid nanoparticle formulation against Leishmania in mice model. *Parasite Immunology*, *38*, 599–608.

Hrkach, J., Von Hoff, D., Ali, M. M., Andrianova, E., Auer, J., Campbell, T., ... Horhota, A. (2012). Preclinical development and clinical translation of a PSMA targeted docetaxel nanoparticle with a differentiated pharmacological profile. *Science Translational Medicine*, *4*(128), 128–139.

Jebali, A., & Kazemi, B. (2013). Nano-based antileishmanial agents: a toxicological study on nanoparticles for future treatment of cutaneous leishmaniasis. *Toxicology In Vitro*, *27*, 1896–1904.

Kalangi, S. K., Dayakar, A., Gangappa, D., Sathyavathi, R., Maurya, R. S., & Narayana Rao, D. (2016). Biocompatible silver nanoparticles reduced from Anethum graveolens leaf extract augments the antileishmanial efficacy of miltefosine. *Experimental Parasitology, 170*, 184−192.

Kalishwaralal, K., Barath Mani Kanth, S., Pandian, S. R. K., Deepak, V., & Gurunathan, S. (2010). Silver nanoparticles impede the biofilm formation by Pseudomonas aeruginosa and Staphylococcus epidermidis. *Colloids and Surfaces B: Biointerfaces, 79*, 340−344.

Kaye, P., & Scott, P. (2011). Leishmaniasis: complexity at the hostpathogen interface. *Nature Reviews Microbiology, 9*, 604.

Khatami, M., Alijani, H., Sharifi, I., Sharifi, F., Pourseyedi, S., Kharazi, S., . . . Khatami, M. (2017). Leishmanicidal activity of biogenic Fe_3O_4 nanoparticles. *Scientia Pharmaceutica, 85*, 36.

Kim, K. J., Sung, W. S., Moon, S.-K., Choi, J.-S., Kim, J. G., & Lee, D. G. (2008). Antifungal effect of silver nanoparticles on dermatophytes. *Journal of Microbiology and Biotechnology, 18*, 1482−1484.

Kozako, T., Arima, N., Yoshimitsu, M., Honda, S. I., & Soeda, S. (2012). Liposomes and nanotechnology in drug development: Focus on onco targets. *International Journal of Nanomedicine, 7* (49), 43.

Kumar, A., Pandey, S. C., & Samant, M. (2018). Slow pace of antileishmanial drug development. *Parasitology Open, 4*(4), 1−11.

Kumar, A., Pandey, S. C., & Samant, M. (2020). A spotlight on the diagnostic methods of a fatal disease visceral leishmaniasis. *Parasite Immunology, 42*, e12727.

Kumar, A., Pandey, S. C., & Samant, M. (2020). DNA-based microarray studies in visceral leishmaniasis: identification of biomarkers for diagnostic, prognostic and drug target for treatment. *Acta Trop, 208*, 105512. Available from https://doi.org/10.1016/j.actatropica. 2020.105512. 32389452.

Laniado-Laborin, R., & Cabrales-Vargas, M. N. (2009). Amphotericin B: side effects and toxicity. *Revista Iberoamericana de Micologia, 26*, 223.

Lembo, D., & Cavalli, R. (2010). Nanoparticulate delivery systems for antiviral drugs. *Antiviral Chemistry & Chemotherapy, 21*, 53.

Liu, Z., Chen, K., Davis, C., Sherlock, S., Cao, Q., Chen, X., & Dai, H. (2008). Drug delivery with carbon nanotubes for in vivo cancer treatment. *Canadian Journal of Research, 68*(16), 6652−6660.

Mayelifar, K., Taheri, A. R., Rajabi, O., & Sazgarnia, A. (2015). Ultraviolet B efficacy in improving antileishmanial effects of silver nanoparticles. *Iranian Journal of Basic Medical Sciences, 18*, 677.

Omwoyo, W. N., Ogutu, B., Oloo, F., Swai, H., Kalombo, L., Melariri, P., . . . Gathirwa, J. W. (2014). Preparation, characterization, and optimization of primaquine-loaded solid lipid nanoparticles. *International Journal of Nanomedicine, 11*, 3865−3874.

Pandey, S. C., Dhami, D. S., Jha, A., Shah, G. C., Kumar, A., & Samant, M. (2019). Identification of *trans*-2-*cis*-8-Matricaria-ester from the Essential Oil of *Erigeron multiradiatus* and evaluation of its antileishmanial potential by in vitro and in silico approaches. *ACS Omega, 4*(11), 14640−14649. Available from https://doi.org/10.1021/acsomega.9b02130. 31528820.

Pandey, S. C., Jha, A., Kumar, A., & Samant, M. (2019). Evaluation of antileishmanial potential of computationally screened compounds targeting DEAD-box RNA helicase of Leishmania donovani. *Int J Biol Macromol, 121*, 480−487. Available from 10.1016/j.ijbiomac.2018.10. 053. 30321635.

Pandey, S. C., Kumar, A., & Samant, M. (2020). Genetically modified live attenuated vaccine: a potential strategy to combat visceral leishmaniasis. *Parasite Immunology, 42*, e12732.

Pandey, S. C., Pande, V., & Samant, M. (2020). DDX3 DEAD-box RNA helicase (Hel67) gene disruption impairs infectivity of Leishmania donovani and induces protective immunity against visceral leishmaniasis. *Sci Rep, 10*(1), 18218. Available from https://doi.org/10.1038/s41598-020-75420-y. 33106577.

Peer, D., Karp, J. M., Hong, S., Farokhzad, O. C., Margalit, R., & Langer, R. (2007). Nanocarriers as an emerging platform for cancer therapy. *Nature Nanotechnology, 2,* 751−760.

Pham, T. T., Loiseau, P. M., & Barratt, G. (2013). Strategies for the design of orally bioavailable antileishmanial treatments. *International Journal of Pharmaceutics, 454,* 539−552.

Pinto, M. C., Barbieri, K., Silva, M. C. E., Graminha, M. A. S., Casanova, C., Andrade, A. J., & Eiras, A. E. (2011). Octenol as attractant to nyssomyianeivai (diptera: psychodidae: phlebotominae) in the field. *Journal of Medical Entomology, 48,* 39.

Prajapati, V. K., Awasthi, K., Gautam, S., Yadav, T. P., Rai, M., Srivastava, O. N., & Sundar, S. (2011). Targeted killing of *Leishmania donovani in vivo* and *in vitro* with amphotericin B attached to functionalized carbon nanotubes. *The Journal of Antimicrobial Chemotherapy, 66,* 874−879.

Rahul, S., Chandrashekhar, P., Hemant, B., Bipinchandra, S., Mouray, E., Grellier, P., & Satish, P. (2015). *In vitro* antiparasitic activity of microbial pigments and their combination with phytosynthesized metal nanoparticles. *Parasitology International, 64,* 353−356.

Ribeiro, T. G., Chávez-Fumagalli, M. A., Valadares, D. G., França, J. R., Rodrigues, L. B., Singh, S., & Sivakumar, R. (2004). Challenges and new discoveries in the treatment of leishmaniasis. *Journal of Infection and Chemotherapy, 10,* 307.

Romero, E. L., & Morilla, M. J. (2010). Nanotechnological approaches against Chagas disease. *Advanced Drug Delivery Reviews, 62,* 576.

Saljoughian, N., Zahedifard, F., Doroud, D., Doustdari, F., Vasei, M., Papadopoulou, B., & Rafati, S. (2013). Cationic solid−lipid nanoparticles are as effcient as electroporation in DNA vaccination against visceral leishmaniasis in mice. *Parasite Immunology, 35,* 397−408.

Santos, F. K., Oyafuso, M., Kiill, C., Daflon-Gremiao, M., & Chorilli, M. (2013). Nanotechnology-based drug delivery systems for treatment of hyperproliferative skin diseases—a review. *Current Nanoscience, 9,* 159.

Sazgarnia, A., Taheri, A. R., Soudmand, S., Parizi, A. J., Rajabi, O., & Darbandi, M. S. (2013). Antiparasitic effects of gold nanoparticles with microwave radiation on promastigotes and amastigotes of *Leishmania major*. *International Journal of Hyperthermia, 29,* 79−86.

Sharma, R., Agrawal, U. N., Mody., & Vyas, S. P. (2015). Polymer nanotechnology-based approaches in mucosal vaccine delivery: challenges and opportunities. *Biotechnology Advances, 33,* 64−79.

Singh, N., Mishra, B. B., Bajpai, S., Singh, R. K., & Tiwari, V. K. (2014). Natural product-based leads to fight against leishmaniasis. *Bioorganic & Medicinal Chemistry, 22,* 18−45.

Singh, O. P., Hasker, E., Boelaert, M., & Sundar, S. (2016). Elimination of visceral leishmaniasis on the Indian subcontinent. *The Lancet Infectious Diseases, 16,* 304−309.

Souto, D. E., Fonseca, A. M., Barragan, J. T., de CS Luz, R., Andrade, H. M., Damos, F. S., & Kubota, L. T. (2015). SPR analysis of the interaction between a recombinant protein of unknown function in *Leishmania infantum* immobilised on dendrimers and antibodies of the visceral leishmaniasis: a potential use in immunodiagnosis. *Biosensors & Bioelectronics, 70,* 275−281.

Srivastava, S., Shankar, P., Mishra, J., & Singh, S. (2016). Possibilities and challenges for developing a successful vaccine for leishmaniasis. *Parasites & Vectors, 9,* 277.

Sundar, S., & Chakravarty, J. (2010). Antimony toxicity. *International Journal of Environmental Research and Public Health, 7*, 4267.

Sundar, S., & Rai, M. (2002). Advances in the treatment of leishmaniasis. *Current Opinion in Infectious Diseases, 15*, 593.

Thakur, K., Sharma, G., Singh, B., & Katare, O. P. (2018). Topical drug delivery of anti-infectives employing lipid-based nanocarriers: dermatokinetics as an important tool. *Current Pharmaceutical Design, 24*, 5108−5128.

Tiwari, G., Tiwari, R., Sriwastawa, B., Bhati, L., Pandey, S., Pandey, P., & Bannerjee, S. K. (2012). Drug delivery systems: an updated review. *International Journal of Pharmaceutical Investigation, 2*, 2.

Tyagi, R., Lala, S., Verma, A. K., Nandy, A. K., Mahato, S. B., Maitra, A., & Basu, M. K. (2005). Targeted delivery of arjunglucoside I using surface hydrophilic and hydrophobic nanocarriers to combat experimental leishmaniasis. *Journal of Drug Targeting, 13*, 161−171.

Van Griensven, J., & Diro, E. (2012). Visceral leishmaniasis. *Infectious Disease Clinics of North America, 26*, 309.

Varshosaz, J., Arbabi, B., Pestehchian, N., Saberi, S., & Delavari, M. (2018). Chitosan-titanium dioxide-glucantime nanoassemblies effects on promastigote and amastigote of *Leishmania major*. *International Journal of Biological Macromolecules, 107*, 212−221.

Verma, N. K., & Dey, C. S. (2006). Anti-leishmanial drug miltefosine causes insulin resistance in skeletal muscle cells *in vitro*. *Diabetologia, 49*, 1656.

Wagner, V., Dullaart, A., Bock, K., & Zweck, A. (2006). The emerging nanomedicine landscapes. *Nature Biotechnology, 24*, 1211.

Wu, W., Wieckowski, S., Pastorin, G., Benincasa, M., Klumpp, C., Briand, J. P., . . . Bianco, A. (2005). Targeted delivery of amphotericin B to cells by using functionalized carbon nanotubes. *Angewandte Chemie International, 44*, 6358−6362.

Zampa, M. F., Araújo, I. M., Costa, V., Nery Costa, C. H., Santos, J. R., Zucolotto, V., . . . Leite, J. R. (2009). Leishmanicidal activity and immobilization of dermaseptin 01 antimicrobial peptides in ultrathin films for nanomedicine applications. *Nanomedicine: Nanotechnology, Biology, and Medicine, 5*, 352.

Zhai, Y., & Zhai, G. (2014). Advances in lipid-based colloid systems as drug carrier for topic delivery. *Journal of Controlled Release, 193*, 90.

Chapter 8

Natural products as a novel source for antileishmanial drug development

Vinita Gouri, Satish Chandra Pandey, Diksha Joshi, Veni Pande, Shobha Upreti and Mukesh Samant
Cell and Molecular Biology Laboratory, Department of Zoology, Kumaun University, SSJ Campus, Almora, India

8.1 Introduction

Leishmaniasis is a vector-borne disease, which is transmitted to humans by female sandfly vector belonging to the genus *Phlebotomus*. Based on the clinical symptoms there are three major forms of leishmaniasis, namely cutaneous leishmaniasis (CL) (*Leishmania major, Leishmania mexicana, Leishmania tropica, Leishmania amazonensis, Leishmania aethiopica, Leishmania venezuelensis, Leishmania braziliensis, Leishmania panamensis, Leishmania guyanensis,* and *Leishmania peruviana*), mucocutaneous leishmaniasis (MCL) (*L. mexicana, L. braziliensis, L. amazonensis, L. guyanensis,* and *L. panamensis*) and visceral leishmaniasis (VL) (*Leishmania donovani, Leishmania infantum,* and *Leishmania chagasi*) (Ridley, 1988). This fatal disease comes in the ninth position of the global burden. This disease is regarded as a protozoan zoonotic disease affecting approximately 12 million people in 88 countries around the world along with a mortality rate of 60,000 (Hosseininejad et al., 2012; Machado et al., 2014; Sarkar & Sarkar, 2013). With the advent of the human immunodeficiency virus, leishmaniasis is rapidly becoming an opportunistic infection in AIDS (acquired immunodeficiency syndrome) patients (Diro et al., 2014). On the other hand, an ideal vaccine is also not available to control the disease (Pandey, Kumar, & Samant, 2020; Pandey, Pande, & Samant, 2020). The standard drugs for leishmaniasis are pentavalent antimonials including sodium stibogluconate (SSG) (Pentostam) and meglumine antimoniate (Glucantime) (Diro et al., 2014). However, severe side effects in the patients include arthralgias, myalgias, leukopenia, pancreatitis, liver problems, cardiotoxicity, and cardiac arrhythmia. Moreover prolonged treatment time and

Pathogenesis, Treatment and Prevention of Leishmaniasis. DOI: https://doi.org/10.1016/B978-0-12-822800-5.00011-1

increased parasite resistance are also among the major limitations of these drugs (Chakravarty & Sundar, 2010; Diro et al., 2014; Lage et al., 2013). Therefore amphotericin B, pentamidine, paromomycin, and miltefosine are the recommended alternative drugs to be used instead of antimonials, but they also come with some side effects such as toxicity, high cost, drug resistance, and therapeutic failure (Lage et al., 2013; Machado et al., 2012; Wiwanitkit, 2012). Given the abovementioned reasons, the development of new, less toxic, and more cost-effective drugs with greater efficacy as well as more accessible alternative therapeutic strategies that could become available for low-income populations to treat the disease have become a necessity (Lage et al., 2013). Since victims of leishmaniasis are generally poor, lengthy treatment using expensive drugs with related costs is far beyond the reach of such families (Oryan, Alidadi, & Akbari, 2014). Therefore many patients seek herbal therapy which is cheaper and readily available. However, most of the herbs have still not been evaluated scientifically. In recent years, there has been growing interest in alternative natural products and plant compounds for the treatment of leishmaniasis (Alviano et al., 2012; Pandey et al., 2019a; Pandey, Jha, Kumar, & Samant, 2019b). Among the major problem in the development of effective drugs is that *Leishmania* is showing resistance against the already manufactured drugs (Kumar, Pandey, & Samant, 2018). Diagrammatic presentation of the drug resistance problem is illustrated in Fig. 8.1. To overcome all these

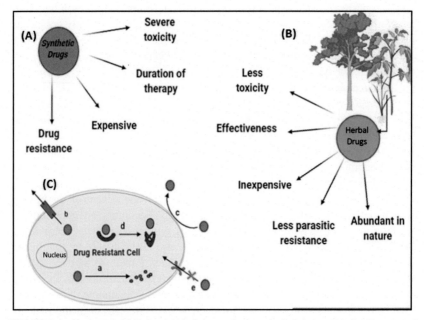

FIGURE 8.1 Reasons behind the switch from synthetic to herbal drugs: (A) disadvantage of synthetic drugs; (B) advantage of herbal drugs; and (C) different modes of drug resistance mechanisms: a., drug inactivation; b., increase drug efflux; c., decrease drug diffusion; d., target modification; e., loss of drug uptake.

limitations, herbal drugs can be an effective alternative to treat leishmaniasis. It has been reported that there are about 250,000 medicinal plant species that have been evaluated for herbal products, but only 15 antiparasitic medicines were approved until 2006 (Newman & Cragg, 2012). Due to the drug resistance problem in chemotherapy herbal-based medicines are usually more acceptable than synthetic chemical medicines (Dhami, Pandey, Shah, Bisht, & Samant, 2020; Zeiman, Greenblatt, Elgavish, Khozin-Goldberg, & Golenser, 2008). The antileishmanial activity of some plants has been attributed to the presence of the compounds such as alkaloids, flavonoids, chalcones, steroids, triterpenoids, naphthoquinones, quinones, lignans, saponins, and terpenes (Lage et al., 2013; Sifaoui et al., 2014). In this chapter, we have attempted to provide some effective alternative herbal compounds with their properties, mechanisms, and significant antileishmanial activity.

8.2   Current antileishmanial chemotherapy

The leishmanial infections have a few remedial choices that contain a limited number of drugs. Until now, there have been no effective vaccines against leishmaniasis, making drugs the only potential method for treatment. The first successful drug against *L. donovani* was launched in 1920 as Urea stibamine (urea salt of stibnic acid). It remained immensely popular for over a decade, after which the use of potassium antimony tartrate (Tartar emetic) was also introduced. Leishmaniasis treatment also includes stibamine and stibactein, which showed some serious side effects. Later, pentavalent antimonials showing less side effect were used as the first-line drug against leishmaniasis (Kumar et al., 2018). Fig. 8.2 represents the time line showing the development of synthetic antileishmanial drug.

8.2.1   Pentavalent antimonials

The pentavalent antimony (V) complexes against leishmaniasis were used in 1945 for the first time and remained popular for several decades. Presently, only two pentavalent antimonials are sold for medical use, namely SSG and meglumine antimoniate (also known as *N*-methylglucamine antimoniate) with trade names Stibanate/Pentostam and Glucantime/Prostib, respectively. However, several cases of parasite resistance have been reported in disease endemic countries, which have lessened its use (Kumar, Boggula, Sundar, Shasany, & Dube, 2009).

8.2.2   Pentamidine

The isethionate salt of pentamidine was used for the treatment of leishmaniasis in patients that showed no response to antimonials. But, pentamidine efficacy is declining in India, indicating that parasite resistance is increasing. Its

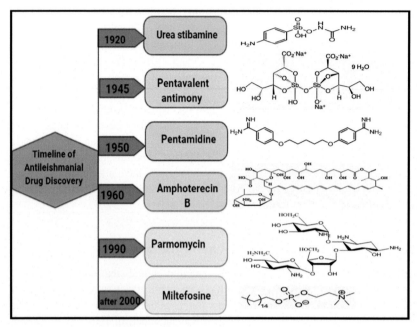

FIGURE 8.2 Time line of synthetic antileishmanial drug.

use for leishmaniasis was finally eliminated due to its reduced efficacy and severe toxicities (Coelho, Beverley, & Cotrim, 2003).

8.2.3 Amphotericin B

Polyunsaturated macrolide antifungal antibiotic was developed in 1960 from bacterium *Streptomyces nodosus* (Lemke, Kiderlen, & Kayser, 2005). Amphotericin B was used to clinically treat patients with SSG/sodium antimony gluconate or pentamidine unresponsiveness. However, its use is highly restricted due to its toxic nature and multiple side effects, for example, high fever, rigor, chills, and renal failure (Berman et al., 1998).

8.2.4 Parmomycin

An aminoglycoside antibiotic isolated from *Streptomyces chrestomyceticus*, is yet another second-line drug, proven to be useful against leishmaniasis. It is also applicable in the treatment of SSG-unresponsive VL and CL in India and Kenya (Moore & Lockwood, 2003). However, poor assimilation and intra muscular route of administration are two major drawbacks of the drug. Paromomycin action mechanism in *Leishmania* spp. is exactly not known but resistance showed a decrease in drug uptake in *L. donovani* (Maarouf,

Adeline, Solignac, Vautrin, & Robert-Gero, 1998). Pentamidine, amphotericin B, and paromomycin are some second-line drugs. A partial number of
drugs (miltefosine, allopurinol, sitamaquine) that are administered orally
have also shown antileishmanial activity.

8.2.5 Oral antileishmanial drugs

8.2.5.1 Miltefosine

It is the first oral drug used against leishmaniasis, chemically, it is hexadecyl, phosphocholine, originally synthesized in 1992 as an anticarcinogenic
agent for treating skin cancer; later in 2000 it was also used against VL. It is
effective against VL and CL, moreover, it is also used against antimony-
resistant infections. Reports show that its use has been restricted nowadays
due to the resistance developed in the parasite resulting in the efflux of drugs
(Pérez-Victoria et al., 2006).

8.2.5.2 Allopurinol

Combination therapy including allopurinol and SSG is being successfully
used to treat leishmaniasis, however allopurinol when used in monotherapy
was ineffective against VL or CL. The drug blocks the purine salvage pathway by specifically targeting the enzyme hypoxanthine-guanine phosphori-
bosyltransferase, which inhibits protein synthesis resulting in the death of the
parasite (Chawla & Madhubala, 2010). Few cases of allopurinol resistance in
L. infantum have been reported leading to disease reoccurrence in dogs
(Singh, Garg, & Ali, 2016; Yasur-Landau et al., 2016).

8.2.5.3 Sitamaquine

Sitamaquine (4-methyl-6-methoxy-8-aminoquinoline) has confined clinical
use. Moreover, until now there were no studies regarding the drug resistance
in *Leishmania*. Sitamaquine is a comparatively less effective compound,
causing nephrotoxicity, therefore this drug cannot be used in monotherapy to
treat leishmaniasis (Singh et al., 2016).

8.3 Plant-derived compounds in the treatment of leishmaniasis

Humans have used medicinal plants in past for the treatment of diverse ail-
ments (Piccoli & Zatti, 1977), still in many developing countries, the rural
population rely on traditional treatment for their primary health care in contrast to synthetic medicine. Herbals can overpower the use of synthetic drugs,
as they aid to overcome parasitic resistances, toxicity, high expenses, and
severe side effects, thus synthetic drugs may be replaced by herbal medication leading to herbal drug discovery. In the majority of therapies, plant

extracts and their bioactive components are used (Craig, 1999; Vayalil, 2002). Different studies have shown that traditional plants including *Polyalthia suaveolens*, *Erigeron multiradiatus*, *Agrimonia pilosa*, *Origanum microphyllum*, *Origanum dictamnus*, *Eryngium ternatum*, and *Piper betel*, etc., have the potential for the development of new agents against leishmaniasis. Some important medicinal plants with potential activity against leishmaniasis are listed in Table 8.1 and various modes of action of plant-derived secondary metabolites have been shown in Fig. 8.3. In the past two or three decades, analysis of potential plant products has progressed a lot by employing modern analytical techniques like chromatography, isotope techniques, and enzymology, etc. Therefore various compounds which are reported to possess antileishmanial activity are described in this chapter.

8.3.1 Flavonoids

Flavonoids are the polyphenolic compounds that are generally present in the plants and while exploring their antiparasitic activity, it was found that compounds like luteolin (Mittra et al., 2000), flavone A (Croft & Coombs, 2003), quercetin (Mittra et al., 2000) and fisetin (Mittra et al., 2000) have significant antileishmanial activity. Luteolin (3′,4′,5,7-tetrahydroxyflavone) derived from *Vitex negundo*, quercetin (3,3′,4′,5,7-pentahydroxyflavanone) derived from *Fagopyrum esculentum* and fisetin (3,7,3′,4′-tetrahydroxyflavone) isolated from *Cotinus coggygria* (smoke tree) are the chief sources of flavonoids and are profusely present in vegetables, fruits, olive oil, tea, and the propolis of apiary (Mittra et al., 2000). Quercetin and luteolin restrain the synthesis of parasitic DNA of *L. donovani* by promoting apoptosis through linearization of the k DNA mediated by topoisomerase II (Mittra et al., 2000). Moreover, Isoquercitrin (quercetin-3-*O*-β-glucoside) and quercitrin (quercetin-3-*O*-rhamnoside) restrain ARG-L of *L. amazonensis* in a noncompetitive manner (Ghodsian, Taghipour, Deravi, Behniafar, & Lasjerdi, 2020). The methanolic and ethanolic extract of *Piper betle* show leishmanicidal action in *L. donovani* (promastigotes and intracellular amastigote) by increasing apoptosis through the production of reactive oxygen species, thus aiming the mitochondria with no cytotoxicity shown towards macrophages (Panche, Diwan, & Chandra, 2016). Epigallocatechin 3-*O*-gallate (EGCG), is the most abundant flavonoid present in ample amount in green tea and has been studied in in vivo and in vitro experiments against *L. infantum*. EGCG has also been accounted to be a novel agent for the treatment of VL (Ghodsian et al., 2020).

Further chalcones, the open-chain flavonoids have two aromatic rings linked by a carbonyl group and two α,β-unsaturated carbon atoms (Cabrera et al., 2007; Chiaradia et al., 2008). Licochalcone A is an oxygenated chalcone that has been examined by various researchers and it was found that licochalcone A, hinders the growth of both *L. major* and *L. donovani* promastigote forms in in vitro condition. It is also evident from their previous studies that it

TABLE 8.1 Various medicinal plants with their crude extract, fractions, isolated compounds, and essential oil evaluated against leishmaniasis (Kolodziej, H. Kiderlen, A. F., 2005).

Plant	Part of Plant	Preparation	Species	Reference
Azadirachta indica	Leaves and seeds	Ethanolic fraction and ethyl	Leishmania donovani	Chouhan et al. (2015)
Asparagus racemosus	Whole plant	Tablets	L. donovani	Kaur, Chauhan, and Sachdeva (2014)
Agrimonia pilosa	Aerial part	Essential oil	L. donovani	Dhami et al. (2020)
Annona squamosa	Leaves	Alkaloid and acetogenic extract	Leishmania chagasi	Vila-Nova et al. (2011)
Annona muricata	Seeds	Alkaloid and acetogenic Extract	L. chagasi	
Aloe vera	Leaves	Extract	Leishmania infantum	Kerkeni et al. (2016)
Allium sativum	Bulb	Methanolic extract	L. donovani	
Annona crassiflora	Stem bark	Exanolic and ethanolic extract	L. donovani	
Artemisia dracunculus	Plant	Ethanolic extract	Leishmania major	
Bidens pilosa Linn	Leaves	Hydroalcoholic extracts	Leishmania amazonensis	Maes et al. (2004)
Casearia arborea	Leaves	Methanolic extract	L. infantum	Santos et al. (2017)
Curcuma longa	Rhizome	Oral formulation based on nanoparticles	L. donovani	Kerkeni et al. (2016)
Cocos nucifera	Husk fiber	Aqueous extract	L. donovani	Rosa et al. (2003)
Coccinia grandis	Leaves	Extract	L. donovani	
Croton caudatus	Leaves	Hexanic extract	L. donovani	
Croton cajucara	Leaves	Essential oil	L. chagasi	
Coriandrum sativum	Seeds	Oleoresin	L. chagasi	Rondon et al. (2012)
Copaifera reticulate	Seeds	Essential oil	L. chagasi	
Chenopodium ambrosioides	Aerial parts	Essential oil	L. donovani	

(Continued)

TABLE 8.1 (Continued)

Plant	Part of Plant	Preparation	Species	Reference
Erigeron multiradiatus	Aerial parts	Essential oil	*L. donovani*	Pandey et al. (2020)
Guarea kunthiana	Roots	Exanolic and ethanolic extracts	*L. donovani*	De Mesquita et al. (2005)
Galipea longiflora	Bark	Alkaloid extract	*Leishmania braziliensis*	Calla-Magariños et al. (2013)
Himatanthus obovatus	Root wood	Exanolic and ethanolic extract	*L. donovani*	De Mesquita et al. (2005)
Lippia sidoides	Not cited	Essential oil	*L. chagasi*	
Moringa oleifera	Flower	Ethyl acetate fraction	*L. donovani*	Rondon et al. (2012)
Momordica charantia	Fruit	Crude extract	*L. donovani*	Kerkeni et al. (2016)
Nuphar lutea	Plant	Methanolic excract	*L. major*	Kaur et al. (2014)
Ocimum sanctum	Leaves	Ethanolic extract	*L. donovani*	Kerkeni et al. (2016)
Piper betle	Leaves	Methanolic extract and essential oil	*L. donovani*	Maes et al. (2004)
Punica granatum	Leaves	Hydroalcoholic extracts	*L. amazonensis*	
Ricinus communis	Leaves	Extract	*L. infantum*	
Syzygium aromaticum	Flower	Essential oil	*L. donovani*	
Solanum torvum	Leaves	Extract	*L. donovani*	Kerkeni et al. (2016)
Spondias mombin	Aerial parts	Ethanolic extract	*L. chagasi*	De Mesquita et al. (2005)
Serjania lethalis	Root bark	Exanolic and ethanolic extract	*L. donovani*	
Tinospora sinensis	Powdered stem	Ethanolic extract	*L. donovani*	
Withania somnifera	Leaves; whole plant	Alcoholic and methanolic extract	*L. donovani*	Hutchinson et al. (2016)

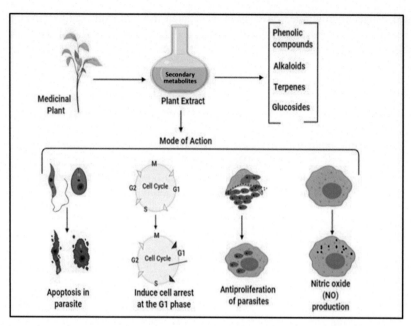

FIGURE 8.3 Various modes of action of plant-derived secondary metabolites.

destroyed the ultrastructure of the promastigote's mitochondria (Chen et al., 1993). Moreover, while further examining the working of parasital mitochondria, they brought up that licochalcone A restrained parasitic respiration in a concentration-dependent way, via the inhibition of CO_2 production and O_2 consumption by the parasites. Also, licochalcone A repressed the activity of the mitochondrial dehydrogenase present in the parasite. These studies established the fact that licochalcone A can modify the ultrastructure and functioning of the leishmanial mitochondria (Zhai, Blom, Chen, Christensen, & Kharazmi, 1995).

8.3.2 Alkaloids

Alkaloids are one of the main herbal compounds with the most significant activity against *Leishmania*. Berberine, the chief analog of quinoline and isoquinoline, is a quaternary isoquinoline alkaloid present in *Berberis* (e.g., *Berberis vulgaris, Berberis aristata, Mahonia aquifolium, Hydrastis canadensis,* and *Tinospora cordifolia*) which is found to have the most elevated level of antileishmanial activity among the alkaloids (Chan-Bacab & Peña-Rodríguez, 2001). Berberine chloride derived from *B. aristata* represses respiration in amastigotes by targeting the mitochondrial proteins thus, triggering a free radical-dependent, caspase-independent apoptosis (Ghodsian et al., 2020). Other isoquinoline alkaloids, that includes anonaine, liriodenine, and isoguattouregidine, have been accounted for showing antileishmanial activity in *L. donovani*, *L. amazonensis*, and *L. braziliensis* (Chan-Bacab & Peña-Rodríguez, 2001).

8.3.3   Lignans

Lignans are also an important group of polyphenolic compounds. Diphyllin, a lignan derived from the plant *Haplophyllum bucharicum* (Rutaceae), which is an endemic plant from Uzbekistan, showed antiproliferative activity in the promastigotes of *L. infantum*. Diphyllin acts by interfering with macromolecules, leading to cell cycle arrest, consequently dropping the intracellular protein content. It acts by preventing the attachment of the parasite to the macrophages, thus restricting the parasite entry into the host cell (Di Giorgio et al., 2004; Salem & Werbovetz, 2006a).

8.3.4   Tannins

Tannins are an extraordinary group of phenolic metabolites derived from various woody and a few herbaceous higher plant species (Ghodsian et al., 2020). Tannins and structurally related compounds were reported for antileishmanial and immunomodulatory properties. These compounds were evaluated against both extra and intracellular leishmania spp. and macrophage activation by release of nitric oxide (NO), interferon (IFN) tumour and necrosis factor (TNF) like activities. Moreover, their positive effect on host macrophage functions were further examined by expression analysis (iNOS, IFN-α, TNF-α, IL-1, IL-10, (Emam et al., 1996) (IL-12, IL-18) (Kolodziej & Kiderlen, 2005). Tannins and their analogs help to increasing the nitric oxide (NO) produced by the nitric oxide synthase (iNOS) enzyme, through host macrophages which is the most important molecule responsible for the leishmanicidal activity. Müller et al. (1997), reported that the release of IFN-α by Leishmania-infected, activated macrophages also seems to play a potential role in antileishmanial defense. Interferon gamma (IFN-γ) cytokines (proinflammatory molecules) in the host cells, and also by upregulating the expression of TNF-α and IFN-γ, interleukin (IL)-12 IL-18, inducible nitric oxide synthase (iNOS), and IL-1 messenger RNA (mRNA) in the host macrophages that are infected with *Leishmania* (Kolodziej & Kiderlen, 2005; Samant, Sahu, Pandey, & Khare, 2021).

8.3.5   Terpenes

Monoterpenes are extracted from the leaves of *Croton cajucara* (Euphorbiaceae), which promotes the production of NO in macrophages infected with *L. amazonensis* and directly targets the parasite via inducing mitochondrial swelling and also by inducing reorganization of the nuclear chromatin and chromatin of the kinetoplast (Ghodsian et al., 2020). Rifolin and piperogalin derived from the plant *Peperomia galioides* (Piperaceae) induce entire lysis in the promastigote form of the various species of *Leishmania* (Chan-Bacab & Peña-Rodríguez, 2001). Besides that espintanol, derived from the plant *Oxandra espintana* (Annonaceae) is highly toxic to the macrophages and display potential leishmanicidal activity against different species of *Leishmania* (Chan-Bacab & Peña-Rodríguez, 2001).

Artemisinin, a sesquiterpene lactone isolated from ethanolic extract of the leaves of *Artemisia indica*. This sesquiterpene amplifies the expression of iNOS mRNA to the levels present in uninfected macrophages and also augments the release of IFN-γ, suggesting that artemisinin can play a significant role in the leishmanicidal activity (Sen et al., 2010). Studies suggest that artemisinin shows significant antileishmanial action against CL, MCL, and VL (Sen et al., 2010). Dehydrozaluzanin C (sesquiterpene lactone) obtained from leaves of *Munnozia maronii* (Asteraceae) inhibit the survival of several promastigote forms of *Leishmania* spp. including *L. mexicana*, *L. amazonensis*, and *L. donovani*, etc. (Chan-Bacab & Peña-Rodríguez, 2001). Compounds such as 12-*O*-tetradecanoyl phorbol-13-acetate, jatrophone and jatrogrossidione obtained from species of Euphorbiaceae family have leishmanicidal effects against the promastigote forms of *L. chagasi*, *L. amazonensis*, and *L. brazilliensis* (Mittal et al., 1998; Ray et al., 1996). Diterpene compounds tanshinones obtained from *Perovskia abrotanoides* and *Salvia miltiorrhiza* have a remarkable potential to cure CL (Salem & Werbovetz, 2006a).

Dihydrobetulinic acid, a triterpene, have shown effective result against *L. donovani* by inducing apoptosis (Alakurtti et al., 2010; Chowdhury et al., 2003). A pentacyclic triterpene, 18-beta-glycyrrhetinic acids, isolated from *Glycyrrhiza glabra* roots has displayed antileishmanial activity by enhancing Th1 (helper T cells) cytokine response associated with the amplified production of iNOS in experimental VL (Ghodsian et al., 2020). Ursolic acid (prevalent triterpenes) and betulinaldehyde derived from the bark of *Jacaranda copaia* and stem of *Doliocarpus dentatus* (Dilleniaceae), respectively, inhibits promastigote and intracellular amastigote form of *L. amazonensis* by manipulating the phagocytic activity of macrophages (Oketch-Rabah et al., 1998; Salem & Werbovetz, 2006a) Moreover, carboxylic acid and epioleanolic acid both isolated from *Celaenodendron mexicanum* have displayed effective activity against *L. donovani* (Tiuman et al., 2005).

8.3.6 Saponins

Saponins including hederagenin, α-hederin and β-hederin are derived from the leaves of *Hedera helix*, these compounds have been reported to possess effective leishmanicidal activity against promastigotes and amastigotes of *L. infantum*, *L. mexicana*, and *L. tropica* (Chan-Bacab & Peña-Rodríguez, 2001; Loukaci et al., 2000; Majester-Savornin et al., 1991). Their prevailing antiproliferative activity is due to their capability to disturb the parasite membrane integrity (Chan-Bacab & Peña-Rodríguez, 2001; Loukaci et al., 2000; Majester-Savornin et al., 1991). Oleane, saponins obtained from the methanolic extract of *Maesa balansae* (Myrsinaceae) leaves have powerful prophylactic and therapeutic effects against VL (Maes et al., 2004). Mimengoside A isolated from the leaves of *Buddleja madagascariensis* (Loganiaceae) and muzanzagenin, derived from the roots of *Asparagus africanus* (Liliaceae) have been reported to show potential activity against promastigotes of *L. infantum* and *L. major*, respectively (Delmas et al. 2000; Emam et al., 1996; Majester-Savornin et al., 1991). Moreover, a steroidal saponin isolated from *Yucca filamentosa* (Agavaceae) has shown inhibitory effects against promastigotes form of *L. mexicana* (Sairafianpour et al., 2001).

8.3.7 Quinones

Diospyrin is a reported naphthoquinones obtained from the bark of *Diospyros montana* (Ebenaceae) with effective antileishmanial activity against the promastigote form of *L. major* and *L. donovani* (Hazra et al., 2013). This compound interacts with topoisomerase I in *Leishmania* and help to stabilize the enzyme−DNA cleavable complex. Plumbagin is another naphthoquinone that is obtained from *Plumbago zeylanica* roots, is effective against *L. donovani*. This compound induces topoisomerase II-mediated mammalian DNA cleavage in vitro and delays the growth of *L. amazonensis* and *L. venezuelensis* in the experimental mice (Torres-Santos et al., 2004). Furthermore, naphthoquinone, lapachol obtained from *Handroanthus* species has displayed leishmanicidal activity against promastigotes of *L. braziliensis* and *L. amazonensis* and amastigotes of *L. donovani* (Araújo et al., 2019; Chan-Bacab & Peña-Rodríguez, 2001; Lima et al., 2004).

Aloe-emodin, an anthraquinone isolated from the aerial parts of *Stephania dinklagei* (Menispermaceae), has displayed potential activity against promastigotes and amastigotes of *L. donovani* (Salem & Werbovetz, 2006b) Emodin, bianthrone A1 and vismione D derived from the stem bark of *Vismia orientalis* (Guttiferae or Clusiaceae) have shown potent activity against protozoan species including *L. donovani*, *Trypanosoma cruzi*, *Plasmodium falciparum* strain K1and *Trypanosoma rhodesiense* (Mbwambo et al., 2004). 4-Hydroxy-1-tetralone obtained from the bark of *Ampelocera edentula* (Ulmaceae) is an active herbal compound against *L. donovani*, *L. braziliensis*, *L. amazonensis* and *L. venezuelensis* (Salem & Werbovetz, 2006b), but the use of this herbal metabolite is limited due to its cytotoxic, carcinogenic effects and mutagenicity in experimental animals (Fournet et al., 1994).

8.3.8 Other metabolites

Acetogenins such as senegalene, squamocine, asimicine, sylvaticin, rolliniastatin-1, annonacin A, molvizarine, and goniothalamicin isolated from the pantropical plants family, acts by inhibiting the growth of promastigotes of *L. amazonensis*, *L. braziliensis*, *L. major*, *L. donovani*, and *L. infantum* (Da Silva et al., 1995; Waechter et al., 1997). Argentilactone excluded from the hexanic extract of *Annona haemantantha* (Annonaceae) has leishmanicidal effects against promastigotes form of *L. donovani*, *L. amazonensis*, and *L. major* and other strains of *Leishmania* spp. (Chan-Bacab & Peña-Rodríguez, 2001; Waechter et al., 1997). Further, crude extract of seeds of the plant *Bixa orellana* (Bixaceae) have shown superior leishmanicidal effects against *L. amazonensis* promastigotes (Ghodsian et al., 2020). *Kalanchoe pinnata* (Crassulaceae) is a medicinal plant used for the cure of cutaneous lesions, aqueous leaf extract of these plants has leishmanicidal activity against *L. amazonensis* in vivo, and reduces the growth of intracellular amastigote by NO production (Ghodsian et al., 2020). Methanolic extract of *Allium sativum* and *Withania somnifera* has shown potent activity against *L. donovani* (Ghodsian et al., 2020). Further, compound withaferin A isolated from *W. somnifera* induces apoptosis in the parasite by inhibiting protein kinase C (Sen et al., 2010; Sharma et al., 2009).

8.4   Conclusion

The currently available studies indicate that chemotherapy is the only effective way to cure and prevent leishmaniasis as no effective vaccine is known to treat this disease. The commonly used synthetic drugs against VL have various negative impacts, such as severe toxicity, long duration of therapy, high cost, development of resistance, etc. Among these, high cost, in rural areas is one of the major drawbacks in the treatment and control of this disease. To overcome these problems medicinal plants can be used successfully, moreover, it is also well established that natural products play an important source of new medications because their derivatives are extremely useful for drug modification and bioactivity optimization. In the present study, we have discussed various metabolic compounds showing promising activity against various forms of leishmaniasis. The main objective of this study is to create awareness about the beneficial role of the plants and their components which can be used against leishmaniasis.

Acknowledgments

The authors are thankful to the Department of Zoology, SSJ Campus, Almora, and Kumaun University for providing a suitable research environment.

Conflict of interest

The authors have declared no conflict of interest.

References

Alakurtti, S., Heiska, T., Kiriazis, A., Sacerdoti-Sierra, N., Jaffe, C. L., & Yli-Kauhaluoma, J. (2010). Synthesis and anti-leishmanial activity of heterocyclic betulin derivatives. *Bioorganic and Medicinal Chemistry, 18*(4), 1573−1582.

Alviano, D. S., Barreto, A. L. S., Dias, F. d A., Rodrigues, I. d A., Rosa, M. d S. d S., Alviano, C. S., & Soares, R. Md. A. (2012). Conventional therapy and promising plant-derived compounds against trypanosomatid parasites. *Frontiers in Microbiology, 3,* 283, Frontiers Research Foundation.

Araújo, I. A. C., de Paula, R. C., Alves, C. L., Faria, K. F., Oliveira, M. M. d, Mendes, G. G., et al. (2019). Efficacy of lapachol on treatment of cutaneous and visceral leishmaniasis. *Experimental Parasitology, 199,* 67−73.

Berman, J. D., Badaro, R., Thakur, C. P., Wasunna, K. M., Behbehani, K., Davidson, R., et al. (1998). Efficacy and safety of liposomal amphotericin B (AmBisome) for visceral leishmaniasis in endemic developing countries. *Bulletin of the World Health Organization, 76*(1), 25−32, World Health Organization.

Cabrera, M., Simoens, M., Falchi, G., Lavaggi, M. L., Piro, O. E., Castellano, E. E., et al. (2007). Synthetic chalcones, flavanones, and flavones as antitumoral agents: biological evaluation and structure-activity relationships. *Bioorganic and Medicinal Chemistry, 15*(10), 3356−3367, Pergamon.

Calla-Magariños, J., Quispe, T., Giménez, A., Freysdottir, J., Troye-Blomberg, M., & Fernández, C. (2013). Quinolinic alkaloids from Galipea longiflora Krause suppress production of proinflammatory cytokines in vitro and control inflammation in vivo upon Leishmania infection in mice. *Scandinavian Journal of Immunology, 77*(1), 30−38.

Chakravarty, J., & Sundar, S. (2010). Drug resistance in leishmaniasis. *Journal of Global Infectious Diseases, 2*(2), 167.

Chan-Bacab, M. J., & Peña-Rodríguez, L. M. (2001). Plant natural products with leishmanicidal activity. *Natural Product Reports, 18*(6), 674 688.

Chawla, B., & Madhubala, R. (2010). Drug targets in Leishmania. *Journal of Parasitic Diseases, 34,* 1−13.

Chen, M., Christensen, S. B., Blom, J., Lemmich, E., Nadelmann, L., Fich, K., et al. (1993). Licochalcone A, a novel antiparasitic agent with potent activity against human pathogenic protozoan species of Leishmania. *Antimicrobial Agents and Chemotherapy, 37*(12), 2550−2556.

Chiaradia, L. D., dos Santos, R., Vitor, C. E., Vieira, A. A., Leal, P. C., Nunes, R. J., et al. (2008). Synthesis and pharmacological activity of chalcones derived from 2,4,6-trimethoxyacetophenone in RAW 264.7 cells stimulated by LPS: quantitative structure-activity relationships. *Bioorganic and Medicinal Chemistry, 16*(2), 658−667.

Chouhan, G., Islamuddin, M., Want, M. Y., Abdin, M. Z., Ozbak, H. A., Hemeg, H. A., et al. (2015). Apoptosis mediated leishmanicidal activity of Azadirachta indica bioactive fractions is accompanied by Th1 immunostimulatory potential and therapeutic cure in vivo. *Parasites and Vectors, 8*(1), 183.

Chowdhury, A. R., Mandal, S., Goswami, A., Ghosh, M., Mandal, L., Chakraborty, D., et al. (2003). Dihydrobetulinic acid induces apoptosis in Leishmania donovani by targeting DNA topoisomerase I and II: implications in antileishmanial therapy. *Molecular Medicine, 9*(1−2), 26−36. Available from https://link.springer.com/articles/10.1007/BF03402104.

Coelho, A. C., Beverley, S. M., & Cotrim, P. C. (2003). Functional genetic identification of PRP1, an ABC transporter superfamily member conferring pentamidine resistance in Leishmania major. *Molecular and Biochemical Parasitology, 130*(2), 83−90, Elsevier.

Craig, W. J. (1999). Health-promoting properties of common herbs. *The American Journal of Clinical Nutrition, 70*(3), 491s−499s.

Croft, S. L., & Coombs, G. H. (2003). Leishmaniasis—current chemotherapy and recent advances in the search for novel drugs. *Trends in Parasitology, 19*(11), 502−508.

Da Silva, S. A. G., Costa, S. S., Mendonça, S. C. F., Silva, E. M., Moraes, V. L. G., & Rossi-Bergmann, B. (1995). Therapeutic effect of oral Kalanchoe pinnata leaf extract in murine leishmaniasis. *Acta Tropica, 60*(3), 201−210.

Delmas, F., di Giorgio, C., Elias, R., Gasquet, M., Azas, N., Mshvildadze, V., Dekanosidze, G., Kemertelidze, E., & Timon-David, P. (2000). Antileishmanial activity of three saponins isolated from ivy, alphahederin, beta-hederin and hederacolchiside A1, as compared to their action on mammalian cells cultured in vitro. *Planta Medica, 66*(4), 343−347.

De Mesquita, M. L., Desrivot, J., Bories, C., Fournet, A., De Paula, J. E., Grellier, P., & Espindola, L. S. (2005). Antileishmanial and trypanocidal activity of Brazilian Cerrado plants. *Memorias do Instituto Oswaldo Cruz, 100*(7), 783−787.

Dhami, D. S., Pandey, S. C., Shah, G. C., Bisht, M., & Samant, M. (2020). In vitro antileishmanial activity of the essential oil from Agrimonia pilosa. *National Academy Science Letters,* 1−4.

Di Giorgio, C., Delmas, F., Ollivier, E., Elias, R., Balansard, G., & Timon-David, P. (2004). In vitro activity of the β-carboline alkaloids harmane, harmine, and harmaline toward parasites of the species Leishmania infantum. *Experimental Parasitology, 106*(3−4), 67−74.

Diro, E., Lynen, L., Mohammed, R., Boelaert, M., Hailu, A., & van, G. J. (2014). High parasitological failure rate of visceral leishmaniasis to sodium stibogluconate among HIV Co-infected adults in Ethiopia. *PLoS Neglected Tropical Diseases, 8*(5), e2875, H. Louzir (Ed.) Public Library of Science.

Emam, A. M., Moussa, A. M., Faure, R., Favel, A., Delmas, F., Elias, R., & Balansard, G. (1996). Isolation and biological study of a triterpenoid saponin, mimengoside A, from the leaves of Buddleja madagascariensis. *Planta Medica, 62*(1), 92−93.

Fournet, A., Barrios, A., Muñoz, V., Hocquemiller, R., Roblot, F., & Cavé, A. (1994). Antileishmanial activity of a tetralone isolated from Ampelocera edentula, a Bolivian Plant used as a treatment for cutaneous leishmaniasis. *Planta Medica, 60*(01), 8−12.

Ghodsian, S., Taghipour, N., Deravi, N., Behniafar, H., & Lasjerdi, Z. (2020). Recent researches in effective antileishmanial herbal compounds: narrative review. *Parasitology Research, 119* (12), 3929−3946.

Hazra, S., Ghosh, S., Sarma, M. D., Sharma, S., Das, M., Saudagar, P., et al. (2013). Evaluation of a diospyrin derivative as antileishmanial agent and potential modulator of ornithine decarboxylase of Leishmania donovani. *Experimental Parasitology, 135*(2), 407−413.

Hosseininejad, M., Mohebali, M., Hosseini, F., Karimi, S., Sharifzad, S., & Akhoundi, B. (2012). Seroprevalence of canine visceral leishmaniasis in asymptomatic dogs in Iran. *Iranian Journal of Veterinary Science, 13*(1), 54−57.

Hutchinson, R., Akhtar, A., Haridas, J., Bhat, D., Roehrborn, C., Lotan, Y., et al. (2016). PD09-02 prostate cancer screening and referral patterns in the years surrounding the United States Preventative Services Task Force recommendation against PSA screening in all men USPSTF PSA screening guidelines result in higher Gleason score diagnoses. *American Urological Association,* 195.

Kaur, S., Chauhan, K., & Sachdeva, H. (2014). Protection against experimental visceral leishmaniasis by immunostimulation with herbal drugs derived from Withania somnifera and Asparagus racemosus. *Journal of Medical Microbiology, 63*(10), 1328−1338.

Kerkeni, L., Ruano, P., Delgado, L.L., Picco, S., Villegas, L., Tonelli, F., et al. (2016). We are IntechOpen, the world's leading publisher of Open Access books Built by scientists, for scientists TOP 1 %. *Intech* (tourism), 13. Retrieved from https://www.intechopen.com/books/advanced-biometric-technologies/liveness-detection-in-biometrics.

Kolodziej, H., & Kiderlen, A. F. (2005). Antileishmanial activity and immune modulatory effects of tannins and related compounds on Leishmania parasitised RAW 264.7 cells. *Phytochemistry*, *66*(17 SPEC. ISS.), 2056−2071.

Kumar, A., Boggula, V. R., Sundar, S., Shasany, A. K., & Dube, A. (2009). Identification of genetic markers in sodium antimony gluconate (SAG) sensitive and resistant Indian clinical isolates of Leishmania donovani through amplified fragment length polymorphism (AFLP). *Acta Tropica*, *110*(1), 80−85.

Kumar, A., Pandey, S. C., & Samant, M. (2018). Slow pace of antileishmanial drug development. *Parasitology Open*, *4*.

Lage, P. S., De, A. P. H. R., Lopes, A. D. S., Chávez, F. M. A., Valadares, D. G., Duarte, M. C., et al. (2013). Strychnos pseudoquina and its purified compounds present an effective in vitro antileishmanial activity. *Evidence-Based Complementary and Alternative Medicine*, *2013*, 304354.

Lemke, A., Kiderlen, A. F., & Kayser, O. (2005). Amphotericin B. *Applied Microbiology and Biotechnology*, *68*(2), 151−162, Springer.

Lima, N. M. F., Correia, C. S., Leon, L. L., Machado, G. M. C., De Fátima Madeira, M., Santana, A. E. G., & Goulart, M. O. F. (2004). Antileishmanial activity of lapachol analogues. *Memorias do Instituto Oswaldo Cruz*, *99*(7), 757−761.

Loukaci, A., Kayser, O., Bindseil, K. U., Siems, K., Frevert, J., & Abreu, P. M. (2000). New trichothecenes isolated from Holarrhena floribunda. *Journal of Natural Products*, *63*(1), 52−56.

Maarouf, M., Adeline, M. T., Solignac, M., Vautrin, D., & Robert-Gero, M. (1998). Development and characterization of paromomycin-resistant Leishmania donovani promastigotes. *Parasite*, *5*(2), 167−173.

Machado, M., Dinis, A. M., Santos-Rosa, M., Alves, V., Salgueiro, L., Cavaleiro, C., & Sousa, M. C. (2014). Activity of Thymus capitellatus volatile extract, 1,8-cineole and borneol against Leishmania species. *Veterinary Parasitology*, *200*(1-2), 39−49, Elsevier.

Machado, M., Pires, P., Dinis, A. M., Santos-Rosa, M., Alves, V., Salgueiro, L., et al. (2012). Monoterpenic aldehydes as potential anti-Leishmania agents: activity of Cymbopogon citratus and citral on L. infantum, L. tropica and L. major. *Experimental Parasitology*, *130*(3), 223−231, Academic Press.

Maes, L., Vanden Berghe, D., Germonprez, N., Quirijnen, L., Cos, P., De Kimpe, N., & Van Puyvelde, L. (2004). In vitro and in vivo activities of a triterpenoid saponin extract (PX-6518) from the plant Maesa balansae against visceral leishmania species. *Antimicrobial Agents and Chemotherapy*, *48*(1), 130−136.

Majester-Savornin, B., Elias, R., Diaz-Lanza, A., Balansard, G., Gasquet, M., & Delmas, F. (1991). Saponins of the ivy plant, Hedera helix, and their leishmanicidic activity. *Planta Medica*, *57*(03), 260−262.

Mbwambo, Z. H., Apers, S., Moshi, M. J., Kapingu, M. C., Van Miert, S., Claeys, M., et al. (2004). Anthranoid compounds with antiprotozoal activity from Vismia orientalis. *Planta Medica*, *70*(8), 706−710.

Mittal, N., Gupta, N., Saksena, S., Goyal, N., Roy, U., & Rastogi, A. K. (1998). Protective effect of Picroliv from Picrorhiza kurroa against Leishmania donovani infections in Mesocricetus auratus. *Life Sciences*, *63*(20), 1823−1834.

Mittra, B., Saha, A., Chowdhury, A. R., Pal, C., Mandal, S., Mukhopadhyay, S., et al. (2000). Luteolin, an abundant dietary component is a potent anti-leishmanial agent that acts by inducing topoisomerase II-mediated kinetoplast DNA cleavage leading to apoptosis. *Molecular Medicine (Cambridge, Mass.)*, *6*(6), 527−541, BioMed Central.

Moore, E. M., & Lockwood, D. N. (2003). Treatment of visceral leishmaniasis. *Turkish Journal of Pediatrics*, *45*(3), 280, Wolters Kluwer -- Medknow Publications.

Müller, I., Freudenberg, M., Kropf, P., Kiderlen, A. F., & Galanos, C. (1997). Leishmania major infection in C57BL/10 mice differing at the Lps locus: a new non-healing phenotype. *Medical Microbiology and Immunology*, *186*, 75−81.

Newman, D. J., & Cragg, G. M. (2012). Natural products as sources of new drugs over the 30 years from 1981 to 2010. *Journal of Natural Products*, *75*(3), 311−335, American Chemical Society and American Society of Pharmacognosy.

Oketch-Rabah, H., Christensen, S., Frydenvang, K., Dossaji, S., Theander, T., Cornett, C., et al. (1998). Antiprotozoal properties of 16,17-dihydroxybrachycalyxolide from Vernonia brachycalyx. *Planta Medica*, *64*(06), 559−562.

Oryan, A. A. S., Alidadi, M., & Akbari, M. (2014). Risk factors associated with leishmaniasis. *Tropical Medicine & Surgery*, *02*(03).

Panche, A. N., Diwan, A. D., & Chandra, S. R. (2016). Flavonoids: an overview. *Journal of Nutritional Science*, *5*, e47.

Pandey, S. C., Dhami, D. S., Jha, A., Shah, G. C., Kumar, A., & Samant, M. (2019a). Identification of *trans-2-cis-8-*Matricaria-ester from the essential oil of *Erigeron multiradiatus* and evaluation of its antileishmanial potential by in vitro and in silico approaches. *ACS Omega*, *4*(11), 14640.

Pandey, S. C., Jha, A., Kumar, A., & Samant, M. (2019b). Evaluation of antileishmanial potential of computationally screened compounds targeting DEAD-box RNA helicase of *Leishmania donovani*. *International Journal of Biological Macromolecules*, *121*, 480−487.

Pandey, S. C., Kumar, A., & Samant, M. (2020). Genetically modified live attenuated vaccine: a potential strategy to combat visceral leishmaniasis. *Parasite Immunology*, e12732.

Pandey, S. C., Pande, V., & Samant, M. (2020). DDX3 DEAD-box RNA helicase (Hel67) gene disruption impairs infectivity of Leishmania donovani and induces protective immunity against visceral leishmaniasis. *Scientific Reports, 10*(1), 18218. Available from https://doi. org/10.1038/s41598-020-75420-y. 33106577.

Pérez-Victoria, F. J., Sánchez-Cañete, M. P., Seifert, K., Croft, S. L., Sundar, S., Castanys, S., & Gamarro, F. (2006). Mechanisms of experimental resistance of Leishmania to miltefosine: implications for clinical use. *Drug Resistance Updates*, *9*(1-2), 26−39.

Piccoli, A., & Zatti, C. (1977). Attuali Orientamenti Terapeutici Nelle Ipoacusie Improvvise. *Minerva Otorinolaringologica*, *27*(2), 81−90.

Ray, S., Majumder, H. K., Chakravarty, A. K., Mukhopadhyay, S., Gil, R. R., & Cordell, G. A. (1996). Amarogentin, a naturally occurring secoiridoid glycoside and a newly recognized inhibitor of topoisomerase I from Leishmania donovani. *Journal of Natural Products*, *59*(1), 27−29.

Ridley, D. S. (1988). Pathogenesis of Leprosy and Related Diseases. *Histological diagnosis*, 146−151.

Rondon, F. C. M., Bevilaqua, C. M. L., Accioly, M. P., de Morais, S. M., de Andrade-Júnior, H. F., de Carvalho, C. A., et al. (2012). In vitro efficacy of Coriandrum sativum, Lippia sidoides and Copaifera reticulata against Leishmania chagasi. *Revista Brasileira de Parasitologia Veterinaria*, *21*(3), 185−191.

Rosa, Md. S. S., Mendonça-Filho, R. R., Bizzo, H. R., Rodrigues, I. d A., Soares, R. M. A., Souto-Padrón, T., et al. (2003). Antileishmanial activity of a linalool-rich essential oil from Croton cajucara. *Antimicrobial Agents and Chemotherapy*, *47*(6), 1895−1901.

Sairafianpour, M., Christensen, J., Steerk, D., Budnik, B. A., Kharazmi, A., Bagherzadeh, K., & Jaroszewski, J. W. (2001). Leishmanicidal, antiplasmodial, and cytotoxic activity of novel diterpenoid 1,2-quinones from Perovskia abrotanoides: new source of tanshinones. *Journal of Natural Products, 64*(11), 1398−1403.

Salem, M., & Werbovetz, K. (2006a). Natural products from plants as drug candidates and lead compounds against leishmaniasis and trypanosomiasis. *Current Medicinal Chemistry, 13*(21), 2571−2598.

Salem, M., & Werbovetz, K. (2006b). Natural products from plants as drug candidates and lead compounds against leishmaniasis and trypanosomiasis. *Current Medicinal Chemistry, 13*(21), 2571−2598, Bentham Science Publishers Ltd.

Samant, M., Sahu, U., Pandey, S. C., & Khare, P. (2021). Role of Cytokines in Experimental and Human Visceral Leishmaniasis. *Front Cell Infect Microbiol, 11*, 624009. Available from https://doi.org/10.3389/fcimb.2021.624009.

Santos, A. L., Yamamoto, E. S., Passero, L. F. D., Laurenti, M. D., Martins, L. F., Lima, M. L., et al. (2017). Antileishmanial activity and immunomodulatory effects of tricin isolated from leaves of Casearia arborea (Salicaceae). *Chemistry & Biodiversity, 14*(5), e1600458.

Sarkar, M., & Sarkar, B. (2013). An economic manufacturing quantity model with probabilistic deterioration in a production system. *Economic Modelling, 31*(1), 245−252, North-Holland.

Sharma, U., Velpandian, T., Sharma, P., & Singh, S. (2009). Evaluation of anti-leishmanial activity of selected Indian plants known to have antimicrobial properties. *Parasitology Research, 105*(5), 1287−1293.

Sen, R., Ganguly, S., Saha, P., & Chatterjee, M. (2010). Efficacy of artemisinin in experimental visceral leishmaniasis. *Journal of Antimicrobial Agents, 36*(1), 43−49.

Sifaoui, I., López-Arencibia, A., Martín-Navarro, C. M., Ticona, J. C., Reyes-Batlle, M., Mejri, M., et al. (2014). In vitro effects of triterpenic acids from olive leaf extracts on the mitochondrial membrane potential of promastigote stage of Leishmania spp. *Phytomedicine, 21*(12), 1689−1694.

Singh, K., Garg, G., & Ali, V. (2016). Current therapeutics, their problems and thiol metabolism as potential drug targets in leishmaniasis. *Current Drug Metabolism, 17*(9), 897−919.

Tiuman, T. S., Ueda-Nakamura, T., Garcia Cortez, D. A., Dias Filho, B. P., Morgado-Díaz, J. A., De Souza, W., & Vataru Nakamura, C. (2005). Antileishmanial activity of partheno-lide, a sesquiterpene lactone isolated from Tanacetum parthenium. *Antimicrobial Agents and Chemotherapy, 49*(1), 176−182.

Torres-Santos, E. C., Lopes, D., Rodrigues Oliveira, R., Carauta, J. P. P., Bandeira Falcao, C. A., Kaplan, M. A. C., & Rossi-Bergmann, B. (2004). Antileishmanial activity of isolated triterpenoids from Pourouma guianensis. *Phytomedicine, 11*(2-3), 114−120.

Vayalil, P. K. (2002). Antioxidant and antimutagenic properties of aqueous extract of date fruit (Phoenix dactylifera L. Arecaceae). *Journal of Agricultural and Food Chemistry, 50*(3), 610−617.

Vila-Nova, N. S., de Morais, S. M., Falcão, M. J. C., Machado, L. K. A., Beviláqua, C. M. L., Costa, I. R. S., et al. (2011). Atividade leishmanicida e citotoxicidade de constituintes quí-micos de duas especies de annonaceae cultivadas no Nordeste do Brasil. *Revista da Sociedade Brasileira de Medicina Tropical, 44*(5), 567−571.

Waechter, A. I., Ferreira, M. E., Fournet, A., Rojas De Arias, A., Nakayama, H., Torres, S., et al. (1997). Experimental treatment of cutaneous leishmaniasis with Argentilactone iso-lated from Annona haernatantha. *Planta Medica, 63*(5), 433−435.

Wiwanitkit, V. (2012). Interest in paromomycin for the treatment of visceral leishmaniasis (Kala-azar). *Therapeutics and Clinical Risk Management*, Dove Press.

Yasur-Landau, D., Jaffe, C. L., David, L., & Baneth, G. (2016). Allopurinol resistance in Leishmania infantum from dogs with disease relapse. *PLoS Neglected Tropical Diseases, 10*(1), e0004341.

Zeiman, E., Greenblatt, C. L., Elgavish, S., Khozin-Goldberg, I., & Golenser, J. (2008). Mode of action of fenarimol against Leishmania spp. *Journal of Parasitology, 94*(1), 280−286.

Zhai, L., Blom, J., Chen, M., Christensen, S. B., & Kharazmi, A. (1995). The antileishmanial agent licochalcone A interferes with the function of parasite mitochondria. *Antimicrobial Agents and Chemotherapy, 39*(12), 2742−2748.

Chapter 9

Evaluation of biomarkers to monitor therapeutic intervention against visceral leishmaniasis

Ankita H. Tripathi[1], Priyanka H. Tripathi[1,2] and Anupam Pandey[1,2]

[1]*Department of Biotechnology, Kumaun University, Sir J C Bose Technical Campus, Bhimtal, India,* [2]*ICAR-Directorate of Coldwater Fisheries Research, Nainital, India*

9.1 Introduction

The emergence of any life-threatening infectious disease, affects complex economic, social, political, ecological, and environmental factors (Smolinski, Hamburg, & Lederberg, 2003). Efforts are made to fight against these infectious diseases (pandemic influenza or severe acute respiratory syndrome) by providing funds, well-established research authorities, etc. But sometimes few infectious diseases remain accentuated and neglected (Guerin et al., 2002; Murray, 2002) and Leishmaniasis is one of the infectious diseases that remains neglected despite affecting, about 350 million people worldwide (Srivastava, Dayama, Mehrotra, & Sundar, 2011). Every year about 1.5 million new cases of leishmaniasis occur worldwide with about 20,000−40,000 deaths (Osman et al., 2017). Leishmaniasis is a tropical disease, endemic in countries like Africa, America, Asia, and Mediterranean regions (Reithinger et al., 2007). Poverty is considered as the major reason for the widespread of leishmaniasis. Worsened environment, low income, malnutrition, poor housing, gender inequality, no access to healthcare, displacement, and war are the main factors responsible for the transmission and spread of leishmaniasis (Alvar, Yactayo, & Bern, 2006).

Leishmaniasis characterizes a group of diverse diseases caused by protozoans of *Leishmania* genus. The disease is transmitted to humans through the bite of female sand flies *Phlebotomus* spp. (Osman et al., 2017). Once released into the blood stream, the flagellated parasite called promastigote enters into phagocytic cells where it multiplies and converts into the

Pathogenesis, Treatment and Prevention of Leishmaniasis. DOI: https://doi.org/10.1016/B978-0-12-822800-5.00010-X
161

nonflagellated amastigote form and, thereby avoiding and escaping from the actions of complement immune components. The amastigotes come out by rupturing the phagocytic cell and entering a new macrophage (Alvar & Arana, 2017) (Fig. 9.1). Leishmaniasis has three clinical manifestations which includes cutaneous leishmaniasis (CL), mucocutaneous leishmaniasis (ML), and visceral leishmaniasis (VL). In humans, leishmaniasis have two clinical forms: CL and VL.

9.1.1   Cutaneous leishmaniasis

CL is responsible for causing skin ulcers. The infection generally starts at the site of bite by sandfly, forming a papule which increases and forms crusts, eventually converting into ulcerates. The incubation period persists from 2 to few months. The clinical manifestations in case of CL include development of one to many skin ulcers, nodular lymphangitis, and satellite lesions (de Vries, Reedijk, & Schallig, 2015).

9.1.2   Mucocutaneous leishmaniasis

ML occurs posthealing of ulcers caused by CL. It generally involves forma-tion of ulcers around the oral cavity, nose, and pharynx causing pain and uneasiness and trouble eating. It may also lead to the occurrence of second-ary infection. The incubation period usually lasts from 1 month to 2−3 months (Piscopo, Mallia, & Azzopardi, 2007).

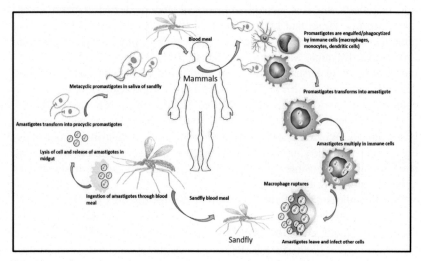

FIGURE 9.1   Life cycle of leishmaniasis.

9.1.3 Visceral leishmaniasis

VL is also known as kala-azar. It is a fatal disease (if untreated) affecting vital body organs including, bone marrow, spleen, and liver (de Vries et al., 2015). VL is a tropical and subtropical disease caused by *Leishmania donovani*, a protozoan (Al-Salem, Herricks, & Hotez, 2016). Depending upon the susceptibility of species, VL are of two types: anthroponotic visceral leishmaniasis (AVL) and zoonotic visceral leishmaniasis (ZVL). AVL spreads to humans through a bite of a sandfly and caused by *L. donovani* (Postigo, 2010). ZVL is transmitted to humans and dogs and caused by *L. donovani*, *Leishmania infantum*, and *Leishmania archibaldi* (Jain & Jain, 2015).

The incubation period lasts from 3to 8 months. The clinical manifestation includes loss of appetite, weight loss, fever, night sweat, hypergammaglobulinemia, enlargement of spleen and liver, pancytopenia, lymphadenopathy, skin pigmentation (dark coloration). VL involves both asymptomatic and subclinical cases, severity extending from chronic, acute, and subacute course.

9.2 Immune response against *Leishmania*

The basic foundation in designing and developing a vaccine depends upon understanding the biological immune response against the infection. The primary response against *Leishmania* is mediated by both immunity (innate and adaptive) responses. Innate immunity involves dendritic cells, macrophages, and neutrophils while adaptive immunity involves both B lymphocytes and T lymphocytes. Leishmanial parasites usually reside inside macrophages (Fig. 9.1) (Duthie, Raman, Piazza, & Reed, 2012). A seditious activity of these parasites is that they have the ability to inhibit cytokine [interleukin 12 (IL-12)] production of macrophages, which is very necessary for inhibiting the parasite. IL-12 activates production of interferons (IFNs), nitric oxide synthase and nitric oxide, further recruit macrophages, neutrophils, and mast cells (proinflammatory cytokines) at the site of infection. Dendritic cells also uptake the parasite, stimulate the production of IL-12, and activate major histocompatibility complex (MHC) I and MHC II pathways, thereby activating the adaptive immune cells and the B cells and T cells (CD4 + and CD8 +) providing resistance against *Leishmania* (Duthie et al., 2012).

In CL, the immune cells activated in response to the infection are T lymphocytes. Induced T cells activates Th1 (type 1 helper cell) (Müller & Kropf, 2012) subpopulations, which on activation release lymphokines, gamma interferon (IFN-γ), and IL-2. These cells activate macrophages, oxygen-dependent processes, and pathways involved in fusion of suicidal bag lysosomes with parasitophorus vacuole of parasite. In counteract, the parasite uses inhibitors to inactivate lysosomal enzymes, free radicals, and reactive nitrogen species (Kaye & Scott, 2011).

In VL, T lymphocytes (CD4 +) get induced by the infection, and activate Th2 (type 2 helper cell) subpopulations which stimulate the release of IL-10, IL-4, and IL-5. The cytokines eventually activate B cells for induction of humoral immunity, for production of antibodies against *Leishmania* (Kaye & Scott, 2011).

9.3 Traditional diagnostic methods for leishmaniasis

VL is a lethal disease, caused by migration of parasite and the infested cells from the primary site of infection, and invade the phagocytic cells present inside the reticulum-endothelial system. *L. donovani* is the causative agent of VL in Africa, Asia, and south Europe while *L. infantum* is responsible for causing the disease in Latin America (Faleiro, Kumar, Hafner, & Engwerda, 2014; Rodrigues, Cordeiro-da-Silva, Laforge, Silvestre, & Estaquier, 2016).

With advancement in research, our knowledge in understanding the physiology, pathology, and immunological processes related to the deadly parasitic infection caused by *Leishmania* has been enhanced. World Health Organization (WHO) has initiated programs for treatment and prevention of leishmaniasis by renewing programs such as OneWorld Health, Special Programme for Research and Training in Tropical Diseases, and the Drugs for Neglected Diseases initiative (DNDi). These programs deal with development of vaccines and drug discovery (Chatelain & Ioset, 2011; Croft & Olliaro, 2011; Ioset & Chang, 2011).

Conventionally, two types of methods (direct and indirect) have been used for the detection of VL (Pandey, Kumar, & Samant, 2020; Pandey, Pande, & Samant, 2020). Direct method involves detection of parasites using microscopic techniques. Indirect method involves detection of antibodies using assays such as direct agglutination test (DAT), enzyme-linked immunosorbent assay (ELISA), and immunochromatography-based assay (Srivastava et al., 2011). Polymerase chain reaction (PCR)-based methods are also used for detection of parasites nucleic acid in asymptomatic affected individuals. The assay is highly sensitive and can detect very low amounts of infectious DNA (Cota, De Sousa, Demarqui, & Rabello, 2012; Kumar, Pandey, & Samant, 2020a, 2020b).

9.3.1 Parasitological diagnosis

The major standard diagnostic method for initial treatment (primary cure) of VL involves analysis of aspirates of bone marrow and lymph nodes and the presence of amastigotes in the spleen through microscopic techniques (Srivastava et al., 2011). The amastigotes present in aspirates of the spleen, lymph nodes, and bone marrow are called *Leishmania donovani* (LD) bodies. In this process, the tissues are stained with Giemsa stain. During analysis, the nucleus appears red, cytoplasm pale blue, and kinetoplast deep red/violet in color. Sensitivity of this assay varies greatly, highest in splenic smear (93.1%−98.7%), less in lymph nodes (52%−58%), and bone marrow (52%−85%), respectively (Ho, Soong, & Li, 1948; Siddig, Ghalib, Shillington, & Petersen, 1988; Zijlstra et al., 1992). However, the major disadvantage of this method is, it requires long periods and experts to handle, tedious, high cost, and well-established research laboratories (Srivastava et al., 2011).

9.3.2 Serological diagnosis

There are several serological methods available for detection of visceral leishmaniasis. These serological methods are specific and nonspecific. Specific test includes immunochromatographic (ICT) strip test, indirect fluorescent antibody test (IFAT), immunoblotting, DAT, ELISA, and antigen detection.

9.3.2.1 ELISA

Detection of VL involves binding of antigen rK39 to the antibody titer. The results have shown 100% sensitivity and 96% specificity of antigen rK39 with the antibodies. This technique helps in envisaging reversion of disease, and also helps in monitoring the treatment (chemotherapy) (Kumar, Pai, Pathak, & Sundar, 2001).

9.3.2.2 Immunochromatographic (ICT) strip test

ICT method has become a very popular test, as the strip is coated by a K39 antigen isolated from *Leishmania chagasi*. The K39 antigen is a 117 base pair gene present in the kinesin region encoding for 39 amino acids. In this assay, one drop of blood is added to the strip and incubated in suitable buffer. The results are obtained within 10−15 minutes (Srivastava et al., 2011).

9.3.2.3 Immunoblotting

Immunoblotting is a highly sensitive technique in comparison to ELISA. It involves binding of all the activated antibodies in response to leishmanial antigens (Srivastava et al., 2011).

9.3.2.4 Indirect fluorescent antibody test assay (IFAT)

The test is based on the detection of antibodies activated initially against leishmaniasis. The test is extremely sensitive (96%) and specific (98%) (Sassi et al., 1999). The only drawback with this technique is that it requires experts to handle the test.

9.3.2.5   Direct agglutination test (DAT)

DAT is a highly sensitive technique, where the stained promastigotes (with Coomassie stain) are incubated with the patient's serum for overnight. The technique has shown 86% specificity and 95% sensitivity. But the technique is tedious, costly, requires greater incubation time, and experts to handle the assays (Chappuis, Rijal, Soto, Menten, & Boelaert, 2006).

9.3.3   Molecular diagnosis

PCR-based methods form the main methodology for detection of VL and coinfection of human immunodeficiency virus (HIV). Studies have shown that PCR-based amplification of genes of different leishmanial species has helped in detection of actual disease-causing species. The species-specific PCR has shown relatively high sensitivity and specificity in comparison to conventional methods (Antinori et al., 2007).

9.4   Diagnostic methods and need for vaccines for leishmaniasis

The conventional clinical indications that are usually evaluated for an individual with VL undergoing treatment involves changes in the size of liver/spleen (usually reduction in size), subsiding of fever, and blood count normalization, which indicates recovery and improvement in bone marrow and the spleen (Boelaert et al., 2007; Chulay & Bryceson, 1983; Kager, Rees, Manguyu, Bhatt, & Bhatt, 1983; Sundar & Rai, 2002; Thakur, 1997). The final cure confirmation of VL, involves long time durations between the primary cure and final cure, because of the risk of recurrence of parasites, thereby extending the follow-up periods (about 6–12 months) to achieve the final cure. While, in the case of serological assays, a few shortcomings are associated with the use of these methods as serology is unable to discriminate between affected and unaffected individuals, asymptomatic individuals having infection, and the test remains positive for many years even after treatment (Savoia, 2015).

For decades, the treatment of VL, has been dependent upon the use of pentavalent antimonials [e.g., sodium stibogluconate (SSG)] (Zijlstra & El-Hassan, 2001), paromomycin (PM), oral miltefosine, and amphotericin B. But there are many issues related with the use of these compounds such as toxicity (cardiotoxicity), administration route, and a duration of about 4 weeks is required for the treatment, development of multidrug resistance, high cost causing an increase in economic burden (Chávez-Fumagalli et al., 2015; Kumar, Pandey, & Samant, 2018), etc. In Eastern Africa, it was found that administration of intramuscular PM for 3 weeks was less effective (Hailu et al., 2010), but when given in combination with SSG for 17 days, the therapy showed active results and is now a first-line treatment against VL. The cons of this therapy are that, the time duration of the treatment is long and requires two times administration of an injection daily (Van Griensven et al., 2010).

Presently, AmBisomeH is the WHO approved antileishmanial drug. It is a nontoxic, liposomal amphotericin B preparation (Bern & Chowdhury, 2006). According to data of trials in India, a single dose (5 mg/kg) of AmBisomeH was effective in curing about 90% of affected patients. While, the percent was high (about 95%) on increasing the doses to 10 mg/kg and also when given along with PM or miltefosine (Sundar et al., 2011). While improved drug treatments are becoming available, exclusion of VL can be accomplished through extensive vaccination. For limiting transmission, long-term protection through vaccination could be one approach (Duthie et al., 2012).

The major problem with vaccine studies and development in the case of VL is the nonavailability/lack of animal models like golden hamster that imitates human disease (Pandey, Kumar, et al., 2020; Pandey, Pande, et al., 2020). Dogs infected naturally by *L. chagasi* or *L. infantum* and golden hamster infected with *L. donovani* serve as the best models in vaccine studies for VL (Melby, Chandrasekar, Zhao, & Coe, 2001) (Tables 9.1–9.3).

9.4.1   First-generation vaccines against leishmaniasis

During ancient times, leishmanization was made into practice to deal with leishmaniasis. In this procedure, live contagious parasites were directly injected into children's skin. After causing mild infection, children use to become immune against the infection. This practice has been done using live *Leishmania major*. But being unsafe, the practice has been abandoned (Badaro et al., 2001).

Trails for developing vaccines using live, killed, whole parasites have been conducted since the 1970s. Many researches have shown that using crude antigens/parasites with suitable adjuvants, provide protection to many animals having leishmaniasis. This formulation has been effective against canine VL in dogs in Iran (Mayrink et al., 2006). Since the strategy involves the use of crude antigen preparation which cannot be optimized or standardized, to initiate proper immune response, resulting medical outcomes have been inconsistent. Therefore there is a need for production of more refined vaccines that are sustainable and can have widespread use (Duthie et al., 2012).

9.4.2   Second-generation vaccines against leishmaniasis

For widespread use and mass campaigns, development of more refined second-generation vaccines is necessary. The strategy used in second-generation

TABLE 9.1 Different diagnostic methods for identification of visceral leishmaniasis.

S. no.	Assay	Specificity	Sensitivity	Time required	Reference(s)
1.	Enzyme-linked immunosorbent assay	96%	100%	Hours	Sassi et al. (1999)
2.	Immunochromatographic strip test	95.3%	93.9%	10–15 minutes	Srivastava et al. (2011)
3.	Direct agglutination test	97.1%	94.8%	Few hours	Chappuis et al. (2006)
4.	Polymerase chain reaction	85%–99%	70%–100%	4–5 hours	Antinori et al. (2007)
5.	Microscopy		(Aspirates) Lymph node 52%–58% Spleen 93.1%–98.7% Bone marrow 52%–85%	Hours	Ho et al. (1948), Siddig et al. (1988), Zijlstra et al. (1992)
6.	Indirect fluorescent antibody test	98%	96%	Hours	Sassi et al. (1999)

TABLE 9.2 List showing drugs and vaccines trial against leishmaniasis.

S. no.	Drugs and vaccines against leishmaniasis	Reference(s)
1.	Sodium stibogluconate (Pentostam)	Gallin, Farber, Holland, and Nutman (1995)
2.	Liposomal amphotericin B (AmBisome)	Kip et al. (2014)
3.	IMPAVIDO (miltefosine)	Sundar et al. (2000)
4.	Aminoglycoside paromomycin (aminosidine)	Jha et al. (1999)
5.	Fluconazole, ketoconazole	Saenz, Paz, and Berman (1990)
6.	Leishmune FML-QuilA vaccine	Borja-Cabrera et al. (2002)
7.	First-generation vaccine—autoclaved *Leishmania major* with BCG (adjuvant): ALM + BCG	Duthie et al. (2012)
8.	(Second-generation vaccine) LEISH-F1 + MPL-SE vaccine	Campos-Neto et al. (2001), Coler, Goto, Bogatzki, Raman, and Reed (2007), Skeiky et al. (2002), Vélez et al. (2009)
9.	ChAd63-KH vaccine (third-generation vaccine in clinical)	Osman et al. (2017)

vaccines involves use of recombinant proteins in conjugation with an adjuvant or elevated expression of recombinant protein in plasmids (Reed, Bertholet, Coler, & Friede, 2009). The major advantage of using recombinant proteins in vaccines is that they are cost-effective, large scale production, can be improved/refined using combinatorial therapy, or mixing with appropriate adjuvant. DNA-based vaccines or recombinant protein have proven effective in trials (Duthie et al., 2012). The search for leishmanial antigens as potential vaccine candidates has been carried out and a number of recombinant proteins have been tested on different animal models.

Leishmaniolysin, a surface glycoprotein (gp63) of *Leishmania* was used as a vaccine candidate and has shown promising results in animal models but was unable to activate and generate T-cell-mediated response in humans (Russo et al., 1991; Burns et al., 1991). In another research, surface antigen of *Leishmania*, PSA-2 polypeptides were used for immunization of an infected mice (Duthie et al., 2012). Until now, very few leishmanial antigens have entered into clinical trials. Recombinant proteins have potential but alone they produce a weak T-cell response. Hence, refinement in the procedure is required, using or developing proper adjuvant that can synergistically

TABLE 9.3 Leishmanial antigens as potential vaccine candidates.

S. no.	Antigen	Leishmanial species	Reference(s)
1.	Centrin knockdown	Leishmania donovani	Fiuza et al. (2015), Selvapandiyan et al. (2009)
2.	Centrin deletion	Leishmania major	Selvapandiyan, Croft, Rijal, Nakhasi, & Ganguly, 2019
3.	ChAd63-KH vaccine KMP-11 antigen HASPB antigen		Osman et al. (2017)
4.	F3 + /GLA-SE vaccine (LEISH-F3 recombinant protein antigen formulated with GLA-SE)	L. major Leishmania braziliensis	Campos-Neto et al. (2001), Coler et al. (2007), Skeiky et al. (2002), Vélez et al. (2009)
5.	Surface-expressed glycoprotein leishmaniolysin (gp63)	Leishmania amazonensis	Russo et al. (1991)
6.	Surface antigen (PSA)-2 polypeptides	L. major	Handman, Symons, Baldwin, Curtis, and Scheerlinck (1995)

or additively enhance the immune response (T-cell activation and response) against *Leishmania*. This could play an important role in controlling the disease (Duthie et al., 2012; Garcon & Van Mechelen, 2011).

The first vaccine against leishmaniasis was a combination of leishmanial recombinant fusion protein (L111f) accompanied by monophosphoryl lipid A (MPL-SE) prepared in an oil-in-water emulsion. MPL is monophosphoryl lipid A isolated from *Salmonella* cell wall. It is an approved TLR4 (Toll-like receptor 4) agonist which is used in vaccines. L111f is a recombinant fusion protein that has the stress inducible protein-1 (LmSTI1) from *L. major*, thiol-specific antioxidant homolog isolated from eukaryotes, and *Leishmania braziliensis* elongation and initiation factor. LEISH-F1 + MPL-SE vaccine was the initial demarcated vaccine against leishmaniasis to go into clinical trials and was also found effective against hamsters, mice, and rhesus monkey (Campos-Neto et al., 2001; Coler et al., 2007; Skeiky et al., 2002; Vélez et al., 2009).

9.4.3 Vaccination of humans

In clinical trials, a vaccine named LEISH-F1 + MPL-SE was examined for CL and VL. For CL, it was found that the vaccine was able to induce IFN response and type IV hypersensitivity which is a delayed type hypersensitivity on administration of LEISH-F1, in many candidates receiving the vaccine (Vélez et al., 2009). In the case of VL, candidates having a history of previous infection by *L. donovani* were chosen for the evaluation. It was found that the vaccine showed induction of different cytokines and T-cell production of IFN. The vaccine showed no toxicity and was safe (Chakravarty et al., 2011).

9.4.4 Third-generation vaccines against leishmaniasis

Until now, both first- and second-generation vaccines against leishmaniasis have been functioning in inducing CD4 + T-cell response, and no vaccines have been developed for inducing the cytotoxic T-cell response (CD8 +) (Duthie et al., 2012; Noazin et al., 2009). Many studies have shown the CD8 + T cells, host protective role. There are many efforts being done for the identification of CD8 + exhaustion or anergy in post-kala-azar dermal leishmaniasis (PKDL) patients (Ganguly et al., 2010; Mukherjee et al., 2016), in understanding the adaptive CD8 + T-cell immunotherapy (Polley et al., 2006), and finding the correlation of CD8 + T cell effector role with vaccine-induced immunity (Osman et al., 2017). In a recent study, a novel vaccine to induce CD8 + T-cell response in patients with PKDL/VL has been designed. The vaccine is adenoviral based having ChAd63, a simian adenovirus synthetically constructed to coexpress KMP-11 and HASPB (two leishmanial antigens) (O'Hara et al., 2012; Sheehy et al., 2011; Sheehy, Duncan, Elias, Biswas, et al., 2012; Sheehy, Duncan, Elias, Choudhary, et al., 2012). The study has reported that the vaccine is safe, and capable of inducing large number of CD8 + T cells and activating immune cells having an important role in innate immunity (dendritic cells, macrophages). This is the first clinical trial of the third-generation vaccine against leishmaniasis (Osman et al., 2017).

9.5 Biomarkers for evaluating the response of treatment against visceral leishmaniasis

Identification of biomarkers for the assessment and evaluation of interventions of leishmanial infections and for early identification of increasing resistance towards antileishmanial drugs is very necessary (Pandey, Kumar, et al., 2020; Pandey, Pande, et al., 2020). The National Institutes of Health of the United States has defined biomarkers as "an attribute that is quantitatively measured and estimated as an indicator of standard physiological pharmacological, pathogenic, biological processes, or a reaction to a therapeutic intercession" (Atkinson et al., 2001). Despite various efforts made to fight against leishmaniasis, development of resistance towards conventional drugs has developed in various areas of the world. The increasing drug resistance has forced the requirement of developing and refining first- and second-line treatments against leishmaniasis. For development of a drug and vaccine, identification of a suitable and appropriate biomarker is necessary. The use of biomarkers for identification of leishmaniasis has many advantages: (1) Biomarkers allow designing smaller, competent clinical studies, decreasing the number of individuals involved as subjects in the experimental treatment thus accelerating the evaluation process and consent of experimental medications (Strimbu & Tavel, 2010). (2) Biomarkers are used for early detection and analysis of disease. (3) They are useful for detection of disease in asymptomatic individuals. (4) And also, in the initial clinical phases of development of treatments, the assessment of biomarkers is observed as an imperative and suitable addition to the evaluation of primary scientific endpoints, and could be used as surrogate endpoints of clinical toxicity or efficiency (Gobburu, 2009). Biomarkers are generally grouped into two categories: direct biomarkers and indirect biomarkers.

9.5.1 Direct biomarkers

Direct biomarkers include parasite detection and antigen detection methods for evaluation of leishmaniasis.

9.5.1.1 Parasite detection

This method involves evaluation of live/viable parasite load inside a patient. Parasite detection is a direct method to estimate the status of leishmanial infection. It helps in monitoring the effects of a treatment by estimating the reduction in biomass of the parasite. The markers identified for molecular identification of leishmaniasis involve, small subunit RNA (SSU—18S rRNA, 7SL RNA), the mini- and maxicircles of kinetoplast DNA (Kip et al., 2014). For the diagnosis of patients with VL, quantitative/real-time PCR has been used. In a study, quantitative PCR was performed using the blood of East African (Khalil et al., 2014) and Indian (Sudarshan, Weirather, Wilson, & Sundar, 2011) VL patients to monitor the effect of different concentration of AmBisome drug on the patients. the assay clearly reflected the response of drug against leishmanial infection. While, in case of CL, microscopy and PCR-based tools are used as the main diagnostic methods. In CL, presence of the parasite load in the upper layer of skin dermis causes inflammation (Dorlo et al., 2011). So, the ulcer can be removed through lesion biopsy and assessed for parasite load. Also, assessment of the RNA in lesions through real-time PCR has been demonstrated as a method for evaluating parasite load in CL ulcers/lesions (Van der Meide et al., 2005). Quantitative PCR has been used to detect spread of infection in CL patients. After treating the patients with miltefosine drug, the treatment response was evaluated and quantified and it was found that there was a decline ($\sim$1 log/week) in of *L. major* parasite burden (Van der Meide et al., 2008).

9.5.1.2 Antigen detection

Generally, antigens specifically associated with a disease are used as a prognostic biomarker, for example, different types of antigens have been classified to identify various cancer types (Sawyers, 2008). In the case of leishmaniasis, a urine-based latex agglutination method known as katex is used as a diagnostic tool. In this method, a heat stable carbohydrate-based antigen having low molecular weight is detected from the urine of VL patients (Attar et al., 2001; Salam, Khan, & Mondal, 2011; Sarkari, Chance, & Hommel, 2002; Hatam, Ghatee, Hossini, & Sarkari, 2009). Though, the assay has very high specificity (98%−100%) the sensitivity is moderate ranging from 48% to 95.2% (Kip et al., 2014).

9.5.2 Indirect markers

9.5.2.1 Macrophage-related markers

Leishmania infect and invade macrophages and direct the production of soluble-infected macrophages which can serve as indirect markers for detection of leishmanial infection.

9.5.2.2 Neopterin

Macrophages induced by IFN-γ (Huber et al., 1984) in response to infection cause production of neopterin (pteridine compound; heterocyclic). The levels of neopterin are found high in several infections such as hepatitis C and B and HIV. Studies have shown an increase in serum neopterin levels in patients having VL in comparison to control groups (Schriefer, Barral, Carvalho, & Barral-Netto, 1995). The levels of neopterin decrease significantly in VL patients undergoing treatment, although serum neopterin levels are high in CL patients (Hamerlinck, Van Gool, Faber, & Kager, 2000).

9.5.2.3 Adenosine deaminase (ADA)

ADA is a major enzyme involved in adenosine breakdown. The purine nucleoside is responsible for suppressing the inflammatory responses against infections. Lymphocytes and macrophages releases ADA. In the case study of VL, the levels of serum ADA increased but the levels were back to normal after the treatment in Indian and Nepalese patients. The levels of serum ADA are found relatively higher in VL patients in comparison to patients having diseases like malaria, tuberculosis, and leprosy (Tripathi et al., 2008).

9.5.2.4   Cytokines

The utmost considered cytokines are the proinflammatory interferon (IFN-γ), the regulatory interleukin (IL-10), and tumor necrosis factor alpha (TNF-α) (Samant, Sahu, Pandey, & Khare, 2021).

9.5.2.5   Interleukin 10 (IL-10)

Many studies have shown that the level of IL-10 is significantly higher in patients with VL. They could be detected in the sweat glands and keratinocytes of VL patients (Gasim et al., 1998). Also, on evaluation it was found that the levels decreased with the course of treatment, suggesting that IL-10 could serve as a potential biomarker for detection of VL.

9.5.2.6   Tumor necrosis factor family—TNF alpha (TNF-α)

Activated macrophages produced TNF-α in response to infections. The levels (TNF-α) are upregulated and are significantly high in patients with VL (Khalil et al., 2014), also the expression of TNF-α was found upregulated in biopsies of lesions in CL patients and were positively correlated with the size of the lesions (Louzir et al., 1998). The levels of TNF-α decreased during end of the treatment.

9.5.2.7   Interferon-gamma (IFN-γ)

IFN-γ is a vital cytokine of both adaptive and innate immunity, involved in initiation of macrophages in response to infections. Various studies have shown the elevated levels of IFN-γ in VL patients from different countries like Brazil, India, Bangladesh, Ethiopia, Iran, and Sicily. During the completion of treatment, the levels of IFN-γ returned back to normal (Kip et al., 2014). According to a study, the levels of IL-10, IFN-γ, and TNF-α mRNA were upregulated in PKDL patients, while the levels returned back to normal levels after successful completion of the treatment, indicating their ability to be used as a diagnostic tool (Ansari, Saluja, & Salotra, 2006; Katara, Ansari, Verma, Ramesh, & Salotra, 2011).

9.5.2.8   Cell surface markers and circulating cytokine receptors

Soluble cytokine receptor of IL-2 and IL-4 (sIL2R and sIL4R) are also found elevated in patients with VL. The levels of sIL2R are found high in active VL patients in comparison to patients with other systemic infections (Kip et al., 2014). Studies have shown that mRNA and sIL2R serum levels are significantly higher in PKDL patients while there is significant decline in the levels after completion of treatment response (Gasim et al., 1998).

Similarly, on evaluation of different soluble cell surface molecules, it was found that the levels of circulating soluble molecules CD8 (sCD8) and CD4 (sCD4) were high in leishmaniasis patients, but with ongoing treatment the levels reduced significantly, making these circulating molecules potential pharmacodynamic markers (Kip et al., 2014).

9.5.2.9   Acute phase proteins (ACPs) in leishmaniasis

ACPs such as, C-reactive protein (CRP), alpha-1-acid glycoprotein (AGP), serum amyloid A (SAA) protein are used as therapeutic markers of infection and inflammation. They are found in high levels during infections. During diagnosis the levels of AGP, CRP, and SAA have been found elevated in VL patients, while the level reached to their normal point during or at the end of the treatment. CRP is usually evaluated for VL patients (Wasunna et al., 1995).

9.5.2.10   Antibody detection

Previous studies carried on VL infection have shown differences in the immunoglobin G (IgG) subclasses (Mukhopadhyay et al., 2012; Saha et al., 2005). Elevated levels of IgG3 and IgG1 have been found in patients with VL in comparison to control groups (noninfected) (Bhattacharyya et al., 2014; Gidwani, Rai, Chakravarty, Boelaert, & Sundar, 2009). In an immuno-proteomic study performed in amastigotes and promastigotes of *L. infantum*, a set of proteins from the parasite were identified using antibodies from the serum of dogs (CVL) produced against VL (Coelho et al., 2012). Among these proteins, few known and unknown proteins were identified namely HRF (IgE-dependent histamine-releasing factor) and hypothetical proteins (LiHyV, LiHyT, LiHyp6, LiHyD). The recombinant counterparts of these identified proteins were investigated for protein- response and parasite- specific response in VL active patients by evaluating the levels of IL-10, IFN-γ, total IgG and IgG2 and IgG1 subclasses before and after treatment (Portela et al., 2018). The results were promising and due to the presence of conserved B- and T-cell epitopes and similar amino acid sequences in proteins of different *Leishmania* species, the study suggested that these proteins could likely be evaluated as prognostic biomarkers for identification of human VL.

9.6   Conclusion

Precise analysis of leishmaniasis still remains a major obstacle for clinicians, researchers, and coordinators of different programs including Special Program for Research and Training in Tropical Diseases, OneWorld Health, and the DNDi initiated by WHO for treatment and prevention of leishmaniasis. Vaccination, identification of drugs and various biological markers for initial identification, diagnosis, and treatment of leishmaniasis hold a great potential in regulating leishmanial infections. Different biomarkers have been regularly assessed as an indicator of normal physiological and biological processes, also they can be assayed for identification of infective progressions, or pharmacological responses towards any therapeutic interventions. DNA/RNA-based direct biomarkers have been considered as the most potential targets for early diagnosis of leishmanial infections. Apart from biomarkers, prophylactic vaccines hold the ultimate goal for fighting against leishmaniasis. To fight against established infection, therapeutic vaccines/drugs should inhibit and target the possible ways of parasite survival. Vaccines can provide long-term protection against the endemic leishmaniasis. Vaccination altogether with chemotherapy and immunotherapy can work against different manifestations of *Leishmania* infection. Overall, future research must emphasis on refining and modification of conventional treatments, assessment of pharmacodynamic markers for monitoring and comparing response of treatments against leishmaniasis with a prominence on assessing the correlation between identified biomarkers and clinical parameters.

References

Al-Salem, W., Herricks, J. R., & Hotez, P. J. (2016). A review of visceral leishmaniasis during the conflict in South Sudan and the consequences for East African countries. *Parasites & Vectors*, 9(1), 460.

Alvar, J., & Arana, B. (2017). I. Appraisal of Leishmaniasis Chemotherapy, Current Status and Pipeline Strategies. Chapter 1 Leishmaniasis, Impact and Therapeutic Needs, pp. 1−23.

Alvar, J., Yactayo, S., & Bern, C. (2006). Leishmaniasis and poverty. *Trends in Parasitology*, 22 (12), 552−557.

Ansari, N. A., Saluja, S., & Salotra, P. (2006). Elevated levels of interferon-γ, interleukin-10, and interleukin-6 during active disease in Indian kala azar. *Clinical Immunology*, 119(3), 339−345.

Antinori, S., Calattini, S., Longhi, E., Bestetti, G., Piolini, R., Magni, C., ... Corvasce, S. (2007). Clinical use of polymerase chain reaction performed on peripheral blood and bone marrow samples for the diagnosis and monitoring of visceral leishmaniasis in HIV-infected and HIV-uninfected patients: a single-center, 8-year experience in Italy and review of the literature. *Clinical Infectious Diseases*, 44(12), 1602−1610.

Atkinson, A. J., Jr, Colburn, W. A., DeGruttola, V. G., DeMets, D. L., Downing, G. J., ... Spilker, B. A. (2001). Biomarkers and surrogate endpoints: preferred definitions and conceptual framework. *Clinical Pharmacology & Therapeutics*, 69(3), 89−95.

Attar, Z. J., Chance, M. L., el-Safi, S., Carney, J., Azazy, A., El-Hadi, M., ... Hommel, M. (2001). Latex agglutination test for the detection of urinary antigens in visceral leishmaniasis. *Acta Tropica*, 78(1), 11−16.

Badaro, R., Lobo, I., Nakatani, M., Muiños, A., M Netto, E., Coler, R. N., & Reed, S. G. (2001). Successful use of a defined antigen/GM-CSF adjuvant vaccine to treat mucosal leishmaniasis refractory to antimony: a case report. *Brazilian Journal of Infectious Diseases*, 5(4), 223−232.

Bern, C., & Chowdhury, R. (2006). The epidemiology of visceral leishmaniasis in Bangladesh: prospects for improved control. *Indian Journal of Medical Research*, 123(3), 275.

Bhattacharyya, T., Ayandeh, A., Falconar, A. K., Sundar, S., El-Safi, S., Gripenberg, M. A., . . . Ahmed, O. (2014). IgG1 as a potential biomarker of post-chemotherapeutic relapse in visceral leishmaniasis, and adaptation to a rapid diagnostic test. *PLoS Neglected Tropical Diseases*, *8*(10), e3273.

Boelaert, M., Bhattacharya, S., Chappuis, F., El Safi, S. H., Hailu, A., Mondal, D., . . . Peeling, R. W. (2007). Evaluation of rapid diagnostic tests: visceral leishmaniasis. *Nature Reviews Microbiology*, *5*(11), S31–S39.

Borja-Cabrera, G. P., Pontes, N. C., Da Silva, V. O., De Souza, E. P., Santos, W. R., Gomes, E. M., . . . De Sousa, C. P. (2002). Long lasting protection against canine kala-azar using the FML-QuilA saponin vaccine in an endemic area of Brazil (Sao Goncalo do Amarante, RN). *Vaccine*, *20*(27-28), 3277–3284.

Burns, J. M., Scott, J. M., Carvalho, E. M., Russo, D. M., March, C. J., Van Ness, K. P., & Reed, S. G. (1991). Characterization of a membrane antigen of Leishmania amazonensis that stimulates human immune responses. *The Journal of Immunology*, *146*(2), 742–748.

Campos-Neto, A., Porrozzi, R., Greeson, K., Coler, R. N., Webb, J. R., Seiky, Y. A., . . . Grimaldi, G. (2001). Protection against cutaneous leishmaniasis induced by recombinant antigens in murine and nonhuman primate models of the human disease. *Infection and Immunity*, *69*(6), 4103–4108.

Chakravarty, J., Kumar, S., Trivedi, S., Rai, V. K., Singh, A., Ashman, J. A., . . . Cowgill, K. D. (2011). A clinical trial to evaluate the safety and immunogenicity of the LEISH-F1 + MPL-SE vaccine for use in the prevention of visceral leishmaniasis. *Vaccine*, *29*(19), 3531–3537.

Chappuis, F., Rijal, S., Soto, A., Menten, J., & Boelaert, M. (2006). A meta-analysis of the diagnostic performance of the direct agglutination test and rK39 dipstick for visceral leishmaniasis. *British Medical Journal*, *333*(7571), 723.

Chatelain, E., & Ioset, J. R. (2011). Drug discovery and development for neglected diseases: the DNDi model. *Drug Design, Development and Therapy*, *5*, 175.

Chávez-Fumagalli, M. A., Ribeiro, T. G., Castilho, R. O., Fernandes, S. O. A., Cardoso, V. N., Coelho, C. S. P., . . . Coelho, E. A. F. (2015). New delivery systems for amphotericin B applied to the improvement of leishmaniasis treatment. *Revista da Sociedade Brasileira de Medicina Tropical*, *48*(3), 235–242.

Chulay, J. D., & Bryceson, A. D. (1983). Quantitation of amastigotes of Leishmania donovani in smears of splenic aspirates from patients with visceral leishmaniasis. *The American Journal of Tropical Medicine and Hygiene*, *32*(3), 475–479.

Coelho, V. T., Oliveira, J. S., Valadares, D. G., Chavez-Fumagalli, M. A., Duarte, M. C., Lage, P. S., . . . Coelho, E. A. (2012). Identification of proteins in promastigote and amastigote-like Leishmania using an immunoproteomic approach. *PLoS Neglected Tropical Diseases*, *6* (1), e1430.

Coler, R. N., Goto, Y., Bogatzki, L., Raman, V., & Reed, S. G. (2007). Leish-111f, a recombinant polyprotein vaccine that protects against visceral Leishmaniasis by elicitation of CD4 + T cells. *Infection and Immunity*, *75*(9), 4648–4654.

Cota, G. F., De Sousa, M. R., Demarqui, F. N., & Rabello, A. (2012). The diagnostic accuracy of serologic and molecular methods for detecting visceral leishmaniasis in HIV infected patients: meta-analysis. *PLoS Neglected Tropical Diseases*, *6*(5), e1665.

Croft, S. L., & Olliaro, P. (2011). Leishmaniasis chemotherapy—challenges and opportunities. *Clinical Microbiology and Infection*, *17*(10), 1478–1483.

de Vries, H. J., Reedijk, S. H., & Schallig, H. D. (2015). Cutaneous leishmaniasis: recent developments in diagnosis and management. *American Journal of Clinical Dermatology*, *16*(2), 99–109.

Dorlo, T. P., van Thiel, P. P., Schoone, G. J., Stienstra, Y., van Vugt, M., Beijnen, J. H., & de Vries, P. J. (2011). Dynamics of parasite clearance in cutaneous leishmaniasis patients treated with miltefosine. *PLoS Neglected Tropical Diseases, 5*(12), e1436.

Duthie, M. S., Raman, V. S., Piazza, F. M., & Reed, S. G. (2012). The development and clinical evaluation of second-generation leishmaniasis vaccines. *Vaccine, 30*(2), 134−141.

Faleiro, R. J., Kumar, R., Hafner, L. M., & Engwerda, C. R. (2014). Immune regulation during chronic visceral leishmaniasis. *PLoS Neglected Tropical Diseases, 8*(7), e2914.

Fiuza, J. A., Gannavaram, S., da Costa Santiago, H., Selvapandiyan, A., Souza, D. M., Passos, L. S. A., . . . Giunchetti, R. C. (2015). Vaccination using live attenuated Leishmania donovani centrin deleted parasites induces protection in dogs against Leishmania infantum. *Vaccine, 33*(2), 280−288.

Gallin, J. I., Farber, J. M., Holland, S. M., & Nutman, T. B. (1995). Interferon-γ in the management of infectious diseases. *Annals of Internal Medicine, 123*(3), 216−224.

Ganguly, S., Mukhopadhyay, D., Das, N. K., Chaduvula, M., Sadhu, S., Chatterjee, U., . . . Mallik, S. (2010). Enhanced lesional Foxp3 expression and peripheral anergic lymphocytes indicate a role for regulatory T cells in Indian post-kala-azar dermal leishmaniasis. *Journal of Investigative Dermatology, 130*(4), 1013−1022.

Garcon, N., & Van Mechelen, M. (2011). Recent clinical experience with vaccines using MPL- and QS-21-containing adjuvant systems. *Expert Review of Vaccines, 10*(4), 471−486.

Gasim, S., Elhassan, A. M., Khalil, E. A. G., Ismail, A., Kadaru, A. M. Y., Kharazmi, A., & Theander, T. G. (1998). High levels of plasma IL-10 and expression of IL-10 by keratinocytes during visceral leishmaniasis predict subsequent development of post-kala-azar dermal leishmaniasis. *Clinical and Experimental Immunology, 111*(1), 64.

Gidwani, K., Rai, M., Chakravarty, J., Boelaert, M., & Sundar, S. (2009). Evaluation of leishmanin skin test in Indian visceral leishmaniasis. *The American Journal of Tropical Medicine and Hygiene, 80*(4), 566−567.

Gobburu, J. V. S. (2009). Biomarkers in clinical drug development. *Clinical Pharmacology & Therapeutics, 86*(1), 26−27.

Guerin, P. J., Olliaro, P., Sundar, S., Boelaert, M., Croft, S. L., Desjeux, P., . . . Bryceson, A. D. (2002). Visceral leishmaniasis: current status of control, diagnosis, and treatment, and a proposed research and development agenda. *The Lancet Infectious Diseases, 2*(8), 494−501.

Hailu, A., Musa, A., Wasunna, M., Balasegaram, M., Yifru, S., Mengistu, G., . . . Makonnen, E. (2010). Geographical variation in the response of visceral leishmaniasis to paromomycin in East Africa: a multicentre, open-label, randomized trial. *PLoS Neglected Tropical Diseases, 4*(10), e709.

Hamerlinck, F. F. V., Van Gool, T., Faber, W. R., & Kager, P. A. (2000). Serum neopterin concentrations during treatment of leishmaniasis: useful as test of cure? *FEMS Immunology & Medical Microbiology, 27*(1), 31−34.

Handman, E., Symons, F. M., Baldwin, T. M., Curtis, J. M., & Scheerlinck, J. P. (1995). Protective vaccination with promastigote surface antigen 2 from Leishmania major is mediated by a TH1 type of immune response. *Infection and Immunity, 63*(11), 4261−4267.

Hatam, G. R., Ghatee, M. A., Hossini, S. M. H., & Sarkari, B. (2009). Improvement of the newly developed latex agglutination test (Katex) for diagnosis of visceral leishmaniasis. *Journal of Clinical Laboratory Analysis, 23*(4), 202−205.

Ho, E. A., Soong, T. H., & Li, Y. (1948). Comparative merits of sternum, spleen and liver punctures in the study of human visceral leishmaniasis. *Transactions of the Royal Society of Tropical Medicine and Hygiene, 41*(5), 629−636.

Huber, C., Batchelor, J. R., Fuchs, D., Hausen, A., Lang, A., Niederwieser, D., ... Wachter, H. (1984). Immune response-associated production of neopterin. Release from macrophages primarily under control of interferon-gamma. *The Journal of Experimental Medicine, 160* (1), 310−316.

Ioset, J. R., & Chang, S. (2011). Drugs for Neglected Diseases initiative model of drug development for neglected diseases: current status and future challenges. *Future Medicinal Chemistry, 3*(11), 1361−1371.

Jain, K., & Jain, N. K. (2015). Vaccines for visceral leishmaniasis: a review. *Journal of Immunological Methods, 422,* 1−12.

Jha, T. K., Sundar, S., Thakur, C. P., Bachmann, P., Karbwang, J., Fischer, C., ... Berman, J. (1999). Miltefosine, an oral agent, for the treatment of Indian visceral leishmaniasis. *New England Journal of Medicine, 341*(24), 1795−1800.

Kager, P. A., Rees, P. H., Manguyu, F. M., Bhatt, K. M., & Bhatt, S. M. (1983). Splenic aspiration; experience in Kenya. *Tropical and Geographical Medicine, 35*(2), 125−131.

Katara, G. K., Ansari, N. A., Verma, S., Ramesh, V., & Salotra, P. (2011). Foxp3 and IL-10 expression correlates with parasite burden in lesional tissues of post kala azar dermal leishmaniasis (PKDL) patients. *PLoS Neglected Tropical Diseases, 5*(5), e1171.

Kaye, P., & Scott, P. (2011). Leishmaniasis: complexity at the host−pathogen interface. *Nature Reviews Microbiology, 9*(8), 604−615.

Khalil, E. A., Weldegebreal, T., Younis, B. M., Omollo, R., Musa, A. M., Hailu, W., ... Haleke, W. (2014). Safety and efficacy of single dose versus multiple doses of AmBisome® for treatment of visceral leishmaniasis in eastern Africa: a randomised trial. *PLoS Neglected Tropical Diseases, 8*(1), e2613.

Kip, A. E., Balasegaram, M., Beijnen, J. H., Schellens, J. H., de Vries, P. J., & Dorlo, T. P. (2014). Biomarkers to monitor therapeutic response in leishmaniasis: a systematic review. *Antimicrobial Agents and Chemotherapy, 59,* 1−14.

Kumar, A., Pandey, S. C., & Samant, M. (2018). Slow pace of antileishmanial drug development. *Parasitology Open, 4*(4), 1−11.

Kumar, R., Pai, K., Pathak, K., & Sundar, S. (2001). Enzyme-linked immunosorbent assay for recombinant K39 antigen in diagnosis and prognosis of Indian visceral leishmaniasis. *Clinical and Diagnostic Laboratory Immunology, 8*(6), 1220−1224.

Kumar, A., Pandey, S. C., & Samant, M. (2020). A spotlight on the diagnostic methods of a fatal disease visceral leishmaniasis. *Parasite Immunology, 42*(10), e12727.

Kumar, A., Pandey, S. C., & Samant, M. (2020). DNA-based microarray studies in visceral leishmaniasis: identification of biomarkers for diagnostic, prognostic and drug target for treatment. *Acta Tropica, 208,* 105512.

Louzir, H., Melby, P. C., Ben Salah, A., Marrakchi, H., Aoun, K., Ben Ismail, R., & Dellagi, K. (1998). Immunologic determinants of disease evolution in localized cutaneous leishmaniasis due to Leishmania major. *Journal of Infectious Diseases, 177*(6), 1687−1695.

Mayrink, W., Botelho, A. C. D. C., Magalhães, P. A., Batista, S. M., Lima, A. D. O., Genaro, O., ... Dias, M. (2006). Immunotherapy, immunochemotherapy and chemotherapy for American cutaneous leishmaniasis treatment. *Revista da Sociedade Brasileira de Medicina Tropical, 39*(1), 14−21.

Melby, P. C., Chandrasekar, B., Zhao, W., & Coe, J. E. (2001). The hamster as a model of human visceral leishmaniasis: progressive disease and impaired generation of nitric oxide in the face of a prominent Th1-like cytokine response. *The Journal of Immunology, 166*(3), 1912−1920.

Mukherjee, S., Mukhopadhyay, D., Ghosh, S., Barbhuiya, J. N., Das, N. K., & Chatterjee, M. (2016). Decreased frequency and secretion of CD26 promotes disease progression in Indian post kala-azar dermal leishmaniasis. *Journal of Clinical Immunology, 36*(1), 85−94.

Mukhopadhyay, D., Das, N. K., De Sarkar, S., Manna, A., Ganguly, D. N., & Barbhuiya, J. N. (2012). Evaluation of serological markers to monitor the disease status of Indian post kala-azar dermal leishmaniasis. *Transactions of the Royal Society of Tropical Medicine and Hygiene, 106*(11), 668−676.

Müller, I., & Kropf, P. (2012). *Immunity to Parasitic Infection* (pp. 153−164). T. J. LambWiley-Blackwell.

Murray, H. W. (2002). Kala-azar—progress against a neglected disease. *New England Journal Medicine, 347*, 1793−1794.

Noazin, S., Khamesipour, A., Moulton, L. H., Tanner, M., Nasseri, K., Modabber, F., ... Smith, P. G. (2009). Efficacy of killed whole-parasite vaccines in the prevention of leishmaniasis—a meta-analysis. *Vaccine, 27*(35), 4747−4753.

O'Hara, G. A., Duncan, C. J., Ewer, K. J., Collins, K. A., Elias, S. C., Halstead, F. D., ... Rowland, R. (2012). Clinical assessment of a recombinant simian adenovirus ChAd63: a potent new vaccine vector. *Journal of Infectious Diseases, 205*(5), 772−781.

Osman, M., Mistry, A., Keding, A., Gabe, R., Cook, E., Forrester, S., ... Cortese, R. (2017). A third generation vaccine for human visceral leishmaniasis and post kala azar dermal leish-maniasis: first-in-human trial of ChAd63-KH. *PLoS Neglected Tropical Diseases, 11*(5), e0005527.

Pandey, S. C., Kumar, A., & Samant, M. (2020). Genetically modified live attenuated vaccine: a potential strategy to combat visceral leishmaniasis. *Parasite Immunology,* e12732.

Pandey, S. C., Pande, V., & Samant, M. (2020). DDX3 DEAD-box RNA helicase (Hel67) gene disruption impairs infectivity of Leishmania donovani and induces protective immunity against visceral leishmaniasis. *Scientific Reports, 10*(1), 1−10.

Piscopo, T. V., Mallia., & Azzopardi, C. (2007). Leishmaniasis. *Postgraduate Medical Journal, 83*(976), 649−657.

Polley, R., Stager, S., Prickett, S., Maroof, A., Zubairi, S., Smith, D. F., & Kaye, P. M. (2006). Adoptive immunotherapy against experimental visceral leishmaniasis with CD8 + T cells requires the presence of cognate antigen. *Infection and Immunity, 74*(1), 773−776.

Portela, Á. S., Costa, L. E., Salles, B. C., Lima, M. P., Santos, T. T., Ramos, F. F., ... Silva, F. R. (2018). Identification of immune biomarkers related to disease progression and treat-ment efficacy in human visceral leishmaniasis. *Immunobiology, 223*(3), 303−309.

Postigo, J. A. R. (2010). Leishmaniasis in the World Health Organization eastern Mediterranean region. *International Journal of Antimicrobial Agents, 36*, S62−S65.

Reed, S. G., Bertholet, S., Coler, R. N., & Friede, M. (2009). New horizons in adjuvants for vac-cine development. *Trends in Immunology, 30*(1), 23−32.

Reithinger, R., Dujardin, J. C., Louzir, H., Pirmez, C., Alexander, B., & Brooker, S. (2007). Cutaneous leishmaniasis. *The Lancet Infectious Diseases, 7*(9), 581−596.

Rodrigues, V., Cordeiro-da-Silva, A., Laforge, M., Silvestre, R., & Estaquier, J. (2016). Regulation of immunity during visceral Leishmania infection. *Parasites & Vectors, 9*(1), 118.

Russo, D. M., Burns, J. M., Carvalho, E. M., Armitage, R. J., Grabstein, K. H., Button, L. L., ... Reed, S. G. (1991). Human T cell responses to gp63, a surface antigen of Leishmania. *The Journal of Immunology, 147*(10), 3575−3580.

Saenz, R. E., Paz, H., & Berman, J. D. (1990). Efficacy of ketoconazole against Leishmania braziliensis panamensis cutaneous leishmaniasis. *The American Journal of Medicine, 89*(2), 147−155.

Saha, S., Mazumdar, T., Anam, K., Ravindran, R., Bairagi, B., Saha, B., & Banerjee, D. (2005). Leishmania promastigote membrane antigen-based enzyme-linked immunosorbent assay and immunoblotting for differential diagnosis of Indian post-kala-azar dermal leishmaniasis. *Journal of Clinical Microbiology, 43*(3), 1269−1277.

Salam, M. A., Khan, M. G., & Mondal, D. (2011). Urine antigen detection by latex agglutination test for diagnosis and assessment of initial cure of visceral leishmaniasis. *Transactions of the Royal Society of Tropical Medicine and Hygiene, 105*(5), 269−272.

Samant, M., Sahu, U., Pandey, S. C., & Khare, P. (2021). Role of cytokines in experimental and human visceral leishmaniasis. *Front Cell Infect Microbiol, 11*, 624009. Available from https://doi.org/10.3389/fcimb.2021.624009.

Sarkari, B., Chance, M., & Hommel, M. (2002). Antigenuria in visceral leishmaniasis: detection and partial characterisation of a carbohydrate antigen. *Acta Tropica, 82*(3), 339−348.

Sassi, A., Louzir, H., Ben Salah, A., Mokni, M., Ben Osman, A., & Dellagi, K. (1999). Leishmanin skin test lymphoproliferative responses and cytokine production after symptomatic or asymptomatic Leishmania major infection in Tunisia. *Clinical & Experimental Immunology, 116*(1), 127−132.

Savoia, D. (2015). Recent updates and perspectives on leishmaniasis. *The Journal of Infection in Developing Countries, 9*(06), 588−596.

Sawyers, C. L. (2008). The cancer biomarker problem. *Nature, 452*(7187), 548−552.

Schriefer, A., Barral, A., Carvalho, E. M., & Barral-Netto, M. (1995). Serum soluble markers in the evaluation of treatment in human visceral leishmaniasis. *Clinical & Experimental Immunology, 102*(3), 535−540.

Selvapandiyan, A., Croft, S. L., Rijal, S., Nakhasi, H. L., & Ganguly, N. K. (2019). *Innovations for the elimination and control of visceral leishmaniasis, 13*(9), e0007616.

Selvapandiyan, A., Dey, R., Nylen, S., Duncan, R., Sacks, D., & Nakhasi, H. L. (2009). Intracellular replication-deficient Leishmania donovani induces long lasting protective immunity against visceral leishmaniasis. *The Journal of Immunology, 183*(3), 1813−1820.

Sheehy, S. H., Duncan, C. J., Elias, S. C., Biswas, S., Collins, K. A., O'Hara, G. A., . . . Miura, K. (2012). Phase Ia clinical evaluation of the safety and immunogenicity of the Plasmodium falciparum blood-stage antigen AMA1 in ChAd63 and MVA vaccine vectors. *PLoS One, 7*(2), e31208.

Sheehy, S. H., Duncan, C. J., Elias, S. C., Choudhary, P., Biswas, S., Halstead, F. D., . . . Ewer, K. J. (2012). ChAd63-MVA−vectored blood-stage malaria vaccines targeting MSP1 and AMA1: assessment of efficacy against mosquito bite challenge in humans. *Molecular Therapy, 20*(12), 2355−2368.

Sheehy, S. H., Duncan, C. J., Elias, S. C., Collins, K. A., Ewer, K. J., Spencer, A. J., . . . Epp, C. (2011). Phase Ia clinical evaluation of the Plasmodium falciparum blood-stage antigen MSP1 in ChAd63 and MVA vaccine vectors. *Molecular Therapy, 19*(12), 2269−2276.

Siddig, M., Ghalib, H., Shillington, D. C., & Petersen, E. A. (1988). Visceral leishmaniasis in the Sudan: comparative parasitological methods of diagnosis. *Transactions of the Royal Society of Tropical Medicine and Hygiene, 82*(1), 66−68.

Skeiky, Y. A., Coler, R. N., Brannon, M., Stromberg, E., Greeson, K., Crane, R. T., . . . Reed, S. G. (2002). Protective efficacy of a tandemly linked, multi-subunit recombinant leishmanial vaccine (Leish-111f) formulated in MPL® adjuvant. *Vaccine, 20*(27-28), 3292−3303.

Smolinski, M. S., Hamburg, M. A., & Lederberg, J. (2003). *Addressing the threats: conclusions and recommendations. In: M.S. Smolinski, M.A. Hamburg and J. Lederberg, eds. Microbial Threats to Health: Emergence, Detection, and Response* (pp. 149−226). Institute of Medicine.

Srivastava, P., Dayama, A., Mehrotra, S., & Sundar, S. (2011). Diagnosis of visceral leishmaniasis. *Transactions of the Royal Society of Tropical Medicine and Hygiene, 105*(1), 1−6.

Strimbu, K., & Tavel, J. A. (2010). What are biomarkers? *Current Opinion in HIV and AIDS, 5* (6), 463.

Sudarshan, M., Weirather, J. L., Wilson, M. E., & Sundar, S. (2011). Study of parasite kinetics with antileishmanial drugs using real-time quantitative PCR in Indian visceral leishmaniasis. *Journal of Antimicrobial Chemotherapy, 66*(8), 1751−1755.

Sundar, S., & Rai, M. (2002). Laboratory diagnosis of visceral leishmaniasis. *Clinical and Diagnostic Laboratory Immunology, 9*(5), 951−958.

Sundar, S., Makharia, A., More, D. K., Agrawal, G., Voss, A., Fischer, C., ... Murray, H. W. (2000). Short-course of oral miltefosine for treatment of visceral leishmaniasis. *Clinical Infectious Diseases, 31*(4), 1110−1113.

Sundar, S., Sinha, P. K., Rai, M., Verma, D. K., Nawin, K., Alam, S., ... Kumari, P. (2011). Comparison of short-course multidrug treatment with standard therapy for visceral leishmaniasis in India: an open-label, non-inferiority, randomised controlled trial. *The Lancet, 377*(9764), 477−486.

Thakur, C. P. (1997). A comparison of intercostal and abdominal routes of splenic aspiration and bone marrow aspiration in the diagnosis of visceral leishmaniasis. *Transactions of the Royal Society of Tropical Medicine and Hygiene, 91*(6), 668−670.

Tripathi, K., Kumar, R., Bharti, K., Kumar, P., Shrivastav, R., Sundar, S., & Pai, K. (2008). Adenosine deaminase activity in sera of patients with visceral leishmaniasis in India. *Clinica Chimica Acta, 388*(1-2), 135−138.

Van der Meide, W. F., Peekel, I., Van Thiel, P. P. A. M., Schallig, H. D. F. H., De Vries, H. J. C., Zeegelaar, J. E., & Faber, W. R. (2008). Treatment assessment by monitoring parasite load in skin biopsies from patients with cutaneous leishmaniasis, using quantitative nucleic acid sequence-based amplification. *Clinical and Experimental Dermatology, 33*(4), 394−399.

Van der Meide, W. F., Schoone, G. J., Faber, W. R., Zeegelaar, J. E., de Vries, H. J., Özbel, Y., ... Schallig, H. D. (2005). Quantitative nucleic acid sequence-based assay as a new molecular tool for detection and quantification of Leishmania parasites in skin biopsy samples. *Journal of Clinical Microbiology, 43*(11), 5560−5566.

Van Griensven, J., Balasegaram, M., Meheus, F., Alvar, J., Lynen, L., & Boelaert, M. (2010). Combination therapy for visceral leishmaniasis. *The Lancet Infectious Diseases, 10*(3), 184−194.

Vélez, I. D., Gilchrist, K., Martínez, S., Ramírez-Pineda, J. R., Ashman, J. A., Alves, F. P., ... Cowgill, K. D. (2009). Safety and immunogenicity of a defined vaccine for the prevention of cutaneous leishmaniasis. *Vaccine, 28*(2), 329−337.

Wasunna, K. M., Raynes, J. G., Were, J. B. O., Muigai, R., Sherwood, J., Gachihi, G., ... McAdam, K. P. W. J. (1995). Acute phase protein concentrations predict parasite clearance rate during therapy for visceral leishmaniasis. *Transactions of the Royal Society of Tropical Medicine and Hygiene, 89*(6), 678−681.

Zijlstra, E. E., Ali, M. S., El-Hassan, A. M., El-Toum, I. A., Satti, M., Ghalib, H. W., & Kager, P. A. (1992). Kala-azar: a comparative study of parasitological methods and the direct agglutination test in diagnosis. *Transactions of the Royal Society of Tropical Medicine and Hygiene, 86*(5), 505−507.

Zijlstra, E. E., & El-Hassan, A. M. (2001). Leishmaniasis in Sudan. 3. Visceral leishmaniasis. *Transactions of the Royal Society of Tropical Medicine and Hygiene, 95*(Suppl. 1), S27−S58.

Chapter 10

Development of a successful vaccine for leishmaniasis: possibilities and challenges

Keerti[1] and Vivek Kumar[2]
[1]Molecular Biology and Genetics Unit, Jawaharlal Nehru Centre for Advanced Scientific Research, Bengaluru, India, [2]Department of Botany, Government Post Graduate College, Champawat, India

10.1 Introduction

Leishmaniasis, a heterogeneous group of vector-borne diseases established by an obligate intracellular protozoan parasite belongs to the genus *Leishmania* transmitted through the bite of sandflies (Dostálová & Volf, 2012). Nearly, 20 species of *Leishmania* are identified to be pathogenic for humans that produced a varied spectrum of clinical manifestations ranging from self-healing ulcers to severe massive tissue destruction and ultimately lead to death if left untreated (Torres-Guerrero, Quintanilla-Cedillo, Ruiz-Esmenjaud, & Arenas, 2017). It is commonly considered as a disease of poor communities, mostly prevalent in the tropical areas of East Africa and the Americas, Indian subcontinent, Mediterranean countries, and South-West Asian regions (Ready, 2014). Due to upsurge in anthropogenic activities, number of leishmaniasis cases rises, that further enhances the likelihoods of human exposure to the sandfly vector (Gebremichael Tedla, Bariagabr, & Abreha, 2018). Besides, environmental risk factors such as population migration, structuring irrigation systems, and human risk factors such as human immunodeficiency virus infection, malnutrition, and genetic vulnerability also render leishmaniasis a significant problem for public health (Desjeux, 2004; Lindoso, Cunha, Queiroz, & Moreira, 2016). Presently, chemotherapeutics are the only available means of controlling visceral leishmaniasis (VL), though it is associated with several demerits such as invasive route of injection, extended treatment regimens, severe side effects, expensive, unresponsiveness to parasite and variation in response with geographical distribution (Chakravarty & Sundar, 2010; Kumar, Pandey, & Samant, 2018;

Pathogenesis, Treatment and Prevention of Leishmaniasis. DOI: https://doi.org/10.1016/B978-0-12-822800-5.00006-8

Singh, Singh, Chakravarty, & Sundar, 2016). Hence, due to these downsides of available antileishmanials, there is a need to search for other alternative strategies or new chemotherapeutic agents to control VL (Roatt et al., 2014) (Pandey et al., 2019; Pandey, Jha, Kumar, & Samant, 2019). Vaccination protocols possibly represent one of the best effective means of controlling leishmaniasis including different levels of parasite transmission and parasite ecologies (Gillespie et al., 2016; Rezvan & Moafi, 2015).

10.2 Immune response to *Leishmania* infection

Induction of broad-spectrum immune responses against any *Leishmania* parasite infection varies from one species to another. However, invasion of parasite primarily activates innate immune defenses, succeeded by cell-mediated immunity. Both arms of immunity are of utmost importance for an effective control of leishmaniasis. In early hours of parasite entry, neutrophils, dendritic cells, or macrophages are recruited to the primary site of infection. Further they stimulate complementation and production of proinflammatory cytokines such as Interleukin-12 (IL-12), Tumor Necrosis Factor-α (TNF-α), Interferon-γ (IFN-γ) mediating downstream signaling pathways in response to parasite-specific surface molecules sensed through pattern recognition receptors. It leads to generation of reactive oxygen species or nitric oxide antioxidant molecules capable of killing parasite during early stages. Also recruit natural killer cells restrict parasite spreading and induces early IFN-γ levels for activating CD4+ T cells. Subsequently, these cytokines or antiparasitic molecules induce T-cell branch of immunity particularly Type I T helper (Th1) subtype required for resolution of leishmaniasis. Alongside, B-cell-based antiparasitic humoral response appears detrimental during early stage of *Leishmania* infection (Rossi & Fasel, 2018). Besides, stimulation of such robust immune defensive mechanisms, pathogen still capable to sustain and replicates within hostile environment. For achieving so, it employs various strategies to bypass host-mediated clearance process like resistance to complement-mediated lysis, altering toll like receptor (TLR) signaling to subvert proactive inflammatory responses and promoting antiinflammatory pathways, preventing phagosomal fusion to lysosome or modifying acidic environment of endosomes, etc. Moreover, it enables antigen sequestration or interference with antigen loading to major histocompatibility complex (MHC-I/II) molecules and impairment of host signaling cascades to circumvent active T-cell-mediated immunity (Gupta, Oghumu, & Satoskar, 2013). Therefore *Leishmania* parasite manages to evade from host defensive responses leading to pathogenesis. Such settings, prerequisites in-depth studies from mouse to human infection for identifying a potent immune target inducing robust and long-lasting immune responses to subside parasite's intricate evasion machinery with complete eradication (Samant, Sahu, Pandey, & Khare, 2021).

10.3   Current status of *Leishmania* vaccine development

Considering feasibility of vaccine is believable as prior studies proved that any infected individual recovering from leishmaniasis becomes gradually resistant to later clinical infection (Faleiro, Kumar, Hafner, & Engwerda, 2014). Also supported with older practices of inoculating *Leishmania* parasites in individuals hidden region to prevent occurrence of natural cutaneous leishmaniasis (CL) infection in the exposed area especially facial regions. Thus efforts required to put forward for an ideal vaccine candidate capable of conferring long-lasting immunity through activating both arms of immune defenses, that is, cellular responses (T-cell-dependent immunity) and humoral immunity against *Leishmania* infection. So far, various vaccine candidates as recombinant protein-based, DNA-based constructs, inactivated/killed or other forms have been trialed against leishmaniasis for their prophylactic and therapeutic efficacies. Although development of a few polyprotein vaccine candidates such as Leish-F1 (or its variants F2 and F3), ChAD63KH, etc., reach phase I and II trials, not approved beyond clinical trials resulted in a sustained *Leishmania* pandemic state (Coler et al., 2015; Llanos-Cuentas et al., 2010; Osman et al., 2017).

10.4   Strategy of immunization/vaccination against leishmaniasis

Various strategies have been employed for addressing this primary concern in the present scenario, including useful diagnostic kits, drug development programs for better improvement, vector control measures, etc. (Kumar, Pandey, & Samant, 2020a, 2020b). Additionally, there has been extensive research on developing a multispecies *Leishmania* vaccine, which is still underway. Identification of appropriate vaccine candidates for a successful vaccine development program could be possible by improving the understanding of the disease's immunobiology and pathogenesis (Handman, 2001; Kumar & Engwerda, 2014). In the last few decades, different groups made several attempts to develop a productive vaccine as an alternative cost-effective treatment approach. Even so, there is no commercially approved vaccine made available until now. With such considerations, various immunization protocols employed so far towards developing an effective vaccine are enlisted below (Fig. 10.1).

10.4.1   Live attenuated vaccines

One of the primitive ways of immunization in the early 1900s is vaccinating person with a low dose of live virulent parasites at specific sites termed as leishmaniazation, conveying substantial protective immunity (Soto et al., 2015). However, later on, such practices were abandoned due to safety

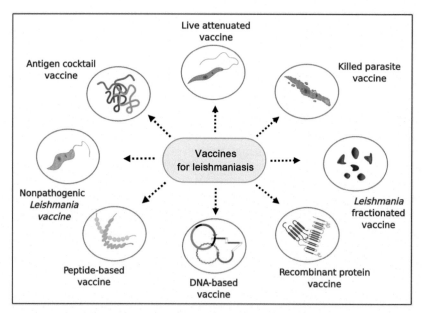

FIGURE 10.1 An illustration of different types of vaccine for leishmaniasis.

issues. Many reports showed that vaccines comprised of live attenuated strains cannot cause any pathology. At the same time, it allows the host system to encounter enough repertoires of antigens to build-up a long-lasting immunity. Usually, a generation of live attenuated strains through irreversible genetic deletion or mutation are safer and do not require adjuvants like that for other vaccine types (Pandey, Kumar, & Samant, 2020). Different methodologies have attempted to manipulate the *Leishmania* parasite and target mostly *Leishmania mexicana* and *Leishmania major* for CL, while *Leishmania infantum* and *Leishmania donovani* for VL. Furthermore, development of live attenuated parasites could be classified based on the attenuation strategy use, that is, undefined and defined genetic modification (Selvapandiyan et al., 2012). Undefined attenuation is generally induced through long-term irradiation or chemical mutagenesis in in vitro culture, with or without any evident selection. For instance, chemically induced mutagenesis in *L. major*, generated a parasite with diminished lipophosphoglycan expression (Svárovská et al., 2010). Similarly, gentamicin antibiotic treatment has been used to attenuate *L. major*, *L. mexicana*, and *L. infantum* parasites (Daneshvar, Coombs, Hagan, & Phillips, 2003). Additionally, a recent study showed that $LdHel67^{-/-}$ null mutant-based live attenuated candidate vaccine exhibited immunogenic response and a higher degree of protection against *L. donovani* in comparison to the infected control group (Pandey, Pande, & Samant, 2020). Similarly immunization with attenuated

L. infantum lacking hsp70-II gene initially confers protection by reducing burden and inducing parasite-specific response but fails to reciprocate the same effect at chronic stage of infection (Solana et al., 2020). Therefore immunization with these parasites provides a potent immunogenicity against virulent *Leishmania* infection, but their regimes need to be optimized.

10.4.2   Killed parasite vaccine

In the late 1930s a few scientists started employing whole-cell killed *Leishmania* parasites for vaccination, passing on adequate protection against CL and VL cases. As a first-generation vaccine candidate, killed *Leishmania* appears more stable with considerable immunogenicity, safety, low-cost production, and no pathologies development. Besides, these could be easily mass-produced even in *Leishmania* affected low-income countries under moderate facilities. Of those, autoclaved *L. major* has given with Bacille Calmette-Guerin (BCG) adjuvant reached phase I clinical trials and found to be effective against both VL and Post-Kala Azar dermal leishmaniasis (PKDL) forms (Khalil, Musa, Modabber, & El-Hassan, 2006). Another approach includes treating parasites with psoralen and amotosalen compounds along with low doses of ultraviolet radiation to generate killed but metabolically active vaccines (Bruhn et al., 2012). Over the last epochs, various killed parasite preparations have been trialed with appropriate adjuvant systems, still there is no commercial *Leishmania* vaccine in market offering considerable efficacy comprehensively. Since, killed parasite-based vaccination was not prophylactically active; it yet warrants further investigation because of cost-effectiveness and minimal risk of reversal effect.

10.4.3   *Leishmania* fractionated vaccines

Another vaccine subtype, comprised of partially or fully purified components of any pathogen responsible for convening strong protection against the disease. In the case of leishmaniasis, Leishmune is one of the first certified *L. donovani* fractionated vaccine composed of fructose mannose ligand (FML) and saponin as adjuvant against Canine visceral leishmaniasis (CVL). FML expressed in almost all stages of *Leishmania* sp., has been isolated from *L. donovani* promastigote and exhibited an efficacy of near about 92%−97% against CVL in the endemic regions of Brazil. There is one more vaccine prototype, named as LiESP/QA-21 vaccine or CaniLeish which is now commercially available as *Leishmania* vaccine in Europe. It consists of secreted proteins of *L. infantum* (LiESP) along with the purified fraction of saponin, that is, QA-21, processed by Institute de Recherche pour le Dévelopement (Moreno et al., 2012). Altogether, these outcomes suggested that *Leishmania* fractionated vaccines could be an active candidate for controlling human leishmaniasis too.

10.4.4 Recombinant protein vaccines (as second-generation vaccine)

Administration of single or multiple defined antigens derived from pathogens together with an adjuvant stimulates immune system against infection. Preparations under this category designated as a second-generation vaccine, synthesized through genetic engineering practices. Several recombinant vaccines have been trialed in animal or human models against different forms of leishmaniasis (Moafi, Rezvan, Sherkat, & Taleban, 2019). Amongst them, antigens could be broadly characterized as two subtypes, that is, membranous proteins, for example, kinetoplastid membrane protein-11 (KMP11), hydrophilic acylated surface protein B1 (HASPB1), nucleoside hydrolase (NH36), etc., and nonmembranous proteins, for example, ribosomal proteins (e.g., P0), metabolic enzymes (e.g., enolase, Triose phosphate isomerase (TPI)), stress-related proteins (e.g., heat shocking protein (HSP)), antioxidant-machinery components (e.g., trypanothione reductase (TPR)), etc. So far, LEISH-F1, a polyprotein construct encoding thiol-specific antioxidant, stress-inducible protein-1 (LmSTI1) of *L. major* and elongation and initiation factor from *Leishmania braziliensis* along with monophosphoryl lipid A plus squalene (MPL-SE) have reached the phase II clinical trials (Llanos-Cuentas et al., 2010). Another multicomponent vaccine variant LEISH-F3 comprises of NH from *L. donovani* and sterol 24-c-methyltransferase from *L. infantum* also displayed promising efficacy against VL (Coler et al., 2015). In the same line, a licensed vaccine composed of *L. infantum* A2 antigen with saponin in Brazil has efficiently prevented the development of active disease state in dogs preexposed to the parasite (Grimaldi et al., 2017). As, of these, few reach clinical trials, but there remains a significant gap towards the development of commercial vaccine for human VL.

10.4.5 DNA vaccine (or third-generation vaccine)

After protein-based vaccines, DNA has been extensively utilized as an antigen delivery tool, contributing as a new arm in the vaccinology field. Immunization with genetically modified mammalian plasmid constructs expressing pathogen-specific antigens eventually induces T-cell-based cellular response considered as DNA vaccine (Kumar & Samant, 2016). However, it was not much accepted earlier like the ones described above due to the inoculation of foreign genetic material and associated risk of generating autoantibodies to the host system. But at present, as from various preclinical trials, the capability to generate humoral and cellular immunity with recent advancements in their preparation, renders them safer and more immunogenic. These could be further categorized as follows:

10.4.5.1 DNA vaccine

It is the most explored subtype vaccine candidate in context to CL and VL. Like recombinant ones, it also consists of membranous (gp63 and KMP11) and nonmembranous (A2, HSPB, NH, HSP70, and TPI) proteins as well as second-generation-based polyprotein antigens for stimulating effective prophylaxis. For instance, LEISHDNAVAX a pan-immunogenic construct composed of plasmids encoding for five different genes (KMP11, thiol-specific-antioxidant protein (TSA), cysteine proteinase A (CPA), cysteine proteinase B (CPB), and P74) belongs to VL interspecies, corroborated considerable protection in *L. donovani* challenged mice (Riede et al., 2015). Likewise, incorporation of heterologous DNA-prime protein-boost (HPB) strategies enhances T-cell-specific immune response against that particular antigen. Such as, HPB stratagem used for CPA and CPB immunization provides an accountable efficacy in both mice and dog models (Rafati et al., 2005; Rafati, Zahedifard, & Nazgouee, 2006). A recent study showed that administration of sirolimus with polyprotein DNA vaccine (comprising LACK, TRYP, PAPLE22, and KMPII genes) yields a promising resistance against *L. infantum* in hamster model (Martínez-Flórez et al., 2020). On the other hand, Dey, Kumar, Sharma, and Singh (2009) research group opted for a chimeric DNA vaccine acting against VL and tuberculosis infection. Vaccine comprises esat-6 gene from *Mycobacterium tuberculosis* and the kinesin motor domain gene of *L. donovani* together as a novel chimera. Results presented that both proteins exhibited an adjuvant effect over one another and offer an alternative option for treating coinfection of VL and tuberculosis (Dey et al., 2009).

10.4.5.2 Viral vector expression system

Another class of DNA vaccine indulges in *in situ* expressions of the parasite antigens within the viral vector system. Up to the present time, modified vaccinia, influenza, and nonreplicative adenoviruses expressing KMP11, LACK, Leish-F3, and HASPB antigens have been employed preclinically against both CL and VL cases. Out of them, semian adenovirus−based (ChAd63) vaccine encoding KMP11 and HASPB (KH) genes made it to phase II trials, evoking CD8$^+$ T-cell-mediated immune response, IFN-γ production, and Dendritic cell (DC) activation in immunized individuals (Osman et al., 2017). Due to generation of such an impactful cellular response, ChAD63KH is also evaluating against PKDL for its therapeutic efficacy.

10.4.5.3 Bacterial expression system

Like viral vector constructs, live bacterial systems have also been tried as antileishmania vaccine candidates, but are not much effective. Of these, gp63 and LACK antigens expressing in recombinant *Salmonella typhimurium* and attenuated *Listeria monocytogenes* strains are recognized to be effective against CL/VL murine models (Gholami, Zahedifard, & Rafati, 2016).

10.4.6 Synthetic peptide vaccine

With recent improvements in bioinformatics tools, small amino acid sequences, or peptides (epitope) of potent immunogen could be predicted, responsible for generating a strong protective immune response. It proposes several leads over the classical vaccine approaches as they are more stable, not infectious, possess low complexity, multiple epitopes could be fused, easy to scale up, and have minimal risk of an immune response against self-antigens. In the last few years, many reports suggested that *in silico* predicted epitopes of *Leishmania* antigen as alone or chimera generally belong to MHC class I and II based restricted peptides class. Combination of these peptides with an appropriate adjuvant or delivery system is markedly immunogenic to both *in vitro* and *in vivo* systems. For instance, antigenic epitopes synthesized for NH36 or LiHyp1, LiHyp6, LiHyV, and histamine releasing factor (HRF) proteins observed more protective against *Leishmania amazonensis* challenge in murine models (Alves-Silva, Nico, Morrot, Palatnik, & Palatnik-de-Sousa, 2017; Martins et al., 2017). On similar lines, another group gives a shot of promastigote surface antigen-based multigenic peptide vaccine along with QA-21 generating a substantial protective Th1 response in *L. infantum* infected dogs (Petitdidier et al., 2019). Likewise, HLA-I and HLA-II restricted multiepitope peptides derived from Promastigote Surface Antigen (PSA), Lml RAB, and H2B antigens induce $CD4^+/CD8^+$ T-cell responses in CL recovered people (Hamrouni et al., 2020). In addition, for improvising shelf life and efficacy of chimeric peptide vaccine, nanoparticle-based delivery has been tested. It consists of three immunogenic proteins, that is, CPA, KMP11, and histone 1 (H1) coadministered with monophosphoryl lipid A (MPLA) conferring IFN-γ production and stimulating substantial protection against *L. infantum* infection (Athanasiou et al., 2017).

10.4.7 Nonpathogenic *Leishmania*-based vaccine

In this approach, potent heterologous proteins of virulent *Leishmania* strains were expressed in live nonpathogenic *Leishmania tarentolae* system, which is safer due to its inability to reverse and a worthwhile alternative for the vaccine. These genes were transfected either episomally or integrally within the ribosomal ribo nucleic acid (rRNA) locus of *L. tarentolae* to develop a recombinant strain as a live vaccine candidate. Initially, the A2 gene of *L. donovani* introduced to construct an A2 recombinant *L. tarentolae* parasite stimulating prominent Th1-biased response against *L. infantum* (Mizbani et al., 2009). In the same line, vaccination with live *L. tarentolae* strain expressing tri-fusion gene (A2-CPA-CPB-CTE) construct presented a strong protective immune response against VL (Saljoughian et al., 2013).

10.4.8   Vector-derived vaccine

Based on preliminary findings, a bite of an uninfected sandfly confers protection against CL. Herein, proteins derived from the both old and new world *Leishmania* vector were utilized as vaccine targets against preclinical models of leishmaniasis. Such as, PdSP15 and LJM-19 proteins seemed to be defensive against CL and VL or MCL models, respectively (Katebi et al., 2015). Correspondingly, some groups also emphasize developing a transmission-blocking vaccine wherein the parasite growth impeded within the vector only. For example, PpGalec fed sandflies exhibited a 50% less infectivity rate and reproducibility than the unfed ones.

10.4.9   Antigen cocktail vaccines

The present vaccine type employs a cocktail mix of known multiple *Leishmania* recombinant proteins, reported to be immunogenic, which were explored for their efficacy along with a suitable adjuvant system. For example, immunization of beagle dogs with H1 and HASPB1cocktail in conjunction with Montanide presented partial protection against CVL (Moreno et al., 2007). Likewise, Soto et al. (2015) also utilized a mix of recombinant DNA vaccines expressing three different forms of *L. infantum* poly(A)-binding proteins instead of protein cocktail and results demonstrated that it stimulates Th1-biased response and confers protection in prone murine models of VL.

10.5   Challenges and future perspectives

Vaccine is a cost-effective and innocuous way of controlling any infectious disease. As discussed above, despite enormous efforts and intense research going on vaccinology field, there is no licensed vaccine made available for human leishmaniasis. Hitherto, whatsoever vaccine candidates considered for clinical trials remain limited to animal models only. There is a large gap in elucidating the long-term impact of immunological functions and exploring a unified strategy affecting different arms of immune defenses in a comprehensive manner. Hence, attempting to put forward certain key pitfalls must be addressed for a successful antileishmanial vaccine program (Srivastava, Shankar, Mishra, & Singh, 2016):

- Failure of vaccine mediated immunity in human trials;
- Improved knowledge of host−parasite pathobiology;
- Demands antigen targets capable of stimulating different arms of the immune system;
- Appropriateness of efficacious adjuvant system;
- Optimization of delivery system or route of administration;
- Variation in the virulence of *Leishmania* across the species;
- Insufficient fund investments for these programs.

So, advancement towards an effective vaccine remains a challenging task but it could be the utmost way of rescuing thousands of lives worldwide. Although the journey towards the development of a commercial human vaccine for leishmaniasis has not succeeded, improvised adjuvant formulations and better understanding of complex host–pathogen biology along with complicated immune responses were anticipated for near-term success. Hence, progression made in vaccine development program is highly commendable and ensures an effectual parasite clearance. Further recent improvements in technology and discoveries in the field of vaccination encourage the quest to produce a safe and successful vaccine for eradicating *Leishmania* infection.

Acknowledgements

This work was supported by the DBT (Department of Biotechnology)—India grant for providing financial assistance in the form of research associate fellowship to Dr. Keerti. The figure was created with BioRender.com under paid subscription.

References

Alves-Silva, M. V., Nico, D., Morrot, A., Palatnik, M., & Palatnik-de-Sousa, C. B. (2017). A chimera containing CD4+ and CD8+ T-cell epitopes of the Leishmania donovani nucleoside hydrolase (NH36) optimizes cross-protection against Leishmania amazonesis infection. *Frontiers in Immunology, 8*(100). Available from https://doi.org/10.3389/fimmu.2017.00100.

Athanasiou, E., Agallou, M., Tastsoglou, S., Kammona, O., Hatzigeorgiou, A., Kiparissides, C., & Karagouni, E. (2017). A poly (lactic-co-glycolic) acid nanovaccine based on chimeric peptides from different Leishmania infantum proteins induces dendritic cells maturation and promotes peptide-specific IFNγ-producing CD8(+) T cells essential for the protection against experimental visceral leishmaniasis. *Frontiers in Immunology, 8*, 684. Available from https://doi.org/10.3389/fimmu.2017.00684.

Bruhn, K. W., Birnbaum, R., Haskell, J., Vanchinathan, V., Greger, S., Narayan, R., ... Craft, N. (2012). Killed but metabolically active Leishmania infantum as a novel whole-cell vaccine for visceral leishmaniasis. *Clinical and Vaccine Immunology, 19*(4), 490–498. Available from https://doi.org/10.1128/cvi.05660-11.

Chakravarty, J., & Sundar, S. (2010). Drug resistance in leishmaniasis. *Journal of Global Infectious Diseases, 2*(2), 167–176. Available from https://doi.org/10.4103/0974-777x.62887.

Coler, R. N., Duthie, M. S., Hofmeyer, K. A., Guderian, J., Jayashankar, L., Vergara, J., ... Reed, S. G. (2015). From mouse to man: safety, immunogenicity and efficacy of a candidate leishmaniasis vaccine LEISH-F3 + GLA-SE. *Clinical & Translational Immunology, 4*(4), e35. Available from https://doi.org/10.1038/cti.2015.6.

Daneshvar, H., Coombs, G. H., Hagan, P., & Phillips, R. S. (2003). Leishmania mexicana and Leishmania major: attenuation of wild-type parasites and vaccination with the attenuated lines. *The Journal of Infectious Diseases, 187*(10), 1662–1668. Available from https://doi.org/10.1086/374783.

Desjeux, P. (2004). Leishmaniasis: current situation and new perspectives. *Comparative Immunology, Microbiology & Infectious Diseases*, 27(5), 305−318. Available from https://doi.org/10.1016/j.cimid.2004.03.004.

Dey, A., Kumar, U., Sharma, P., & Singh, S. (2009). Immunogenicity of candidate chimeric DNA vaccine against tuberculosis and leishmaniasis. *Vaccine*, 27(37), 5152−5160. Available from https://doi.org/10.1016/j.vaccine.2009.05.100.

Dostálová, A., & Volf, P. (2012). Leishmania development in sand flies: parasite-vector interactions overview. *Parasites & Vectors*, 5, 276. Available from https://doi.org/10.1186/1756-3305-5-276.

Faleiro, R. J., Kumar, R., Hafner, L. M., & Engwerda, C. R. (2014). Immune regulation during chronic visceral leishmaniasis. *PLoS Neglected Tropical Diseases*, 8(7), e2914. Available from https://doi.org/10.1371/journal.pntd.0002914.

Gebremichael Tedla, D., Bariagabr, F. H., & Abreha, H. H. (2018). Incidence and trends of leishmaniasis and its risk factors in Humera, Western Tigray. *Journal of Parasitology Research*, 2018, 8463097. Available from https://doi.org/10.1155/2018/8463097.

Gholami, E., Zahedifard, F., & Rafati, S. (2016). Delivery systems for Leishmania vaccine development. *Expert Review of Vaccines*, 15(7), 879−895. Available from https://doi.org/10.1586/14760584.2016.1157478.

Gillespie, P. M., Beaumier, C. M., Strych, U., Hayward, T., Hotez, P. J., & Bottazzi, M. E. (2016). Status of vaccine research and development of vaccines for leishmaniasis. *Vaccine*, 34(26), 2992−2995. Available from https://doi.org/10.1016/j.vaccine.2015.12.071.

Grimaldi, G., Jr., Teva, A., Dos-Santos, C. B., Santos, F. N., Pinto, I. D., Fux, B., ... Falqueto, A. (2017). Field trial of efficacy of the Leish-tec® vaccine against canine leishmaniasis caused by Leishmania infantum in an endemic area with high transmission rates. *PLoS One*, 12(9), e0185438. Available from https://doi.org/10.1371/journal.pone.0185438.

Gupta, G., Oghumu, S., & Satoskar, A. R. (2013). Mechanisms of immune evasion in leishmaniasis. *Advances in Applied Microbiology*, 82, 155−184. Available from https://doi.org/10.1016/b978-0-12-407679-2.00005-3.

Hamrouni, S., Bras-Gonçalves, R., Kidar, A., Aoun, K., Chamakh-Ayari, R., Petitdidier, E., ... Meddeb-Garnaoui, A. (2020). Design of multi-epitope peptides containing HLA class-I and class-II-restricted epitopes derived from immunogenic Leishmania proteins, and evaluation of CD4+ and CD8+ T cell responses induced in cured cutaneous leishmaniasis subjects. *PLoS Neglected Tropical Diseases*, 14(3), e0008093. Available from https://doi.org/10.1371/journal.pntd.0008093.

Handman, E. (2001). Leishmaniasis: current status of vaccine development. *Clinical Microbiology Reviews*, 14(2), 229−243. Available from https://doi.org/10.1128/cmr.14.2.229-243.2001.

Katebi, A., Gholami, E., Taheri, T., Zahedifard, F., Habibzadeh, S., Taslimi, Y., ... Rafati, S. (2015). Leishmania tarentolae secreting the sand fly salivary antigen PpSP15 confers protection against Leishmania major infection in a susceptible BALB/c mice model. *Molecular Immunology*, 67(2 Pt B), 501−511. Available from https://doi.org/10.1016/j.molimm.2015.08.001.

Khalil, E. A., Musa, A. M., Modabber, F., & El-Hassan, A. M. (2006). Safety and immunogenicity of a candidate vaccine for visceral leishmaniasis (Alum-precipitated autoclaved Leishmania major + BCG) in children: an extended phase II study. *Annals of Tropical Paediatrics*, 26(4), 357−361. Available from https://doi.org/10.1179/146532806x152890.

Kumar, A., Pandey, S. C., & Samant, M. (2018). Slow pace of antileishmanial drug development. *Parasitology Open*, 4(4), 1−11.

Kumar, A., Pandey, S. C., & Samant, M. (2020a). A spotlight on the diagnostic methods of a fatal disease visceral leishmaniasis. *Parasite Immunology, 42*(10), e12727.

Kumar, A., Pandey, S. C., & Samant, M. (2020b). DNA-based microarray studies in visceral leishmaniasis: identification of biomarkers for diagnostic, prognostic and drug target for treatment. *Acta Tropica, 208*, 105512.

Kumar, A., & Samant, M. (2016). DNA vaccine against visceral leishmaniasis: a promising approach for prevention and control. *Parasite Immunol, 38*(5), 273−281. Available from https://doi.org/10.1111/pim.12315. 27009772.

Kumar, R., & Engwerda, C. (2014). Vaccines to prevent leishmaniasis. *Clinical & Translational Immunology, 3*(3), e13. Available from https://doi.org/10.1038/cti.2014.4.

Lindoso, J. A., Cunha, M. A., Queiroz, I. T., & Moreira, C. H. (2016). Leishmaniasis-HIV coinfection: current challenges. *HIV AIDS (Auckland, N.Z.), 8*, 147−156. Available from https://doi.org/10.2147/hiv.s93789.

Llanos-Cuentas, A., Calderón, W., Cruz, M., Ashman, J. A., Alves, F. P., Coler, R. N., ... Piazza, F. M. (2010). A clinical trial to evaluate the safety and immunogenicity of the LEISH-F1 + MPL-SE vaccine when used in combination with sodium stibogluconate for the treatment of mucosal leishmaniasis. *Vaccine, 28*(46), 7427−7435. Available from https://doi.org/10.1016/j.vaccine.2010.08.092.

Martínez-Flórez, A., Martori, C., Monteagudo, P. L., Rodriguez, F., Alberola, J., & Rodríguez-Cortés, A. (2020). Sirolimus enhances the protection achieved by a DNA vaccine against Leishmania infantum. *Parasites & Vectors, 13*(1), 294. Available from https://doi.org/10.1186/s13071-020-04165-4.

Martins, V. T., Lage, D. P., Duarte, M. C., Carvalho, A. M., Costa, L. E., Mendes, T. A., ... Coelho, E. A. (2017). A recombinant fusion protein displaying murine and human MHC class I- and II-specific epitopes protects against Leishmania amazonensis infection. *Cellular Immunology, 313*, 32−42. Available from https://doi.org/10.1016/j.cellimm.2016.12.008.

Mizbani, A., Taheri, T., Zahedifard, F., Taslimi, Y., Azizi, H., Azadmanesh, K., ... Rafati, S. (2009). Recombinant Leishmania tarentolae expressing the A2 virulence gene as a novel candidate vaccine against visceral leishmaniasis. *Vaccine, 28*(1), 53−62. Available from https://doi.org/10.1016/j.vaccine.2009.09.114.

Moafi, M., Rezvan, H., Sherkat, R., & Taleban, R. (2019). Leishmania vaccines entered in clinical trials: a review of literature. *International Journal of Preventive Medicine, 10*, 95. Available from https://doi.org/10.4103/ijpvm.IJPVM_116_18.

Moreno, J., Nieto, J., Masina, S., Cañavate, C., Cruz, I., Chicharro, C., ... Alvar, J. (2007). Immunization with H1, HASPB1 and MML Leishmania proteins in a vaccine trial against experimental canine leishmaniasis. *Vaccine, 25*(29), 5290−5300. Available from https://doi.org/10.1016/j.vaccine.2007.05.010.

Moreno, J., Vouldoukis, I., Martin, V., McGahie, D., Cuisinier, A. M., & Gueguen, S. (2012). Use of a LiESP/QA-21 vaccine (CaniLeish) stimulates an appropriate Th1-dominated cell-mediated immune response in dogs. *PLoS Neglected Tropical Diseases, 6*(6), e1683. Available from https://doi.org/10.1371/journal.pntd.0001683.

Osman, M., Mistry, A., Keding, A., Gabe, R., Cook, E., Forrester, S., ... Lacey, C. J. (2017). A third generation vaccine for human visceral leishmaniasis and post kala azar dermal leishmaniasis: First-in-human trial of ChAd63-KH. *PLoS Neglected Tropical Diseases, 11*(5), e0005527. Available from https://doi.org/10.1371/journal.pntd.0005527.

Pandey, S. C., Jha, A., Kumar, A., & Samant, M. (2019). Evaluation of antileishmanial potential of computationally screened compounds targeting DEAD-box RNA helicase of Leishmania donovani. *International journal of biological macromolecules*, *121*, 480−487. Available from https://doi.org/10.1016/j.ijbiomac.2018.10.053. 30321635.

Pandey, S. C., Dhami, D. S., Jha, A., Chandra Shah, G., Kumar, A., & Samant, M. (2019). Identification of trans-2-cis-8-Matricaria-ester from the Essential Oil of Erigeron multiradiatus and Evaluation of Its Antileishmanial Potential by in Vitro and in Silico Approaches. *ACS Omega*, *4*(11), 14640−14649. Available from https://doi.org/10.1021/acsomega. 9b02130. 31528820.

Pandey, S. C., Kumar, A., & Samant, M. (2020). Genetically modified live attenuated vaccine: a potential strategy to combat visceral leishmaniasis. *Parasite Immunology*, *42*(9), e12732.

Pandey, S. C., Pande, V., & Samant, M. (2020). DDX3 DEAD-box RNA helicase (Hel67) gene disruption impairs infectivity of Leishmania donovani and induces protective immunity against visceral leishmaniasis. *Scientific Reports*, *10*(1), 1−10.

Petitdidier, E., Pagniez, J., Pissarra, J., Holzmuller, P., Papierok, G., Vincendeau, P., ... Bras-Gonçalves, R. (2019). Peptide-based vaccine successfully induces protective immunity against canine visceral leishmaniasis. *NPJ Vaccines*, *4*(1), 49. Available from https://doi.org/ 10.1038/s41541-019-0144-2.

Rafati, S., Nakhaee, A., Taheri, T., Taslimi, Y., Darabi, H., Eravani, D., ... Rad, M. A. (2005). Protective vaccination against experimental canine visceral leishmaniasis using a combination of DNA and protein immunization with cysteine proteinases type I and II of L. infantum. *Vaccine*, *23*(28), 3716−3725. Available from https://doi.org/10.1016/j.vaccine.2005.02.009.

Rafati, S., Zahedifard, F., & Nazgouee, F. (2006). Prime-boost vaccination using cysteine proteinases type I and II of Leishmania infantum confers protective immunity in murine visceral leishmaniasis. *Vaccine*, *24*(12), 2169−2175. Available from https://doi.org/10.1016/j. vaccine.2005.11.011.

Ready, P. D. (2014). Epidemiology of visceral leishmaniasis. *Clinical Epidemiology*, *6*, 147−154. Available from https://doi.org/10.2147/clep.s44267.

Rezvan, H., & Moafi, M. (2015). An overview on Leishmania vaccines: a narrative review article. *Veterinary Research Forum*, *6*(1), 1−7.

Riede, O., Seifert, K., Oswald, D., Endmann, A., Hock, C., Winkler, A., ... Juhls, C. (2015). Preclinical safety and tolerability of a repeatedly administered human leishmaniasis DNA vaccine. *Gene Therapy*, *22*(8), 628−635. Available from https://doi.org/10.1038/gt.2015.35.

Roatt, B. M., Aguiar-Soares, R. D., Coura-Vital, W., Ker, H. G., Moreira, N., Vitoriano-Souza, J., ... Reis, A. B. (2014). Immunotherapy and Immunochemotherapy in visceral leishmaniasis: promising treatments for this neglected disease. *Frontiers in Immunology*, *5*, 272. Available from https://doi.org/10.3389/fimmu.2014.00272.

Rossi, M., & Fasel, N. (2018). How to master the host immune system? Leishmania parasites have the solutions!. *International Immunology*, *30*(3), 103−111. Available from https://doi. org/10.1093/intimm/dxx075.

Saljoughian, N., Taheri, T., Zahedifard, F., Taslimi, Y., Doustdari, F., Bolhassani, A., ... Rafati, S. (2013). Development of novel prime-boost strategies based on a tri-gene fusion recombinant L. tarentolae vaccine against experimental murine visceral leishmaniasis. *PLoS Neglected Tropical Diseases*, *7*(4), e2174. Available from https://doi.org/10.1371/journal. pntd.0002174.

Samant, M., Sahu, U., Pandey, S. C., & Khare, P. (2021). Role of Cytokines in Experimental and Human Visceral Leishmaniasis. *Frontiers in Cellular and Infection Microbiology*, *11*, 624009. Available from https://doi.org/10.3389/fcimb.2021.624009. 33680991.

Selvapandiyan, A., Dey, R., Gannavaram, S., Lakhal-Naouar, I., Duncan, R., Salotra, P., & Nakhasi, H. L. (2012). Immunity to visceral leishmaniasis using genetically defined live-attenuated parasites. *Journal of Tropical Medicine*, *2012*, 631460. Available from https://doi.org/ 10.1155/2012/631460.

Singh, O. P., Singh, B., Chakravarty, J., & Sundar, S. (2016). Current challenges in treatment options for visceral leishmaniasis in India: a public health perspective. *Infectious Diseases of Poverty*, *5*, 19. Available from https://doi.org/10.1186/s40249-016-0112-2.

Solana, J. C., Ramírez, L., Cook, E. C., Hernández-García, E., Sacristán, S., Martín, M. E., ... Soto, M. (2020). Subcutaneous immunization of Leishmania HSP70-II null mutant line reduces the severity of the experimental visceral leishmaniasis in BALB/c mice. *Vaccines (Basel)*, *8*(1), 141. Available from https://doi.org/10.3390/vaccines8010141.

Soto, M., Corvo, L., Garde, E., Ramírez, L., Iniesta, V., Bonay, P., ... Iborra, S. (2015). Coadministration of the three antigenic Leishmania infantum poly (a) binding proteins as a DNA vaccine induces protection against Leishmania major infection in BALB/c mice. *PLoS Neglected Tropical Diseases*, *9*(5), e0003751. Available from https://doi.org/10.1371/journal.pntd.0003751.

Srivastava, S., Shankar, P., Mishra, J., & Singh, S. (2016). Possibilities and challenges for developing a successful vaccine for leishmaniasis. *Parasites & Vectors*, *9*(1), 277. Available from https://doi.org/10.1186/s13071-016-1553-y.

Svárovská, A., Ant, T. H., Seblová, V., Jecná, L., Beverley, S. M., & Volf, P. (2010). Leishmania major glycosylation mutants require phosphoglycans (lpg2 −) but not lipophosphoglycan (lpg1 −) for survival in permissive sand fly vectors. *PLoS Neglected Tropical Diseases*, *4*(1), e580. Available from https://doi.org/10.1371/journal.pntd.0000580.

Torres-Guerrero, E., Quintanilla-Cedillo, M. R., Ruiz-Esmenjaud, J., & Arenas, R. (2017). Leishmaniasis: a review. *F1000Research*, *6*, 750. Available from https://doi.org/10.12688/ f1000research.11120.1.

Chapter 11

Interferon-γ: a key cytokine in leishmaniasis

Utkarsha Sahu and Prashant Khare

Department of Microbiology, All India Institute of Medical Sciences, Bhopal, India

11.1 Introduction

Leishmaniasis is a zoonotic disease caused by different species of *Leishmania*, an obligate intracellular protozoan parasite transmitted by female phlebotomine sandflies (Solano-Gallego, Montserrrat-Sangrà, Ordeix, & Martínez-Orellana, 2016). According to the World Health Organization, there are about 350 million people suffering from leishmaniasis around the world. The female sandfly seeks blood meals at dusk and is least active during the day time (Murray, Berman, Davies, & Saravia, 2005). After the sandfly bites, the parasites replicate in the gut of sandfly and are later injected into the skin of human or animal with a subsequent bite (Davies, Kaye, Croft, & Sundar, 2003). *Leishmania* parasite mainly targets and multiplies within different phagocytic cells of the innate immune system such as macrophages, neutrophils, and dendritic cells (Launois, Tacchini-Cottier, Parra-Lopez, & Louis, 1998; Solbach & Laskay, 1999). Uncontrolled parasite replication can result in cell lysis followed by subsequent infection in surrounding cells. In normal conditions, the infection and detection of *Leishmania* parasite leads to migration of inflammatory cells at the site of infection, thereby activating the adaptive immune response (David & Craft, 2009). On the basis of species and host immune response, there are three clinical forms of leishmaniasis: visceral leishmaniasis (VL), cutaneous leishmaniasis (CL), and mucocutaneous leishmaniasis (MCL). VL is also known as kala-azar, and is categorized by irregular stretches of fever, swelling of the liver and spleen, extensive weight loss and anemia (https://www.who.int/leishmaniasis/disease_epidemiology/en/). CL causes skin ulcers on face, legs, arms and on the other exposed parts of the body. The disease can produce severe lesions causing serious disability and leaving permanent scars (https://www.who.int/leishmaniasis/disease_epidemiology/en/). The MCL-associated lesions can lead to partial or complete damage of the mucous membranes of the mouth, nose, and throat cavities, and surrounding tissues (https://www.who.int/leishmaniasis/disease_epidemiology/en/).

Pathogenesis, Treatment and Prevention of Leishmaniasis. DOI: https://doi.org/10.1016/B978-0-12-822800-5.00001-9

Interferon gamma (IFN-γ) is a homodimeric glycoprotein with two subunits of about 21−24 kDa, respectively. It is the most efficient type II interferon involved in the activation of macrophages and subsequent antileishmanial activity (Carvalho et al., 1994). The cytokine IFN-γ is a key cytokine involved in the elimination of *Leishmania* parasites from infected cells (Carneiro et al., 2016). IFN-γ is generally produced in lymphoid organs where the parasite proliferates (Goto & Prianti, 2009). However, a few studies suggest the difficulty in obtaining tissue samples from active patients. The mRNA expression of IFN-γ has also been detected in lymph nodes (Ghalib et al., 1993), spleen (Nylén & Sacks, 2007), and in aspirates of bone marrow (Karp et al., 1993). IFN-γ is mainly produced by activated $CD4^+$ and $CD8^+$ T cells, and natural killer cells via interleukin (IL)-12 signaling (Gough, Levy, Johnstone, & Clarke, 2008). Among different antileishmanial cytokines, IFN-γ is the most crucial cytokine involved in macrophage priming and production of leishmanicidal molecules thereby providing immunity against parasite infection (Mosser & Edwards, 2008; Murray & Nathan, 1999; Taylor & Murray, 1997). IFN-γ acts as monocyte-activating factor (Nathan & Hibbs, 1991) and induces, secretion of proinflammatory cytokines [tumor necrosis factor alpha (TNF-α), IL-l, and IL-6] and release of oxygen radicals (Hart, Whitty, Piccoli, & Hamilton, 1989), major histocompatibility complex class-II expression, and antigen presentation. Also, IFN-γ blocks IL-10 production, which inhibits all the above functions of monocytes (de Waal Malefyt et al., 1991).

Single nucleotide polymorphism (SNP) is the most common type of gene variation. It is a substitution of a single nucleotide by another nucleotide at a specific position. Based on their position in the genome, some SNPs can regulate the expression of associated proteins. The rs2430561 SNP in the IFN-γ gene known as IFN-γ +874 A/T polymorphism is located in the first intron of the human IFN-γ gene and can putatively regulate the expression of IFN-γ (Pravica, Perrey, Stevens, Lee, & Hutchinson, 2000). This SNP results in two genotypes: AT and TT, respectively, and is involved in VL and CL (Ahmed et al., 2020; Kalani, Choopanizadeh, & Rasouli, 2019; Kamali-Sarvestani, Rasouli, Mortazavi, & Gharesi-Fard, 2006). In this chapter, we summarize the role of IFN-γ, a key molecule in leishmaniasis and its SNPs involved in the immune response in three forms of leishmaniasis. Here in this chapter, we discuss the active involvement of IFN-γ in respect to parasite killing and controlling the progression CL, MCL, and VL form of leishmaniasis.

11.2   IFN-γ response in leishmaniasis

11.2.1   IFN-γ response in VL

VL is a systematic fatal disease caused by *Leishmania donovani*, *Leishmania infantum*, and *Leishmania chagasi* strains of *Leishmania* parasite and is characterized by the invasion of lymphoid tissues by the parasite. It is marked with an immunosuppressed state with the impaired T-cell response (Carvalho et al., 1994) that is evident from reduced IFN-γ production (Samant, Sahu, Pandey, & Khare, 2021). The IL-12 primed T cells produce IFN-γ that induces the production of inducible nitric oxide synthase (iNOS) that causes release of microbicidal molecules such as nitric oxide (NO) in macrophages, which is crucial for parasite clearance (Bacellar, D'Oliveira, Jerônimo, & Carvalho, 2000; Engwerda, Murphy, Cotterell, Smelt, & Kaye, 1998). The inhibition of NOS by its inhibitor L-NG monomethylarginine significantly reduced the parasite killing (Brandonisio et al., 2001; Panaro et al., 1998). Similar results were found in the canine model of VL, where the protective immune response in *L. infantum*-infected dogs was mediated by IFN-γ activated macrophages. IFN-γ activated macrophages displayed antiparasitic activity by L-arginine NO pathway leading to intracellular killing of amastigotes after successful chemotherapy (Vouldoukis et al., 1996). The lack of *L. infantum*-specific IFN-γ increased parasite load, clinical manifestation, and humoral response in canines, thereby implying its protective role (Solano-Gallego et al., 2016). Furthermore, supporting these findings, the IFN-γ-mediated NO production and antileishmanial activity is also reported in a canine macrophage cell line infected with *L. infantum* (Pinelli et al., 2000). In humans, the plasma level of IFN-γ is high in patients with active VL as compared to asymptomatic patients and comparatively higher in asymptomatic patients as compared to uninfected people (Ansari, Saluja, & Salotra, 2006; Khoshdel et al., 2009). In vitro study of lymphocytes isolated from VL patients challenged with *Leishmania* antigen showed downregulation of IFN-γ level that was restored after successful chemotherapy (Carvalho, Badaró, Reed, Jones, & Johnson, 1985). This downregulation of IFN-γ in VL is followed by an elevated type 2 T helper cell (Th2) response. On inhibiting the Th2 response, the IFN-γ levels were restored in vitro state (Carvalho et al., 1994). Another evidence of the protective role of IFN-γ was reported by a study performed on peripheral blood mononuclear cells (PBMCs) of children from an endemic area of VL. Children whose antigen stimulated PBMCs produced increased level of IFN-γ exhibited protective immunity while low level of IFN-γ lead to disease progression (Carvalho et al., 1992). Thus the absence or reduced secretion of IFN-γ is a marker of VL susceptibility.

A positive correlation of IL-10 and human VL progression is well documented (Nylén & Sacks, 2007). IL-10 is a key molecule in the downregulation of IFN-γ production in human VL infection (Gautam et al., 2011). Neutralization of IL-10 with anti-IL-10 antibody upregulated the IFN-γ production in splenic aspirate cells of VL patients (Gautam et al., 2011). IL-10 partially suppresses the IFN-γ production but strongly inhibits IFN-γ-mediated macrophage activation required for antileishmanial activity (Bhattacharyya, Ghosh, Jhonson, Bhattacharya, & Majumdar, 2001; de Medeiros, Castelo, &

Salomão, 1998; Ghalib et al., 1993; Melby, Chandrasekar, Zhao, & Coe, 2001) (Pandey, Pande, & Samant, 2020). Similarly, the reduced IFN-γ levels result in higher IL-10 level in human leishmaniasis suggests for the deactivation of macrophages and parasite persistence (de Medeiros et al., 1998). Substitution of a single nucleotide at +874 position in IFN-γ gene results in rs2430561 SNP with AT and TT genotypes. Based on their position in the genome, the SNPs can influence the expression of the associated proteins. The AT genotype of IFN-γ at +874 position may predispose while the TT genotype resists VL in an endemic area of Iran (Kalani et al., 2019). In VL patients, the restriction fragment length polymorphism (RFLP) and allele-specific polymerase chain reaction analysis revealed that AT genotype was more frequent in patients as compared to family and controls while TT genotype was frequently present in families of patients rather than in patients (Kalani et al., 2019).

11.2.2 IFN-γ response in CL

CL is mainly caused by *Leishmania tropica*, *Leishmania major*, and *Leishmania aethiopica* which occurs in India, Iran, Afghanistan, the Middle East, south Russia, north and east Africa, and southern Europe. However, CL of the New World, particularly forested areas of Mexico and Central America, is caused by the species complexes *Leishmania mexicana* and *Leishmania braziliensis* (David & Craft, 2009). CL is not a life-threatening disease; however, the lesions associated with CL can lead to significant disfigurement. In the absence of proper treatment, the CL may progress into life-threatening MCL form (David & Craft, 2009). In contrast to VL, patients with CL have a dominant T-cell response marked with upregulated IFN-γ production and increased lymphocyte proliferation in response to parasite antigen stimulation (Carvalho et al., 1985; Mendonça, Coutinho, Amendoeira, Marzochi, & Pirmez, 1986). There is a dominant type 1 helper cell (Th1) response in CL leading to upregulation of IFN-γ along with other inflammatory cytokine production contributing to the formation of CL lesions (Oliveira et al., 2011). The Th1 and Th2 response against *Leishmania* infection determine the susceptibility and resistance against the parasite. The resistant mouse strain C3H/HeN displays an active Th1 immune response involving IFN-γ and has a self-limiting pattern of disease (Heinzel, Sadick, Mutha, & Locksley, 1991). The *Leishmania amazonensis*-infected C3H mice results in downregulation of IFN-γ production by antigen-specific CD4$^+$ T cells (Jones, Buxbaum, & Scott, 2000). However, the presence of CD4$^+$ T cells was correlated with parasite burden and increased skin lesions. Altogether implying that IFN-γ secreting CD4$^+$ T cells contribute to immunopathology of *L. amazonensis* infection (Soong et al., 1997). In macaques model of *L. braziliensis* infection, the presence of IFN-γ producing CD4$^+$ T cells and CD8$^+$ T cells are crucial for granuloma function, an important step for parasite clearance (de-Campos, Souza-Lemos, Teva, Porrozzi, & Grimaldi, 2010; Souza-Lemos, de-Campos, Teva, Porrozzi, & Grimaldi, 2011). The CD8$^+$ T cells contribute to memory response and resolution of secondary lesions in *L. major* challenged immune mice (Müller, Kropf, Etges, & Louis, 1993). Upon reinfection the lymphocytes marked with presence of secondary IFN-γ secretion in both resistant CBA mice and susceptible BALB/c mice. The BALB/c mice were rendered resistant by anti-CD4 monoclonal antibody during the early phase of infection. Thus the ability of CD8$^+$ T cells to produce IFN-γ during reinfection in the murine model of CL implies their protective role. The neutralization of IFN-γ at the time of reinfection reduced *Leishmania*-specific delayed-type hypersensitivity response, suggesting its role in in vivo memory response to *L. major* (Müller et al., 1993). TNF-α synergizes with IFN-γ for NO-mediated *L. major* killing in macrophages (Liew, Li, & Millott, 1990). In patients with CL the macrophages infected with *L. braziliensis* have upregulated TNF-α production as compared to macrophages with *L. braziliensis* subclinical infection (Giudice et al., 2012). This upregulated TNF-α production induces dysregulated IFN-γ secretion in patients with CL. The neutralization of TNF-α may induce downregulation of IFN-γ. Thus the cytokines involved in parasite killing might also be involved in disease progression of CL. Treatment with TNF-α inhibitor pentoxifylline and antimony promotes healing after parasite infection (Lessa et al., 2001; Machado et al., 2007). Altogether these findings support the idea that TNF-α-induced exaggerated IFN-γ production causes tissue damage in CL. A study performed on in vitro priming with *L. amazonensis* antigen, showed that the cells from different individuals produce high or low IFN-γ (Pompeu et al., 2001). This difference in antiparasite response in vitro was associated with in vivo postvaccination response. People with high IFN-γ production displayed rapid immune response with soluble *Leishmania* antigen vaccination, while individuals with lower IFN-γ production had delayed postvaccination immune response. Thus the pace of IFN-γ production in in vitro condition replicated the in vivo condition and could be used to analyze the pace of immune response after vaccination (Pompeu et al., 2001). In tegumentary leishmaniasis caused by *L. braziliensis*, IFN-γ production is associated with inflammatory response, tissue damage, and development of lesions in CL (Oliveira et al., 2014). The PBMCs stimulated with *L. major* secreted IFN-γ in IL-10 and IL-12 in a dependent manner (Rogers & Titus, 2004).

The PCR analysis of different Saudi CL patients revealed that IFN-γ + 874 A/T polymorphism was found to be associated with the susceptibility of *L. major* infection (Ahmed et al., 2020). The TT versus AA + AT genotypes showed a significant association with *L. major*-infected individuals. Furthermore, the synergistically combined analysis of TNF-α and IFN-γ SNPs TNF-α 308 G/A/IFN-γ 874 A/T resulted in a significant association with CL susceptibility (Ahmed et al., 2020). In SNP analysis on American tegumentary leishmaniasis patients, the IFN-γ + 874 A/T SNP determined the production of IFN-γ level rather than determining the susceptibility (Matos et al., 2007).

11.2.3   IFN-γ response in MCL

MCL is caused by *L. amazonensis*, *L. braziliensis*, *Leishmania guyanensis*, and *Leishmania panamensis* (David & Craft, 2009). The clinical progression of MCL is associated with parasite virulence and cell-mediated immune response of the host. Among a population of *Leishmania*-infected individuals, only in 1%−10% people, the infection progresses to the mucosa (Blum, Desjeux, Schwartz, Beck, & Hatz, 2004; Konecny & Stark, 2007; Weigle & Saravia, 1996). The precise factors determining which patient will develop MCL are unknown (David & Craft, 2009). In contrast to CL, MCL is life threatening and requires proper treatment (Murray et al., 2005). In MCL the stimulation with *Leishmania* antigens induces increased activation and proliferation of lymphocytes and secretion of cytokine as compared to CL, indicating severity of tissue damage in MCL (Carvalho et al., 1985; Ribeiro-de-Jesus, Almeida, Lessa, Bacellar, & Carvalho, 1998). Similar to CL, the IFN-γ production during *L. braziliensis* infection is associated with MCL lesions (Oliveira et al., 2014). In human tegumentary leishmaniasis the macrophages produces TNF-α which increases the secretion of IFN-γ by $CD4^+$ T cells (Bacellar et al., 2002). Neutralization of TNF-α in PBMCs of MCL patients downregulated the IFN-γ production and neutralization of IFN-γ inhibits the TNF-α production. Also IFN-γ and TNF-α decreases the production of IL-10 leading to dysregulated inflammatory response associated with the development of lesions in MCL patients (Bacellar et al., 2002). The synergy between IFN-γ and TNF-α is associated with antiparasitic activity and tissue damage as well. Thus the dysregulation of protective cytokines like IFN-γ can also lead to disease progression and associated pathology in MCL (Ribeiro-de-Jesus et al., 1998). Similar to CL, the *L. braziliensis*-infected macrophages secreted a higher amount of TNF-α, which in turn dysregulated the IFN-γ production leading to disease progression; however, the downregulation of TNF-α with inhibitor pentoxifylline and antimony promoted healing after infection (Lessa et al., 2001; Machado et al., 2007). Therefore similar to other form of leishmaniasis, the TNF-α-induced IFN-γ dysregulation is associated with tissue damage in MCL as well.

11.3   Conclusion

IFN-γ is a proinflammatory cytokine with a wide range of functions. In parasitic infections, especially during *Leishmania* infection, IFN-γ has been reported to be involved in Th1 immune response in the host and its function might vary in different clinical forms of leishmaniasis. For example in VL,

IFN-γ activates the macrophages for the production of microbicidal molecules such as iNOS by induction of NOS. In CL the *Leishmania* infection is followed by an inflammatory response mediated with other proinflammatory cytokines leading to skin lesions. Although CL is not life threatening, negligence can lead to the development of MCL which is a life-threatening form of leishmaniasis. MCL is associated with severe tissue damage and permanent scars. In CL and MCL IFN-γ in synergy with TNF-α causes dysregulated inflammation that leads to lesions.

The interactions between *Leishmania* parasites and host immune response have been widely explored in different animal models. In the murine model of leishmaniasis, the nonhealing severe parasite infection is associated with impaired parasite killing in macrophages and dominance of less-mature macrophages in infiltrate (Kolde, Luger, Sorg, & Sunderkötter, 1996). The Th1-mediated parasite killing and clearance of immature macrophages leads to parasite elimination and disease resolution (Kolde et al., 1996). This response is mediated by IFN-γ that activates macrophages for leishmanicidal killing by NO production (Kolde et al., 1996). In the context of mouse model of *L. major*, the susceptible BALB/c mice displayed a predominant Th2 response resulting in severe clinical outcomes. On the contrary, the resistant C3H/HeN model displays an active IFN-γ-mediated Th1 immune response, which could lead to self-limiting of the disease (Heinzel et al., 1991). Similarly, in the C3H mouse model of *L. amazonensis*, IFN-γ production was reported to be downregulated during infection, which implies the protective role of IFN-γ and induction of Th1 response (Jones et al., 2000). In the canine model of VL, the IFN-γ activated macrophages exhibited antiparasitic activity by L-arginine NO pathway leading to intracellular killing of amastigotes (Vouldoukis et al., 1996) and the study performed on canine macrophage cell line suggested NO-mediated antiparasite activity induced by IFN-γ. In macaques model of *L. braziliensis* the presence of IFN-γ secreting CD4[+] T cells and CD8[+] T cells are crucial for granuloma function which is a major step for parasite clearance (de-Campos et al., 2010; Souza-Lemos et al., 2011). Altogether these studies highlight the active involvement of IFN-γ response in all clinical forms of leishmaniasis. The SNP in IFN-γ arising from one nucleotide variation leads to rs2430561 SNP. The rs2430561 SNP of IFN-γ also called IFN-γ + 874 A/T SNP is involved in tuberculosis (López-Maderuelo et al., 2003; Rossouw, Nel, Cooke, van Helden, & Hoal, 2003), hepatitis C virus infection (El-Bendary et al., 2017), inflammatory diseases like chronic periodontitis (Heidari et al., 2015), cervical cancer (Liu, Song, & Shi, 2015), and *Leishmania* infection (Ahmed et al., 2020; Kalani et al., 2019; Matos et al., 2007). We have discussed the role of this SNP in VL and CL diseases, respectively. The active involvement of IFN-γ response in all forms of leishmaniasis makes it a good marker for leishmaniasis disease. Future research on IFN-γ biology in *Leishmania* infection may provide new insights for better therapeutic options for resolving this parasitic infection.

References

Ahmed, A. A., Rasheed, Z., Salem, T., Al-Dhubaibi, M. S., Al Robaee, A. A., & Alzolibani, A. A. (2020). TNF-α − 308 G/A and IFN-γ + 874 A/T gene polymorphisms in Saudi patients with cutaneous leishmaniasis. *BMC Medical Genetics, 21*(1), 104.

Ansari, N. A., Saluja, S., & Salotra, P. (2006). Elevated levels of interferon-gamma, interleukin-10, and interleukin-6 during active disease in Indian kala azar. *Clinical Immunology, 119*(3), 339−345.

Bacellar, Ov, D'Oliveira, A., Jerônimo, S., & Carvalho, E. M. (2000). IL-10 and IL-12 are the main regulatory cytokines in visceral leishmaniasis. *Cytokine, 12*(8), 1228−1231.

Bacellar, O., Lessa, H., Schriefer, A., Machado, P., Ribeiro de Jesus, A., Dutra, W. O., et al. (2002). Up-regulation of Th1-type responses in mucosal leishmaniasis patients. *Infection and Immunity, 70*(12), 6734−6740.

Bhattacharyya, S., Ghosh, S., Jhonson, P. L., Bhattacharya, S. K., & Majumdar, S. (2001). Immunomodulatory role of interleukin-10 in visceral leishmaniasis: defective activation of protein kinase C-mediated signal transduction events. *Infection and Immunity, 69*(3), 1499−1507.

Blum, J., Desjeux, P., Schwartz, E., Beck, B., & Hatz, C. (2004). Treatment of cutaneous leishmaniasis among travellers. *Journal of Antimicrobial Chemotherapy, 53*(2), 158−166.

Brandonisio, O., Panaro, M. A., Sisto, M., Acquafredda, A., Fumarola, L., Leogrande, D., et al. (2001). Nitric oxide production by Leishmania-infected macrophages and modulation by cytokines and prostaglandins. *Parassitologia, 43*(Suppl 1), 1−6.

Carneiro, M. W., Fukutani, K. F., Andrade, B. B., Curvelo, R. P., Cristal, J. R., Carvalho, A. M., et al. (2016). Gene expression profile of high IFN-γ producers stimulated with Leishmania braziliensis identifies genes associated with cutaneous leishmaniasis. *PLoS Neglected Tropical Diseases, 10*(11), e0005116.

Carvalho, E. M., Bacellar, O., Brownell, C., Regis, T., Coffman, R. L., & Reed, S. G. (1994). Restoration of IFN-gamma production and lymphocyte proliferation in visceral leishmaniasis. *The Journal of Immunology, 152*(12), 5949−5956.

Carvalho, E. M., Badaró, R., Reed, S. G., Jones, T. C., & Johnson, W. D., Jr. (1985). Absence of gamma interferon and interleukin 2 production during active visceral leishmaniasis. *The Journal of Clinical Investigation, 76*(6), 2066−2069.

Carvalho, E. M., Barral, A., Pedral-Sampaio, D., Barral-Netto, M., Badaró, R., Rocha, H., et al. (1992). Immunologic markers of clinical evolution in children recently infected with Leishmania donovani chagasi. *The Journal of Infectious Diseases, 165*(3), 535−540.

David, C. V., & Craft, N. (2009). Cutaneous and mucocutaneous leishmaniasis. *Dermatologic Therapy, 22*(6), 491−502.

Davies, C. R., Kaye, P., Croft, S. L., & Sundar, S. (2003). Leishmaniasis: new approaches to disease control. *British Medical Journal, 326*(7385), 377−382.

de Medeiros, I. M., Castelo, A., & Salomão, R. (1998). Presence of circulating levels of interferon-gamma, interleukin-10 and tumor necrosis factor-alpha in patients with visceral leishmaniasis. *Revista do Instituto de Medicina Tropical de Sao Paulo, 40*(1), 31−34.

de Waal Malefyt, R., Haanen, J., Spits, H., Roncarolo, M. G., te Velde, A., Figdor, C., et al. (1991). Interleukin 10 (IL-10) and viral IL-10 strongly reduce antigen-specific human T cell proliferation by diminishing the antigen-presenting capacity of monocytes via downregulation of class II major histocompatibility complex expression. *Journal of Experimental Medicine, 174*(4), 915−924.

de-Campos, S. N., Souza-Lemos, C., Teva, A., Porrozzi, R., & Grimaldi, G., Jr. (2010). Systemic and compartmentalised immune responses in a Leishmania braziliensis-macaque model of self-healing cutaneous leishmaniasis. *Veterinary Immunology and Immunopathology, 137*(1-2), 149−154.

El-Bendary, M., Neamatallah, M., Elalfy, H., Besheer, T., El-Setouhy, M., Kasim, N., et al. (2017). Association of interferon gamma gene polymorphism and susceptibility to hepatitis C virus infection in Egyptian patients: a multicenter, family-based study. *JGH Open, 1*(4), 140−147.

Engwerda, C. R., Murphy, M. L., Cotterell, S. E. J., Smelt, S. C., & Kaye, P. M. (1998). Neutralization of IL-12 demonstrates the existence of discrete organ-specific phases in the control of Leishmania donovani. *European Journal of Immunology, 28*(2), 669−680.

Gautam, S., Kumar, R., Maurya, R., Nylén, S., Ansari, N., Rai, M., et al. (2011). IL-10 Neutralization promotes parasite clearance in splenic aspirate cells from patients with visceral leishmaniasis. *The Journal of Infectious Diseases, 204*(7), 1134−1137.

Ghalib, H. W., Piuvezam, M. R., Skeiky, Y. A., Siddig, M., Hashim, F. A., el-Hassan, A. M., et al. (1993). Interleukin 10 production correlates with pathology in human Leishmania donovani infections. *The Journal of Clinical Investigation, 92*(1), 324−329.

Giudice, A., Vendrame, C., Bezerra, C., Carvalho, L. P., Delavechia, T., Carvalho, E. M., et al. (2012). Macrophages participate in host protection and the disease pathology associated with Leishmania braziliensis infection. *BMC Infectious Diseases, 12*(1), 75.

Goto, H., & Prianti, M. (2009). Immunoactivation and immunopathogeny during active visceral leishmaniasis. *Revista do Instituto de Medicina Tropical de São Paulo, 51*, 241−246.

Gough, D. J., Levy, D. E., Johnstone, R. W., & Clarke, C. J. (2008). IFNγ signaling—does it mean JAK−STAT? *Cytokine & Growth Factor Reviews, 19*(5), 383−394.

Hart, P. H., Whitty, G. A., Piccoli, D. S., & Hamilton, J. A. (1989). Control by IFN-gamma and PGE2 of TNF alpha and IL-1 production by human monocytes. *Immunology, 66*(3), 376−383.

Heidari, Z., Mahmoudzadeh-Sagheb, H., Hashemi, M., Ansarimoghaddam, S., Moudi, B., & Sheibak, N. (2015). Association between IFN-γ +874A/T and IFN-γR1 (-611A/G, +189T/ G, and +95C/T) gene polymorphisms and chronic periodontitis in a sample of Iranian population. *International Journal of Dentistry, 2015*375359.

Heinzel, F. P., Sadick, M. D., Mutha, S. S., & Locksley, R. M. (1991). Production of interferon gamma, interleukin 2, interleukin 4, and interleukin 10 by CD4 + lymphocytes in vivo during healing and progressive murine leishmaniasis. *Proceedings of the National Academy of Sciences of the United States of America, 88*(16), 7011−7015.

Jones, D. E., Buxbaum, L. U., & Scott, P. (2000). IL-4-independent inhibition of IL-12 responsiveness during Leishmania amazonensis infection. *Journal of Immunology, 165*(1), 364−372.

Kalani, M., Choopanizadeh, M., & Rasouli, M. (2019). Influence of genetic variants of gamma interferon, interleukins 10 and 12 on visceral leishmaniasis in an endemic area, Iran. *Pathogens and Global Health, 113*(1), 14−19.

Kamali-Sarvestani, E., Rasouli, M., Mortazavi, H., & Gharesi-Fard, B. (2006). Cytokine gene polymorphisms and susceptibility to cutaneous leishmaniasis in Iranian patients. *Cytokine, 35*(3-4), 159−165.

Karp, C. L., el-Safi, S. H., Wynn, T. A., Satti, M. M., Kordofani, A. M., Hashim, F. A., et al. (1993). In vivo cytokine profiles in patients with kala-azar. Marked elevation of both interleukin-10 and interferon-gamma. *The Journal of Clinical Investigation, 91*(4), 1644−1648.

Khoshdel, A., Alborzi, A., Rosouli, M., Taheri, E., Kiany, S., & Javadian, M. H. (2009). Increased levels of IL-10, IL-12, and IFN- in patients with visceral leishmaniasis. *The Brazilian Journal of Infectious Diseases, 13*(1), 44–46.

Kolde, G., Luger, T., Sorg, C., & Sunderkötter, C. S. (1996). Successful treatment of cutaneous leishmaniasis using systemic interferon-gamma. *Dermatology (Basel, Switzerland), 192*(1), 56–60.

Konecny, P., & Stark, D. J. (2007). An Australian case of New World cutaneous leishmaniasis. *The Medical Journal of Australia, 186*(6), 315–317.

Launois, P., Tacchini-Cottier, F., Parra-Lopez, C., & Louis, J. A. (1998). Cytokines in parasitic diseases: the example of cutaneous leishmaniasis. *International Reviews of Immunology, 17* (1-4), 157–180.

Lessa, H. A., Machado, P., Lima, F., Cruz, A. A., Bacellar, O., Guerreiro, J., et al. (2001). Successful treatment of refractory mucosal leishmaniasis with pentoxifylline plus antimony. *The American Journal of Tropical Medicine and Hygiene, 65*(2), 87–89.

Liew, F. Y., Li, Y., & Millott, S. (1990). Tumor necrosis factor-alpha synergizes with IFN-gamma in mediating killing of Leishmania major through the induction of nitric oxide. *Journal of Immunology, 145*(12), 4306–4310.

Liu, N., Song, Y., & Shi, W. (2015). IFN-γ +874 T/A polymorphisms contributes to cervical cancer susceptibility: a meta-analysis. *International Journal of Clinical and Experimental Medicine, 8*(3), 4008–4015.

López-Maderuelo, D., Arnalich, F., Serantes, R., González, A., Codoceo, R., Madero, R., et al. (2003). Interferon-gamma and interleukin-10 gene polymorphisms in pulmonary tuberculosis. *American Journal of Respiratory and Critical Care Medicine, 167*(7), 970–975.

Machado, P. R. L., Lessa, H., Lessa, M., Guimarães, L. H., Bang, H., Ho, J. L., et al. (2007). Oral pentoxifylline combined with pentavalent antimony: a randomized trial for mucosal leishmaniasis. *Clinical Infectious Diseases, 44*(6), 788–793.

Matos, G. I., Covas, Cd. J. F., Bittar, Rd. C., Gomes-Silva, A., Marques, F., Maniero, V. C., et al. (2007). IFNG +874T/A polymorphism is not associated with American tegumentary leishmaniasis susceptibility but can influence Leishmania-induced IFN-γ production. *BMC Infectious Diseases, 7*(1), 33.

Melby, P. C., Chandrasekar, B., Zhao, W., & Coe, J. E. (2001). The hamster as a model of human visceral leishmaniasis: progressive disease and impaired generation of nitric oxide in the face of a prominent Th1-like cytokine response. *The Journal of Immunology, 166*(3), 1912–1920.

Mendonça, S. C., Coutinho, S. G., Amendoeira, R. R., Marzochi, M. C., & Pirmez, C. (1986). Human american cutaneous leishmaniasis (Leishmania b. braziliensis) in Brazil: lymphoproliferative responses and influence of therapy. *Clinical and Experimental Immunology, 64*(2), 269–276.

Mosser, D. M., & Edwards, J. P. (2008). Exploring the full spectrum of macrophage activation. *Nature Reviews Immunology, 8*(12), 958–969.

Müller, I., Kropf, P., Etges, R. J., & Louis, J. A. (1993). Gamma interferon response in secondary Leishmania major infection: role of CD8 + T cells. *Infection and Immunity, 61*(9), 3730–3738.

Murray, H. W., Berman, J. D., Davies, C. R., & Saravia, N. G. (2005). Advances in leishmaniasis. *The Lancet, 366*(9496), 1561–1577.

Murray, H. W., & Nathan, C. F. (1999). Macrophage microbicidal mechanisms in vivo: reactive nitrogen versus oxygen intermediates in the killing of intracellular visceral leishmania donovani. *Journal of Experimental Medicine, 189*(4), 741–746.

Nathan, C. F., & Hibbs, J. B. (1991). Role of nitric oxide synthesis in macrophage antimicrobial activity. *Current Opinion in Immunology, 3*(1), 65−70.

Nylén, S., & Sacks, D. (2007). Interleukin-10 and the pathogenesis of human visceral leishmaniasis. *Trends in Immunology, 28*(9), 378−384.

Oliveira, F., Bafica, A., Rosato, A. B., Favali, C. B., Costa, J. M., Cafe, V., et al. (2011). Lesion size correlates with Leishmania antigen-stimulated TNF-levels in human cutaneous leishmaniasis. *The American Journal of Tropical Medicine and Hygiene, 85*(1), 70−73.

Oliveira, W. N., Ribeiro, L. E., Schrieffer, A., Machado, P., Carvalho, E. M., & Bacellar, O. (2014). The role of inflammatory and anti-inflammatory cytokines in the pathogenesis of human tegumentary leishmaniasis. *Cytokine, 66*(2), 127−132.

Pandey, S. C., Pande, V., & Samant, M. (2020). DDX3 DEAD-box RNA helicase (Hel67) gene disruption impairs infectivity of Leishmania donovani and induces protective immunity against visceral leishmaniasis. *Scientific Reports, 10*(1), 18218. Available from https://doi.org/10.1038/s41598-020-75420-y.

Panaro, M. A., Lisi, S., Mitolo, V., Acquafredda, A., Fasanella, A., Carelli, M. G., et al. (1998). Evaluation of killing, superoxide anion and nitric oxide production by Leishmania infantum-infected dog monocytes. *Cytobios, 95*(380), 151−160.

Pinelli, E., Gebhard, D., Mommaas, A. M., van Hoeij, M., Langermans, J. A., Ruitenberg, E. J., et al. (2000). Infection of a canine macrophage cell line with Leishmania infantum: determination of nitric oxide production and anti-leishmanial activity. *Veterinary Parasitology, 92*(3), 181−189.

Pompeu, M. M., Brodskyn, C., Teixeira, M. J., Clarêncio, J., Van Weyenberg, J., Coelho, I. C., et al. (2001). Differences in gamma interferon production in vitro predict the pace of the in vivo response to Leishmania amazonensis in healthy volunteers. *Infection and Immunity, 69*(12), 7453−7460.

Pravica, V., Perrey, C., Stevens, A., Lee, J. H., & Hutchinson, I. V. (2000). A single nucleotide polymorphism in the first intron of the human IFN-gamma gene: absolute correlation with a polymorphic CA microsatellite marker of high IFN-gamma production. *Human Immunology, 61*(9), 863−866.

Ribeiro-de-Jesus, A., Almeida, R. P., Lessa, H., Bacellar, O., & Carvalho, E. M. (1998). Cytokine profile and pathology in human leishmaniasis. *Brazilian Journal of Medical and Biological Research, 31*(1), 143−148.

Rogers, K. A., & Titus, R. G. (2004). Characterization of the early cellular immune response to Leishmania major using peripheral blood mononuclear cells from Leishmania-naive humans. *The American Journal of Tropical Medicine and Hygiene, 71*(5), 568−576.

Rossouw, M., Nel, H. J., Cooke, G. S., van Helden, P. D., & Hoal, E. G. (2003). Association between tuberculosis and a polymorphic NFkappaB binding site in the interferon gamma gene. *Lancet, 361*(9372), 1871−1872.

Samant, M., Sahu, U., Pandey, S. C., & Khare, P. (2021). Role of cytokines in experimental and human visceral leishmaniasis. *Frontiers in Cellular and Infection Microbiology, 11*, 624009. Available from https://doi.org/10.3389/fcimb.2021.624009.

Solano-Gallego, L., Montserrrat-Sangrà, S., Ordeix, L., & Martínez-Orellana, P. (2016). Leishmania infantum-specific production of IFN-γ and IL-10 in stimulated blood from dogs with clinical leishmaniosis. *Parasites & Vectors, 9*(1), 317.

Solbach, W., & Laskay, T. (1999). The host response to Leishmania infection. In F. J. Dixon (Ed.), *Advances in immunology* (74, pp. 275−317). Academic Press.

Soong, L., Chang, C. H., Sun, J., Longley, B. J., Jr., Ruddle, N. H., Flavell, R. A., et al. (1997). Role of CD4 + T cells in pathogenesis associated with Leishmania amazonensis infection. *Journal of Immunology, 158*(11), 5374−5383.

Souza-Lemos, C., de-Campos, S. N., Teva, A., Porrozzi, R., & Grimaldi, G., Jr. (2011). In situ characterization of the granulomatous immune response with time in nonhealing lesional skin of Leishmania braziliensis-infected rhesus macaques (Macaca mulatta). *Veterinary Immunology and Immunopathology, 142*(3-4), 147—155.

Taylor, A. P., & Murray, H. W. (1997). Intracellular antimicrobial activity in the absence of interferon-γ: effect of interleukin-12 in experimental visceral leishmaniasis in interferon-γ gene-disrupted mice. *Journal of Experimental Medicine, 185*(7), 1231—1240.

Vouldoukis, I., Drapier, J. C., Nüssler, A. K., Tselentis, Y., Da Silva, O. A., Gentilini, M., et al. (1996). Canine visceral leishmaniasis: successful chemotherapy induces macrophage antil-eishmanial activity via the L-arginine nitric oxide pathway. *Antimicrobial Agents and Chemotherapy, 40*(1), 253—256.

Weigle, K., & Saravia, N. G. (1996). Natural history, clinical evolution, and the host-parasite interaction in New World cutaneous leishmaniasis. *Clinics in Dermatology, 14*(5), 433—450.

Chapter 12

Apoptosis in *Leishmania*: biochemical footprint and its relevance to surmount leishmaniasis

Shobha Upreti, Veni Pande, Diksha Joshi, Vinita Gouri and Mukesh Samant
Cell and Molecular Biology Laboratory, Department of Zoology, Kumaun University, SSJ Campus, Almora, India

12.1 Introduction

Apoptosis is a significant biological process, playing a crucial role starting from embryogenesis to the management of immune cells. There are several distinct morphological and biochemical features associated with this process (Kerr, Wyllie, & Currie, 1972). The former ones include a reduction in the cell size, disintegration of the nucleus, condensation of chromatin, and blebbing whereas breakdown of DNA into oligonucleotides, localization of phosphatidylserine (PS) in the outer leaflet of the plasma membrane, and protein-mediated breakdown of various intracellular substrates are the latter ones. Earlier, it was believed that apoptosis is the character of multicellular forms only. However, it is now proven apoptotic pathways also occurs in unicellular life forms (Ameisen, 1998; Arnoult et al., 2002). As per now, at least nine different species of single-celled eukaryotes have been described showing visible signs of apoptosis. These species have been believed to diverge from each other from some 2 billion years ago to 1 billion years (Ameisen, 1998). Slime mold *Dictyostelium discoideum* (Olie et al., 1998), kinetoplastid parasites of genus *Trypanosoma* (Welburn, Lillico, & Murphy, 1999) and *Leishmania* (Moreira, Del Portillo, Milder, Balanco, & Barcinski, 1996), the ciliate *Tetrahymena thermophila* (Straarup et al., 1997), and the dinoflagellate *Peridinium gatunense* (Vardi et al., 1999) comes under unicellular eukaryotes showing observable apoptosis. The fact that the kinetoplastid parasite *Leishmania* is capable of apoptosis becomes far more significant

Pathogenesis, Treatment and Prevention of Leishmaniasis. DOI: https://doi.org/10.1016/B978-0-12-822800-5.00008-1

in the context of the dangerous disease caused by it. Genus *Leishmania* includes flagella-bearing protozoa of Trypanosomatidae family and is the infective agent of leishmaniasis.

In 2017 out of the total reported leishmaniasis incidents, 94% corresponds to only seven countries: Brazil, Ethiopia, India, Kenya, Somalia, south Sudan, and Sudan (World Health Organization reports). *Leishmania*, a digenetic parasite, that is, requires two hosts for completion of its life cycle, its intermediate host is sandfly (*Phlebotomus*) and the definitive host is human. In the gut of the sandfly, the parasite multiplies into flagella-bearing promastigote form, which initially differentiates into a noninfectious procyclic form of the promastigotes in the gut and eventually matures to a highly infectious metacyclic form of the promastigotes in the mouthparts of the fly (Bates, 2008). Bite of a female sandfly *Phlebotomus* spp. (a type of sandfly in the dipteran family Psycholidae) transfers the *Leishmania* parasite in humans as metacyclic promastigotes, where they are phagocytosed and adopt an immobile amastigote form, characterized by stunted flagellum. The life cycle of *Leishmania* is very complex and requires successive changes, that is, procyclic, metacyclic, and amastigote form. To accompany these changes, the parasite goes through remarkable shrinkage which is an example of controlled autophagy. Hence, shrinking cells alone cannot act as a constant indicator of programmed cell death (PCD) in *Leishmania* (Besteiro, Williams, Morrison, Coombs, & Mottram, 2006). Studies suggest that a lack of nutrients induces autophagy in *Leishmania*, but if starved for a longer duration they undergo apoptosis.

Therefore the present chapter will bring together information regarding various biochemical events such as PS exposure, cytochrome C release, mitochondrial membrane potential ($\Delta\psi$m) loss, expression of caspases, DNA fragmentation, etc., that occurs during or leads to leishmanial apoptosis (Table 12.1) which further forms the target for various chemotherapies, hence aid in the development of more relevant drugs. It also outlines the conventional occurrence, mechanism, and apoptosis as targets for various antileishmanial drugs.

12.2 Conventional cell death

In 2015 the Nomenclature Committee on Cell Death suggested that a cell is recognized to be dead when the integrity of a cell's plasma membrane is lost, or when there is absolute disintegration of the cell along with the nucleus into "apoptotic bodies," or when there is in vivo phagocytosis of cell fragments by the proximal cell (Kroemer et al., 2005). Regulated cell death (RCD) and accidental cell death (ACD) are the two major forms of cell death (Galluzzi et al., 2015). Severe physical/chemical/mechanical harm like elevated temperatures and pressures, effective detergents, intense alteration in pH induces ACD, which is practically instant and no defined molecular

TABLE 12.1 Cell death markers in *Leishmania* spp. in response to various stimuli.

Leishmania spp.	Cell death stimulus	Cell death marker
Leishmania donovani	Novobiocin (Singh, Jayanarayan, & Dey, 2005); respiratory chain inhibitors (Mehta & Shaha, 2004); miltefosine (Paris, Loiseau, Bories, & Breard, 2004)	PS exposure
	Stationary phase (Lee et al., 2002); flavonoids (Sen et al., 2006); camptothecin (Sen et al., 2004); novobiocin (Singh et al., 2005); amphotericin B (Lee et al., 2002); miltefosine (Paris et al., 2004)	Caspase-like activity
	Stationary phase (Lee et al., 2002); edelfosine (Alzate, Arias, Moreno-Mateos, Alvarez-Barrientos, & Jimenez-Ruiz, 2007)	$\Delta\Psi m$ changes
	Stationary phase (Lee et al., 2002); novobiocin (Singh et al., 2005); miltefosine (Paris et al., 2004); respiratory chain inhibitors (Mehta & Shaha, 2004); H_2O_2 (Das, Mukherjee, & Shaha, 2001)	DNA degradation
	Novobiocin (Singh et al., 2005); miltefosine (Verma, Singh, & Dey, 2007); withaferin A (Sen et al., 2007)	Cytochrome C release
Leishmania major	Serum deprivation/stationary phase (Zangger, Mottram, & Fasel, 2002)	Caspase-like activity
	Serum deprivation/stationary phase (Zangger et al., 2002)	DNA degradation
Leishmania infantum	Heat shock (Alzate, Alvarez-Barrientos, Gonzalez, & Jimenez-Ruiz, 2006)	PS exposure
	Heat shock (Alzate et al., 2006); edelfosine (Alzate et al., 2007)	Caspase-like activity
	Heat shock (Alzate et al., 2006); edelfosine (Alzate et al., 2007)	$\Delta\Psi m$ changes
	Heat shock (Alzate et al., 2006); edelfosine (Alzate et al., 2007)	DNA degradation
Leishmania mexicana	Serum deprivation/stationary phase (Zangger et al., 2002)	Caspase-like activity
	Serum deprivation/stationary phase (Zangger et al., 2002)	DNA degradation
Leishmania amazonensis	Metacyclogenesis (Wanderley et al., 2009);	PS exposure
	nitric oxide (NO) (Holzmuller et al., 2002)	DNA degradation

machinery is associated with this kind of cell death (Galluzzi et al., 2015). Consequently, activation or inhibition of ACD through a particular drug, and genetic manipulation is not applicable. Conversely, RCD having molecular machinery is genetically encoded and can be altered through genetic and pharmacological variation (Galluzzi et al., 2015). The following two situations lead to RCD: in the first case, when a cell is going through microenvironmental interference, in the second case, physiological reasons are being associated with RCD for example, during the development of an embryo, tissue homeostasis, and immune response occurs thus also known as PCD (Galluzzi et al., 2015). Characteristically, necrosis, apoptosis, and autophagy are explained depending upon the morphology of the cell. Morphological characterization of necrosis includes swelling of the organelle, an increase in cell volume, and loss of integrity of the plasma membrane as a result intracellular contents are lost (Kroemer et al., 2005). Earlier necrosis was thought to be an accidental non-RCD that induces ACD but now it is explained to be a probable inducer of RCD because it can be controlled finely due to definite pathways of signal transduction (Kroemer et al., 2005).

Kerr et al. (1972) coined the word "apoptosis" which is identified by numerous morphological features—shrinkage and rounding of a cell, condensation of chromatin, some ultrastructural alteration of organelles of cytoplasm, fragmented DNA, changes in the plasma membrane with its integrity being maintained, and membrane blebbing that leads to the formation of apoptotic bodies (Kroemer et al., 2005). RCD is induced by apoptosis and is mistakenly baffled with PCD which as above mentioned is associated with physiological reasons and therefore also regarded as a physiological form of RCD that happens in a situation like tissue homeostasis and embryo development (Galluzzi et al., 2012). Intracellular/extracellular stimuli instigate apoptosis by the means of two signal transduction pathways namely intrinsic/extrinsic respectively (the two interrelated pathways). Pro- and antiapoptotic molecules belonging to the Bcl-2 family are associated with the intrinsic pathways that depend upon the permeabilization of the outer membrane of the mitochondrion and causing it to release molecules like cytochrome C, thereby activating caspases enzymes (Elmore, 2007). Besides caspases enzymes and molecules belonging to the Bcl-2 family, the extrinsic pathway employs cell death receptors linked with the plasma membrane (Bredesen, 2000). *Leishmania* cell death is shown to be regulated and not accidental by the latest findings of various proteins as cell death effectors (Proto, Coombs, & Mottram, 2013). Though as compared to other eukaryotes, either ancestral or higher eukaryotes like yeast, the understanding of *Leishmania* cell death is not much.

12.3   Relevance of apoptosis in *Leishmania*

Controlled cell suicide in multicellular organisms is the usual method that permits the elimination of extra cells throughout the development of organism;

cells that have been damaged will form the entire organism (Elmore, 2007). Before the explanation of numerous in vivo functions of RCD, the suicide of cells has been a subject of discussion for a long time. In the case of *Leishmania*, RCD proves to control the population of the parasite since the resources in the gut of the sandfly are inadequate (Lee et al., 2002). For example, undifferentiated promastigotes (that have not transformed into an infectious metacyclic form) enter RCD which is advantageous to metacyclic form because the uptake of necessary nutrients are in a limited amount in the gut of the sandfly and would not be hindered by the procyclic form (Lee et al., 2002). Consequently, RCD emerges to be a selfless method for the preference of appropriate parasites for the spread of disease. Moreover, RCD evades hyperparasitism by adjusting the density of the parasite which otherwise would hinder the transmission of the parasite by killing the host (Bruchhaus, Roeder, Rennenberg, & Heussler, 2007). It has been confirmed that the macrophages are induced to secrete molecules which are antiinflammatory like interleukin 10 (IL-10), transforming growth factor beta (TGF-β), or lipids similar to lipoxin A4 in response to the internalization of *Leishmania* and conversely restrains the release of cytokines like tumor necrosis factor alpha and lipids like leukotriene molecules that are proinflammatory (Wanderley et al., 2009) (Samant, Sahu, Pandey, & Khare, 2021). Reduction in the parasitic antigen presentation by macrophages also seems to occur because of the phagocytosis of apoptotic cells (Zangger et al., 2002). Finally, the autophagic mechanism of the host cells also gets activated by the apoptotic cells that decline the proliferation of T cells thereby maintaining the survival of the parasite (Crauwels et al., 2015). "Selfish altruism" has been given for meeting the criteria of RCD in parasitic protozoans: a selfless trend employed for clonal whole population (Smirlis et al., 2010).

In simple words, PS, a ligand exposed to the outer leaflet of the lipid bilayer is crucial for the internalization of amastigotes inside the human host. This whole process of internalization is not harmful to the amastigotes as PS recognition by the macrophage inside the host triggers the release of TGF-β and IL-10 thus suppressing the production of NO and inactivating the macrophages consequently favoring the growth of *Leishmania* in macrophage of the human host (de Freitas Balanco et al., 2001).

The surplus amount of cells growing together may upshot contact inhibition, a process where cells die off as a result of contact established due to excessive division leading to lack of nutrients and other necessities, thus it makes sense that *Leishmania* undergo apoptosis to check its multiplication consequently aiding in its survival. Observing the life cycle of *Leishmania* gives an idea about the site of apoptosis, where the parasite is in close association with each other, namely inside the vector's gut and within the host macrophages. Apoptosis kick starts when the procyclic form of the parasite inside the vector gut starts multiplying their number, which would be fatal for the vector and subsequently for the parasite too as it would halt its

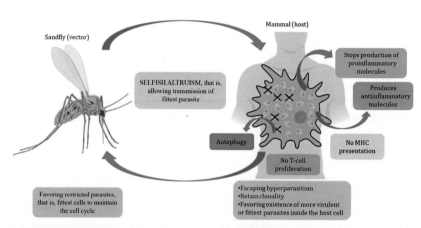

FIGURE 12.1 Diagrammatic illustration of *Leishmania* RCD.

transmission process, likewise in the host macrophages where amastigotes are present (Killick-Kendrick, 1990). Besides, limiting the multiplication of cells, apoptosis is thought to be relevant in limiting the numbers of unfit cells. Consequently, controlling cell count as well, this is an important aspect for the survival of both promastigotes and amastigotes in the insect gut and host macrophage, respectively. These physiological roles associated with *Leishmania* RCD are demonstrated in Fig. 12.1.

12.4 Biochemical footprints in *Leishmania*

12.4.1 Morphological changes

Leishmania show variations in its shape and size both in the insect vector and human host. The parasite undergoes various differentiations in its life cycle. When it transforms from procyclic to metacyclic form in the gut of insect vector there is a significant reduction in its size usually thought to be an autophagic process (Besteiro et al., 2006) which is not a part of apoptosis. Though when the promastigote reaches the stationary phase (when cell number stops increasing) some significant features of apoptosis were observed (Lee et al., 2002).

Studies (Basmaciyan, Berry, Gros, Azas, & Casanova, 2018) suggest that autophagy and apoptosis show some differences among them, namely cells undergoing autophagy become narrower with a decrease in the cellular area while apoptosis is marked by rounding up of cells, area increase, and cell shrinkage. Cells undergoing autophagy showed variation in their motility pattern (ceased movement or moving very fast) while apoptotic cells did not show any signs of defected motility. The study also suggests that the absence of nutrients in autophagic cells results in apoptosis. Autophagy is a self-destruction process, creating metabolic reactants to fulfill the energetic requirements of cells, thus ensuring cell survival in a nutrient starving environment (Basmaciyan et al., 2018; Besteiro et al., 2006; Lum, DeBerardinis, & Thompson, 2005). Despite these observations, morphological changes (i.e., nuclear condensation, reduction in cell size) are still in a great need to be further studied and it is dubious to use morphological changes as an indicator of apoptosis.

12.4.2 Phosphatidylserine

PS is one of the crucial biomarkers of apoptosis placed generally on the inner side of the phospholipid bilayer however it gets exposed to the outer layer during apoptosis as demonstrated in Fig. 12.2. In *Leishmania*, various studies have been carried out where starvation, heat shock, chemical stimuli, and stationary growth phase leads to exposure of PS in promastigotes (refer Table 12.1), which is proved by the binding of annexin V (a marker of apoptosis in them (de Freitas Balanco et al., 2001; Jimenez-Ruiz et al., 2010).

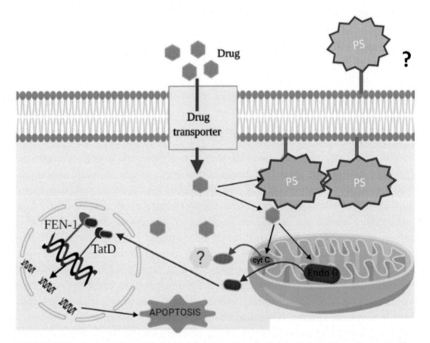

FIGURE 12.2 Action of drugs inside *Leishmania*: drugs in *Leishmania* leads to the externalization of PS (further study required), moreover translocation of cytochrome C (role of cyt C in cytoplasm still needs investigation), as well as endonuclease G (Endo G) from mitochondria to cytosol and nucleus, respectively, have been observed. Inside the nucleus Endo G form complex with nucleases such as FEN-1 (flap endonuclease-1) and TatD (Tat stands for Twin arginine translocation, however, TatD is a nuclease) individually, resulting in the severing of DNA which ultimately leads to apoptosis.

The exposed PS further binds to the receptors present on the host macrophage resulting in the internalization of the parasite and also release of some antiinflammatory cytokines like TGF-β by the host macrophage which suppresses the inflammation (Wanderley et al., 2009).

Despite all the reports available, the presence of PS is still questionable in *Leishmania* (Fig. 12.2). To sort this out various papers have been reviewed and it was found that though Weingartner et al. (2012) questioned the presence of PS, Imbert et al. (2012) showed the presence of PS in promastigotes of *Leishmania donovani*. Further, there were studies carried out, among the interesting one is by Banerjee, Roychoudhury, and Ali (2008) who demonstrated that annexin V incubated promastigotes survived when exposed to PS-specific antibody (PC-SA) liposome (which has a high affinity for PS). This shows that annexin V would have covered all the exposed PS, thus making it difficult for the PC-SA liposome to bind. Annexin V, protein S, and PS-SA were used to confirm the presence of PS is in promastigotes of *Leishmania major* (Zangger et al., 2002). There is much evidence that suggests that amastigotes treated with annexin V at high calcium concentration decreased its contagious power by 50% moreover reduced TGF-β1 released by the infected macrophages (de Freitas Balanco et al., 2001). Also, when macrophages infected with *L. donovani* strains were stimulated by antileishmanial drugs like antimony for about 12 hours, PS gets exposed leading to cell death in the parasite (Sudhandiran & Shaha, 2003). Hence, PS is an apoptotic marker in amastigotes, though the exact mechanism remains unknown.

12.4.3 Mitochondrial modification

Mitochondria, popularly known as the powerhouse of a cell are critical players of cell death, since *Leishmania* possess a single mitochondrion, its whole machinery depends on this mitochondrion for survival, therefore making it an imperative target for potent drugs (Alzate et al., 2006, 2007; Lee et al., 2002; Mehta & Shaha, 2004; Paris et al., 2004; Sen et al., 2007; Zangger et al., 2002). Translocation of cytochrome C from the inter mitochondrial space into the cytosol has been observed in *Leishmania* spp. in response to various stimuli as presented in Table 12.1 and shown in Fig. 12.2. Lack of knowledge regarding the downstream signaling of cytochrome C (i.e., binding to Apaf-1 and caspase-9 activation) makes it a less relevant apoptotic marker (Gannavaram & Debrabant, 2012).

Disruption of $\Delta\psi$m is also one of the markers of apoptosis since maintenance of $\Delta\psi$m is crucial for the viability of a cell (specifically for a cell with a single mitochondrion) (Gottlieb, 2000, 2003). Several studies in *Leishmania* suggest that various stimuli disrupt $\Delta\psi$m leading to cell death (Table 12.1). Experiments have been done where hydrogen peroxide (H_2O_2) was used as a death stimulus in promastigotes and disruption of the membrane potential was observed, also there were areas with variable $\Delta\psi$m inside a particular mitochondrion. This variable $\Delta\psi$m is an important aspect for the protozoans where a single mitochondrion is present compared to the metazoan where energy requirement can be compensated by one or the other mitochondria, thus metazoans can afford the disruption of the membrane potential in a mitochondrion as the active ones would compensate for the energy requirement (Diaz et al., 1999; Overly, Rieff, & Hollenbeck, 1996). Excluding protozoan, where disruption in the membrane potential would lead to complete shut off of the machinery, consequently making this variation in $\Delta\psi$m an imperative marker of protozoan apoptosis (Shaha, 2006).

$\Delta\psi$m can also be targeted by inhibiting the complexes present in the Electron Transport Chain (ETC) of mitochondria (Table 12.1). It was observed, when the first three complexes were inhibited it resulted in cell death of *L. donovani* present in the bloodstream, though variation in $\Delta\psi$m was observed. For instance, inhibition of complex I caused hyperpolarization leading to increased superoxide generation, and inhibition of complex II caused a decrease in $\Delta\psi$m and utmost increase in H_2O_2, but comparatively a mild increase in superoxide levels, lastly inhibition of complex III induced only superoxide production and a decreased $\Delta\psi$m (Mehta & Shaha, 2004).

When mitochondrion of stationary and a log-phase *Leishmania* were observed, the stationary phase had a lower $\Delta\psi$m than the log phase suggesting that with aging there is a drop in $\Delta\psi$m (Table 12.1) (Rosenthal & Marty, 2003). In a nutshell, the incidence of a particular mitochondrion in *Leishmania* plays a significant role in apoptosis.

12.4.4 Apoptotic proteins in *Leishmania*

Despite various studies that confirm cell death in *Leishmania*, its mechanism is still dubious. One of the reasons behind this is the crucial mammalian apoptotic proteins (antiapoptotic molecules, caspases, and cell death receptors) in *Leishmania* are still not recognized (Smirlis et al., 2010). However, there are some proteins which have been acknowledged in *Leishmania* which can be used as targets for potential apoptotic drugs:

12.4.4.1 Endonuclease G

Endo G is an apoptotic protein in metazoans (mammals and *Caenorhabditis elegans*), which normally lies in the mitochondria, but as soon as it confronts any apoptotic stimuli it moves into the nucleus where it shows its nuclease activity by severing the DNA. Two species of *Leishmania* [LINF_100012900 in *Leishmania infantum* and LdBPK_100600.1 in *L. donovani* (BoseDasgupta et al., 2008; Lee et al., 2002; Rico et al., 2009)] are recognized to comprise Endo G with similar functions as in metazoans, and R, G, and H are the three conserved regions in both the species of *Leishmania* which were mentioned to account for their in vitro nuclease activity [1(LINF_100012900 in *L. infantum* and LdBPK_100600.1 in *L. donovani* (BoseDasgupta et al., 2008; Lee et al., 2002; Rico et al., 2009)].

Endo G has been scrutinized in promastigote and amastigote culture (axenic) where it was found to be a crucial protein for their survival and is placed inside the mitochondrion of both the forms (LINF_100012900 in *L. infantum* and LdBPK_100600.1 in *L. donovani* (BoseDasgupta et al., 2008; Lee et al., 2002; Rico et al., 2009, 2014). The mechanism how Endo G acts are well-known and have been illustrated in Fig. 12.2, it is studied that in response to various stimuli, namely edelfosine and H_2O_2, it translocates to the nucleus from the mitochondria where it builds complexes with nucleases such as FEN-1 (flap endonuclease-1) and TatD individually (BoseDasgupta et al., 2008). Consequently, resulting in the severing of DNA (precisely single-stranded DNA) with exonuclease or endonuclease activity, the Table 12.1 shows some of the stimuli which induce degradation of DNA by activating nucleases in *Leishmania* (BoseDasgupta et al., 2008; Lee et al., 2002; Rico et al., 2009, 2014). Therefore taking into account the level of characterization of these particular proteins in apoptosis, makes it a crucial target for antileishmanial drugs.

12.4.4.2 Metacaspases (MCAs)

Some of the crucial regulators of apoptosis in metazoans are the members of the BCl-2 family and caspases. Though in *Leishmania* evidence regarding the presence of BCl-2 members are rare, however, some studies showed the presence of proteins similar to caspases (Alzate et al., 2006; Lee et al., 2002).

MCAs are orthologs of caspases, as both are cysteine proteases although with a distinct site of action, that is, Asp for caspases and Lys (L)/arginine (R) for MCA (Alzate et al., 2006; Meslin, Beavogui, Fasel, & Picot, 2011; Vercammen, Declercq, Vandenabeele, & Van Breusegem, 2007). MCAs has an His/Cys catalytic dyad and a P-rich site at the *C*-terminal similar to the p20 and p10 subunit of caspase, respectively (Alzate et al., 2006; Tsiatsiani et al., 2011; Vercammen et al., 2007; Zalila et al., 2011). Studies in various *Leishmania* spp. confirms that the site of cleavage is particularly R situated at 63, 136, 218, and 298 positions and His147/Cys202 being the catalytic dyad (Basmaciyan et al., 2018). The MCAs in *L. major* are termed as LmjMCA and are coded by the LmjF.35.1580 gene. These MCAs are translated in both stationary and log-phase promastigote forms and also in amastigote forms (Table 12.1) (Alzate et al., 2006; Ambit, Fasel, Coombs, & Mottram, 2008). It has cytoplasmic localization but can also inhabit mitochondrion owing to its *N*-terminal localization signal (Ambit et al., 2008; Zalila et al., 2011). The specific location of LmjMCA is altered throughout the cell cycle as it gets uniformly distributed in the entire cytoplasm during interphase, and remain attached to kinetoplast, at the time of organellar separation or along with mitotic spindles during mitosis (Ambit et al., 2008). LmjMCA does not act similar to caspase but actions very similar to trypsin can be observed against the R residue situated at P1 which rely on the catalytic dyad His147/Cys202(Alzate et al., 2006; Martin, Gonzalez, & Fasel, 2014), though it takes part in PCD as caspases. Moreover, overexpressing LmjMCA causes apoptosis after heat stress, oxidative stress, or after the introduction of an antileishmanial drug (miltefosine or curcumin) in *L. major* (Zalila et al., 2011), while its knock out results into hampering of miltefosine- and curcumin-triggered apoptosis (Casanova et al., 2015). Specifically, apoptotic stimulus triggers the self-processing activity of LmjMCA, which depends on the catalytic dyad, leading to breakdown of the *C*-terminal domain and discharging the catalytic domain, generally from amino acids 136−218, bearing the catalytic dyad His147/Cys202 (Alzate et al., 2006; Zalila et al., 2011). It looks like that the release of catalytic domain causes PCD by the enzymatic breakdown of substrates, whereas the pro-rich domain at *C*-terminus which is discharged in apoptosis, act together with stress regulatory proteins like LmaMPK7 which is a mitogen-activated protein kinase, and LmCALP27.2 which is protease-like calpains (Casanova et al., 2015). Additionally, LmjMCA is also engaged with autophagy in *L. major*, a much-needed process for cell survival (Casanova et al., 2015), elucidating its wider role other than cell death (Djavaheri-Mergny, Maiuri, & Kroemer, 2016; Jeong et al., 2011; Lamkanfi, Festjens, Declercq, Vanden Berghe, & Vandenabeele, 2007). A total of two MCAs have been described till now for *L. donovani* and these are LdMC1 (DQ367530) and LdMC2 (DQ367531) (Lee et al., 2002). Among them, LdMC1 has expression in both amastigotes (axenic) and promastigotes (Lee et al., 2002). However, unlike LmjMCA, it remains unprocessed in PCD and wild-type conditions (Lee et al., 2002). LdMC1 remains localized in acidocalcisomes, where acidic pH keeps a check on its activity (Lee et al., 2002). Lack of caspase-like activity makes it resistant towards caspase inhibitors, although the presence of trypsin-like activity aids in cleaving the sites containing R/K at the P1 position (Lee et al., 2002). Concludingly, LdMC1 has a possible role in H_2O_2-induced apoptosis of *L. donovani* after being released from acidocalcisomes (Lee et al., 2002). In both normal and oxidative stress−induced PCD conditions, LdMC1 and LdMC2, without any proteolytic activation, directly cut R/K containing substrates in *L. donovani*. Acidocalcisomes bearing LdMCs upon treatment with H_2O_2 are secreted out from vesicles (Lee et al., 2002). Susceptibility for hydrogen peroxide increases in leishmanial constructs having an overexpression of LdMC1 indicating its role in PCD (Lee et al., 2002).

Leishmania mexicana is also among the species of *Leishmania* where MCA has been explored for its role in PCD. LmxM.34.1580 gene codes for MCA, the only MCA, present in this species. MCA is predominantly present in the cytosol and is crucial in *L. mexicana* miltefosine-triggered PCD in promastigotes, experimentally designed LmxM.34.1580 gene knock out cells are shown to be less vulnerable to the drug miltefosine (Castanys-Munoz, Brown, Coombs, & Mottram, 2012). MCA could also have an active role in the cell cycle and intracellular amastigote production in *Leishmania* and could be loaded after encountering any proapoptotic stimuli to play its role in PCD. Nevertheless, further research is required to recognize all possible functions MCAs in *Leishmania*.

12.4.4.3 Cathepsin B-like protein

Cysteine proteinase C (CPC), is a cell death effector in *Leishmania* and is a member of the cathepsin B-like protein family (El-Fadili et al., 2010). It is originally transcribed by gene LmjF.29.0820 in *L. major*. CPC functions by binding with pan-caspase inhibitor Z-VAD-FMK (El-Fadili et al., 2010). After getting proper apoptotic stimuli such as miltefosine or heat shock, this enzyme is secreted out from lysosomes into the cytosol, where it triggers *Leishmania* apoptosis (El-Fadili et al., 2010). The release of other cell death effectors, particularly other cathepsins like CPA and CPB could also be held responsible for breaking apart of the lysosomal membrane during *Leishmania* apoptosis (El-Fadili et al., 2010; Zangger et al., 2002).

12.4.4.4 Calpains

Calpains are calcium-dependent cysteine protease (Goll, Thompson, Li, Wei, & Cong, 2003). In the mammalian system, they are engaged in a wide range of cellular roles like proliferation, differentiation, cell survival, PCD, cell migration, and cytoskeletal rearrangements (Perrin & Huttenlocher, 2002). Like other trypanosomatids, *Leishmania* also contains various proteins which are similar to calpains, even greater than that of mammals (Ersfeld, Barraclough, & Gull, 2005). They constitute proteins having a domain with high protease activity called CALP (calpain-like proteins) and short calpain resembling proteins lacking a protease domain but having a well-conserved *N*-terminal domain, known as SKCRP (small kinetoplastid calpain-related proteins) (Ersfeld et al., 2005). All calpain-like sequences present in *Leishmania*, are marked with the absence of calmodulin-related calcium-binding domain at the *C*-terminus generally present in their mammalian counterparts (Ersfeld et al., 2005). Additionally, their protease domain is deficient in cysteine/histidine/asparagine catalytic sequence, crucial for enzymatic action in mammals (Ersfeld et al., 2005).

12.4.4.5 Aquaporin

Aquaporin Li-BH3AQP was first discovered in *L. infantum* and it is coded by the LINF_220020300 gene, possessing BH3, a domain showing Bcl-2 homology. This BH3 domain is generally present in all the members of the Bcl-2 family (Genes, de Lucio, Gonzalez, et al., 2016; Genes, de Lucio,

Sanchez-Murcia, Gago, & Jimenez-Ruiz, 2016). In the mammalian system, it binds to Bcl-XL, an antiapoptotic molecule, and upon expression decreases cell viability (Genes, de Lucio, Gonzalez, et al., 2016; Genes, de Lucio, Sanchez-Murcia, et al., 2016). Li-BH3AQP has a perinuclear localization in *L. infantum* and requires some critical residues of the BH3 domain to trigger its prodeath activity. After stimulating with proapoptotic drugs like staurosporine and antimycin A, it decreases the viability of cells and leads to DNA fragmentation (Genes, de Lucio, Gonzalez, et al., 2016; Genes, de Lucio, Sanchez-Murcia, et al., 2016). Additionally, in the situation of nutrient scarcity or hypotonic stress, Li-BH3AQP has a prosurvival activity, which does not depend on critical residues of the BH3 domain (Genes, de Lucio, Gonzalez, et al., 2016; Genes, de Lucio, Sanchez-Murcia, et al., 2016). Li-BH3AQP is the first and only nonenzymatic member engaged in *Leishmania* cell death. So far, the discovery of Bcl-XL type antiapoptotic molecule has not been made possible which in turn challenges the role of Li-BH3AQP in *Leishmania* (Genes, de Lucio, Sanchez-Murcia, et al., 2016). Hence, more research is required to establish the roles of Li-BH3AQP in leishmanial apoptosis.

12.5   Apoptotic signaling in *Leishmania*

Like caspase-independent and caspase-dependent pathways in mammals (Broker, Kruyt, & Giaccone, 2005), there are pathways in *Leishmania* where MCA is the concerned protein, namely in *L. major* there are three apoptotic pathways related to MCA: first, where LmjMCA is activated (miltefosine as stimulus) known as the "classic pathway." Second, where LmjMCA is inhibited (amphotericin B and H_2O_2 as stimuli), known as the "original pathway." Third, which is LmjMCA independent [pentamidine and curcumin as stimulus (Basmaciyan et al., 2018)], where different proteases like cathepsins and calpains are thought to be involved. It is thought that in the "original pathway" probably apoptosis is induced by inhibiting autophagy caused by inhibition of LmjMCA (Casanova et al., 2015; Marino, Niso-Santano, Baehrecke, & Kroemer, 2014).

How these stimuli bring about downstream signaling which leads to apoptosis has been explained in Fig. 12.3. LmjHYD36 is an effector of is LmjMCA-independent pathway where pentamidine and curcumin are the inducers (Basmaciyan et al., 2018). It has been observed that curcumin amplified the expression of LmjHYD36 in normal strains and also in the strains which lack the LmjMCA gene (Basmaciyan et al., 2018). There have been many investigations which suggest that miltefosine also induces amplified expression of LmjHYD36 but, only in the normal strains, that is, where LmjMCA is present, proving the presence of LmjHYD36 after LmjMCA in the apoptotic pathway (Basmaciyan et al., 2018), so the sequence when miltefosine acts will be, miltefosine will activate LmjMCA which will further

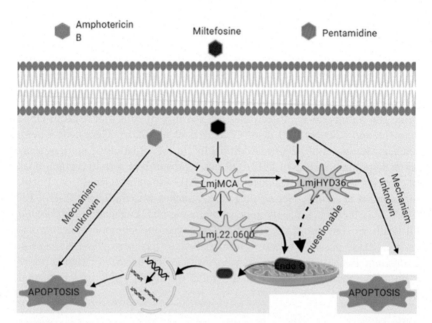

FIGURE 12.3 Modeling apoptotic signaling pathway in *Leishmania major*. By compiling available data from various studies, it can be proposed that different chemical stimuli, namely miltefosine, amphotericin B, and pentamidine activate the apoptotic pathway differently. Miltefosine inside *L. major* activates LmjMCA which leads to amplification of LmjHYD36 and Lmj.22.0600 separately. Both LmjHYD36 (questionable) and Lmj.22.0600 stimulate Endo G in the mitochondrion and in response Endo G is translocated into the nucleus where it acts as a nuclease and starts degrading the DNA which ultimately leads to apoptosis. In contrast, amphotericin B acts by inhibiting LmjMCA. Lastly, pentamidine amplifies the expression of LmjHYD36 and acts in a LmjMCA-independent manner. Both amphotericin B and pentamidine apoptotic pathways are thought to have some unknown proteins which directly lead to apoptosis.

stimulate LmjHYD36 and which will ultimately activate the nuclease Endo G to degrade the DNA, leading to apoptosis, LmjHYD36 whether activates Endo G or not still needs to be investigated, but studies confirm that it does leads to apoptosis (Basmaciyan et al., 2018). While curcumin and pentamidine act in a MCA-independent manner, thus straight away activating LmjHYD36 and further signals downstream similar to miltefosine explained above (Basmaciyan et al., 2018). How curcumin act on LmjMCA (whether inhibits it or independent of it) still needs to be investigated. Miltefosine signals apoptosis by one more pathway, where LmjMCA stimulation leads to expression of LmjF.22.0600 which activates Endo G and which ultimately leads to apoptosis. Endo G is also stimulated by H_2O_2 (Gannavaram, Vedvyas, & Debrabant, 2008), and it has been suggested that Endo G is stimulated after LmjMCA (Chowdhury et al., 2014) thus confirming the Fig. 12.3. However, there are still studies that need to be done for proposing the apoptotic signaling by the antimonials.

12.6   Targeting cell death in *Leishmania* to surmount leishmaniasis

Understanding the significance of apoptosis in parasite biology, the specific nature of proteins, apoptotic pathway, and deficiency of these proteins in humans (lack of host immunological response) has made proteins engaged in leishmanial apoptosis as emerging candidates for discovering some novel remedial tools. To make it possible, the identification of proteins and signaling pathways involved is a prerequisite (Basmaciyan et al., 2018; Kumar et al., 2020a; 2020b). For this objective, two approaches can be proposed. The first approach deals with the identification of overexpressing proteins throughout the cell death in *Leishmania*. This strategy points out the significance of calpains in the same (Ersfeld et al., 2005). The second approach revolves around finding out the substrates. For example, MCA engaged in some leishmanial apoptotic pathways, the identification of immediate neighbors of MCA in the pathway will lead to detection of effectors in apoptosis. Peculiarly, the cutting position of LmjMCA has been traced in vitro, petite peptides like GGR, GRR, RR, and VRPR work as effective LmjMCA substrates: (Alzate et al., 2006; Martin et al., 2014).

Several other restorative strategies include inhibition of leishmanial apoptosis by the use of specific inhibitors. For instance targeting LmjMCA-binding peptides for inhibition of heat stress—mediated apoptosis in *Leishmania amazonensis* (Pena, Cabral, Fotoran, Perez, & Stolf, 2017), this can be made possible by using specific MCA inhibitors which are hardly fatal to the host cells. Various liposome vectors can also be used to target promastigotes and amastigotes, as these would easily pass the lipid bilayer consequently leading to apoptosis (Basmaciyan et al., 2018). Various pathways are interconnected in almost every organism thus inhibiting a particular molecule in a pathway would lead to disruption of other pathways as well. Therefore activating the cell death pathway in *Leishmania* is less complex comparatively. Thanks to the presence of specific pathways in the parasite which decreases the probability of disturbance to the host machinery (Basmaciyan et al., 2018). Moreover, leishmanial apoptosis would not induce an immunological response in the host cells compared to necrosis. But still, as a preventative measure host cell proteins are complexed with proteins involved in leishmanial apoptosis to keep a check on the structural changes (Basmaciyan et al., 2018).

12.6.1   Induction of apoptosis by antileishmanial drugs

One of the existing first-line treatments for visceral leishmaniasis is pentavalent antimony Sb (V), whereas second-line treatment is amphotericin B and pentamidine (Vardi et al., 1999). Antimony act by suppressing the metabolic pathways but its mechanism of action is still unknown (Rosenthal & Marty, 2003). Antimony is now rarely used for treatment due to the toxicity and drug resistance appeared in the host (Kumar, Pandey, & Samant, 2018; Laguna, 2003).

Various studies confirmed that antileishmanial drugs mostly work by inducing apoptosis in the parasite, axenic amastigotes of *L. donovani* in the late log phase treated with an escalating level of Sb (V) resulted in an increased level of protease activity (Lee et al., 2002). At the same time, the promastigotes didn't show any sign of apoptosis even at a higher amount and longer exposure of Sb (V), indicating that different forms of parasite respond differently to a particular drug (Lee et al., 2002). Although, when axenic amastigotes of *L. infantum* were exposed to trivalent antimony Sb (III), cell death characteristics like severed DNA was noticed but no protease activity was observed (Holzmuller et al., 2002; Lee et al., 2002). While in its promastigotes also protease activity was missing but DNA laddering was observed (Lee et al., 2002). Therefore such studies provided the basis for the existence of a MCA-independent pathway in *Leishmania*.

The third line of treatment which would kill *Leishmania* includes amphotericin B which causes cell death by lowering the $\Delta\psi$m which leads to an increase in permeability of the mitochondrial membrane and consequently (refer Table 12.1) enhancing the protease activity (Rosenthal & Marty, 2003). Further, camptothecin has been reported to be topoisomerase I poison leading to disruption in $\Delta\psi$m and ultimately cell death. Some oral drugs like miltefosine induce apoptosis in *L. donovani* through fragmentation and condensation of DNA in its nucleus, associated with ladder formation (Verma et al., 2007). Dihydrobetulinic acid and pentacyclic triterpenoid (topoisomerase poisons) which leads to apoptosis are used to design more drugs to induce cell death in *Leishmania* (Chowdhury et al., 2003), (Chandra Pandey et al., 2019; Pandey, Jha, Kumar, & Samant, 2019). In promastigotes of *L. donovani* some compounds like quercetin and luteolin induce apoptosis by inhibiting the cell cycle progression (Mittra et al., 2000). Therefore targeting apoptosis by antileishmanial drugs can only be successful when both the promastigote and amastigote apoptosis are taken into account.

12.7 Conclusion

After comprehending various studies it can be concluded that *Leishmania* undergoes cell death. Although some proteins like MCAs and nuclease like Endo G have been fairly recognized in *Leishmania*, there is still scope for further investigation, in contrast to a multicellular organism where apoptosis has been well-known. Various forms of *Leishmania* respond differently towards a particular stimulus, thus the cell death pathway cannot be generalized in them. Therefore there is a need to further investigate a general apoptotic pathway in all forms of *Leishmania* spp. specifically inside the host, so that apoptosis could be better targeted in them.

Acknowledgments

The authors are thankful to the Department of Zoology, Kumaun University, SSJ Campus, Almora, for providing a suitable research environment.

References

Alzate, J. F., Alvarez-Barrientos, A., Gonzalez, V. M., & Jimenez-Ruiz, A. (2006). Heat-induced programmed cell death in Leishmania infantum is reverted by Bcl-X(L) expression. *Apoptosis, 11*(2), 161–171.

Alzate, J. F., Arias, A. A., Moreno-Mateos, D., Alvarez-Barrientos, A., & Jimenez-Ruiz, A. (2007). Mitochondrial superoxide mediates heat-induced apoptotic-like death in Leishmania infantum. *Molecular and Biochemical Parasitology, 152*(2), 192–202.

Ambit, A., Fasel, N., Coombs, G. H., & Mottram, J. C. (2008). An essential role for the Leishmania major metacaspase in cell cycle progression. *Cell Death and Differentiation, 15*(1), 113–122.

Ameisen, J. C. (1998). The origin of programmed cell death in the flow of evolution and its role in host-pathogen interactions. *Comptes Rendus des Seances de la Societe de Biologie et de ses Filiales, 192*(6), 1095–1098.

Arnoult, D., Akarid, K., Grodet, A., Petit, P. X., Estaquier, J., & Ameisen, J. C. (2002). On the evolution of programmed cell death: apoptosis of the unicellular eukaryote Leishmania major involves cysteine proteinase activation and mitochondrion permeabilization. *Cell Death and Differentiation, 9*(1), 65–81.

Banerjee, A., Roychoudhury, J., & Ali, N. (2008). Stearylamine-bearing cationic liposomes kill Leishmania parasites through surface exposed negatively charged phosphatidylserine. *Journal of Antimicrobial Chemotherapy, 61*(1), 103–110.

Basmaciyan, L., Berry, L., Gros, J., Azas, N., & Casanova, M. (2018). Temporal analysis of the autophagic and apoptotic phenotypes in Leishmania parasites. *Microbial Cell, 5*(9), 404–417.

Bates, P. A. (2008). Leishmania sand fly interaction: progress and challenges. *Current Opinion in Microbiology, 11*(4), 340–344.

Besteiro, S., Williams, R. A., Morrison, L. S., Coombs, G. H., & Mottram, J. C. (2006). Endosome sorting and autophagy are essential for differentiation and virulence of Leishmania major. *The Journal of Biological Chemistry, 281*(16), 11384–11396.

BoseDasgupta, S., Das, B. B., Sengupta, S., Ganguly, A., Roy, A., Dey, S., et al. (2008). The caspase-independent algorithm of programmed cell death in Leishmania induced by baicalein: the role of LdEndoG, LdFEN-1 and LdTatD as a DNA 'degradesome'. *Cell Death and Differentiation, 15*(10), 1629–1640.

Bredesen, D. E. (2000). Apoptosis: overview and signal transduction pathways. *Journal of Neurotrauma, 17*(10), 801–810.

Broker, L. E., Kruyt, F. A., & Giaccone, G. (2005). Cell death independent of caspases: a review. *Clinical Cancer Research, 11*(9), 3155–3162.

Bruchhaus, I., Roeder, T., Rennenberg, A., & Heussler, V. T. (2007). Protozoan parasites: programmed cell death as a mechanism of parasitism. *Trends in Parasitology, 23*(8), 376–383.

Casanova, M., Gonzalez, I. J., Sprissler, C., Zalila, H., Dacher, M., Basmaciyan, L., et al. (2015). Implication of different domains of the Leishmania major metacaspase in cell death and autophagy. *Cell Death & Disease, 6*, e1933.

Castanys-Munoz, E., Brown, E., Coombs, G. H., & Mottram, J. C. (2012). Leishmania mexicana metacaspase is a negative regulator of amastigote proliferation in mammalian cells. *Cell Death & Disease, 3*, e385.

Chandra Pandey, S., Dhami, D. S., Jha, A., Chandra Shah, G., Kumar, A., & Samant, M. (2019). Identification of trans-2-cis-8-Matricaria-ester from the essential oil of Erigeron multiradiatus and evaluation of its antileishmanial potential by in vitro and in silico approaches. *ACS Omega*, *4*(11), 14640–14649.

Chowdhury, A. R., Mandal, S., Goswami, A., Ghosh, M., Mandal, L., Chakraborty, D., et al. (2003). Dihydrobetulinic acid induces apoptosis in Leishmania donovani by targeting DNA topoisomerase I and II: implications in antileishmanial therapy. *Molecular Medicine*, *9*(1-2), 26–36.

Chowdhury, S., Mukherjee, T., Chowdhury, S. R., Sengupta, S., Mukhopadhyay, S., Jaisankar, P., & Majumder, H. K. (2014). Disuccinyl betulin triggers metacaspase-dependent endonuclease G-mediated cell death in unicellular protozoan parasite Leishmania donovani. *Antimicrobial Agents and Chemotherapy*, *58*(4), 2186–2201.

Crauwels, P., Bohn, R., Thomas, M., Gottwalt, S., Jackel, F., Kramer, S., et al. (2015). Apoptotic-like Leishmania exploit the host's autophagy machinery to reduce T-cell-mediated parasite elimination. *Autophagy*, *11*(2), 285–297.

Das, M., Mukherjee, S. B., & Shaha, C. (2001). Hydrogen peroxide induces apoptosis-like death in Leishmania donovani promastigotes. *Journal of Cell Science*, *114*(Pt 13), 2461–2469.

de Freitas Balanco, J. M., Moreira, M. E., Bonomo, A., Bozza, P. T., Amarante-Mendes, G., Pirmez, C., et al. (2001). Apoptotic mimicry by an obligate intracellular parasite downregulates macrophage microbicidal activity. *Current Biology*, *11*(23), 1870–1873.

Diaz, G., Setzu, M. D., Zucca, A., Isola, R., Diana, A., Murru, R., et al. (1999). Subcellular heterogeneity of mitochondrial membrane potential: relationship with organelle distribution and intercellular contacts in normal, hypoxic and apoptotic cells. *Journal of Cell Science*, *112*(Pt 7), 1077–1084.

Djavaheri-Mergny, M., Maiuri, M. C., & Kroemer, G. (2016). Cross talk between apoptosis and autophagy by caspase-mediated cleavage of Beclin 1. *Oncogene*, *29*(12), 1717–1719.

El-Fadili, A. K., Zangger, H., Desponds, C., Gonzalez, I. J., Zalila, H., Schaff, C., et al. (2010). Cathepsin B-like and cell death in the unicellular human pathogen Leishmania. *Cell Death & Disease*, *1*, e71.

Elmore, S. (2007). Apoptosis: a review of programmed cell death. *Toxicologic Pathology*, *35*(4), 495–516.

Ersfeld, K., Barraclough, H., & Gull, K. (2005). Evolutionary relationships and protein domain architecture in an expanded calpain superfamily in kinetoplastid parasites. *Journal of Molecular Evolution*, *61*(6), 742–757.

Galluzzi, L., Bravo-San Pedro, J. M., Vitale, I., Aaronson, S. A., Abrams, J. M., Adam, D., et al. (2015). Essential versus accessory aspects of cell death: recommendations of the NCCD 2015. *Cell Death and Differentiation*, *22*(1), 58–73.

Galluzzi, L., Vitale, I., Abrams, J. M., Alnemri, E. S., Baehrecke, E. H., Blagosklonny, M. V., et al. (2012). Molecular definitions of cell death subroutines: recommendations of the Nomenclature Committee on Cell Death 2012. *Cell Death and Differentiation*, *19*(1), 107–120.

Gannavaram, S., & Debrabant, A. (2012). Programmed cell death in Leishmania: biochemical evidence and role in parasite infectivity. *Frontiers in Cellular and Infection Microbiology*, *2*, 95.

Gannavaram, S., Vedvyas, C., & Debrabant, A. (2008). Conservation of the pro-apoptotic nuclease activity of endonuclease G in unicellular trypanosomatid parasites. *Journal of Cell Science*, *121*(Pt 1), 99–109.

Genes, C. M., de Lucio, H., Gonzalez, V. M., Sanchez-Murcia, P. A., Rico, E., Gago, F., et al. (2016). A functional BH3 domain in an aquaporin from Leishmania infantum. *Cell Death Discovery*, *2*, 16043.

Genes, C. M., de Lucio, H., Sanchez-Murcia, P. A., Gago, F., & Jimenez-Ruiz, A. (2016). Pro-death activity of a BH3 domain in an aquaporin from the protozoan parasite Leishmania. *Cell Death & Disease, 7*(7), e2318.

Goll, D. E., Thompson, V. F., Li, H., Wei, W., & Cong, J. (2003). The calpain system. *Physiological Reviews, 83*(3), 731−801.

Gottlieb, R. A. (2000). Role of mitochondria in apoptosis. *Critical Reviews in Eukaryotic Gene Expression, 10*(3-4), 231−239.

Gottlieb, R. A. (2003). Mitochondrial signaling in apoptosis: mitochondrial daggers to the breaking heart. *Basic Research in Cardiology, 98*(4), 242−249.

Holzmuller, P., Sereno, D., Cavaleyra, M., Mangot, I., Daulouede, S., Vincendeau, P., et al. (2002). Nitric oxide-mediated proteasome-dependent oligonucleosomal DNA fragmentation in Leishmania amazonensis amastigotes. *Infection and Immunity, 70*(7), 3727−3735.

Imbert, L., Ramos, R. G., Libong, D., Abreu, S., Loiseau, P. M., & Chaminade, P. (2012). Identification of phospholipid species affected by miltefosine action in Leishmania donovani cultures using LC-ELSD, LC-ESI/MS, and multivariate data analysis. *Analytical and Bioanalytical Chemistry, 402*(3), 1169−1182.

Jeong, H. S., Choi, H. Y., Lee, E. R., Kim, J. H., Jeon, K., Lee, H. J., et al. (2011). Involvement of caspase-9 in autophagy-mediated cell survival pathway. *Biochimica et Biophysica Acta, 1813*(1), 80−90.

Jimenez-Ruiz, A., Alzate, J. F., Macleod, E. T., Luder, C. G., Fasel, N., & Hurd, H. (2010). Apoptotic markers in protozoan parasites. *Parasites & Vectors, 3*, 104.

Kerr, J. F., Wyllie, A. H., & Currie, A. R. (1972). Apoptosis: a basic biological phenomenon with wide-ranging implications in tissue kinetics. *British Journal of Cancer, 26*(4), 239−257.

Killick-Kendrick, R. (1990). The life-cycle of Leishmania in the sandfly with special reference to the form infective to the vertebrate host. *Annales de Parasitologie Humaine et Comparee, 65*(Suppl 1), 37−42.

Kroemer, G., El-Deiry, W. S., Golstein, P., Peter, M. E., Vaux, D., Vandenabeele, P., et al. (2005). Classification of cell death: recommendations of the Nomenclature Committee on Cell Death. *Cell Death and Differentiation, 12*(Suppl 2), 1463−1467.

Kumar, A., Pandey, S. C., & Samant, M. (2018). Slow pace of antileishmanial drug development. *Parasitology Open, 4*, 1−11.

Kumar, A., Pandey, S. C., & Samant, M. (2020a). A spotlight on the diagnostic methods of a fatal disease visceral leishmaniasis. *Parasite Immunology, 42*(3), e12727.

Kumar, A., Pandey, S. C., & Samant, M. (2020b). DNA-based microarray studies in visceral leishmaniasis: identification of biomarkers for diagnostic, prognostic and drug target for treatment. *Acta Tropica, 208*, 105512.

Laguna, F. (2003). Treatment of leishmaniasis in HIV-positive patients. *Annals of Tropical Medicine and Parasitology, 97*(Suppl 1), 135−142.

Lamkanfi, M., Festjens, N., Declercq, W., Vanden Berghe, T., & Vandenabeele, P. (2007). Caspases in cell survival, proliferation and differentiation. *Cell Death and Differentiation, 14*(1), 44−55.

Lee, N., Bertholet, S., Debrabant, A., Muller, J., Duncan, R., & Nakhasi, H. L. (2002). Programmed cell death in the unicellular protozoan parasite Leishmania. *Cell Death and Differentiation, 9*(1), 53−64.

Lum, J. J., DeBerardinis, R. J., & Thompson, C. B. (2005). Autophagy in metazoans: cell survival in the land of plenty. *Nature Reviews Molecular Cell Biology, 6*(6), 439−448.

Marino, G., Niso-Santano, M., Baehrecke, E. H., & Kroemer, G. (2014). Self-consumption: the interplay of autophagy and apoptosis. *Nature Reviews Molecular Cell Biology, 15*(2), 81−94.

Martin, R., Gonzalez, I., & Fasel, N. (2014). Leishmania metacaspase: an arginine-specific peptidase. *Methods in Molecular Biology, 1133,* 189−202.

Mehta, A., & Shaha, C. (2004). Apoptotic death in Leishmania donovani promastigotes in response to respiratory chain inhibition: complex II inhibition results in increased pentamidine cytotoxicity. *The Journal of Biological Chemistry, 279*(12), 11798−11813.

Meslin, B., Beavogui, A. H., Fasel, N., & Picot, S. (2011). Plasmodium falciparum metacaspase PfMCA-1 triggers a z-VAD-fmk inhibitable protease to promote cell death. *PLoS One, 6*(8), e23867.

Mittra, B., Saha, A., Chowdhury, A. R., Pal, C., Mandal, S., Mukhopadhyay, S., et al. (2000). Luteolin, an abundant dietary component is a potent anti-leishmanial agent that acts by inducing topoisomerase II-mediated kinetoplast DNA cleavage leading to apoptosis. *Molecular Medicine, 6*(6), 527−541.

Moreira, M. E., Del Portillo, H. A., Milder, R. V., Balanco, J. M., & Barcinski, M. A. (1996). Heat shock induction of apoptosis in promastigotes of the unicellular organism Leishmania (Leishmania) amazonensis. *Journal of Cellular Physiology, 167*(2), 305−313.

Olie, R. A., Durrieu, F., Cornillon, S., Loughran, G., Gross, J., Earnshaw, W. C., et al. (1998). Apparent caspase independence of programmed cell death in Dictyostelium. *Current Biology, 8*(17), 955−958.

Overly, C. C., Rieff, H. I., & Hollenbeck, P. J. (1996). Organelle motility and metabolism in axons vs dendrites of cultured hippocampal neurons. *Journal of Cell Science, 109*(Pt 5), 971−980.

Pandey, S. C., Jha, A., Kumar, A., & Samant, M. (2019). Evaluation of antileishmanial potential of computationally screened compounds targeting DEAD-box RNA helicase of Leishmania donovani. *International Journal of Biological Macromolecules, 121,* 480−487.

Paris, C., Loiseau, P. M., Bories, C., & Breard, J. (2004). Miltefosine induces apoptosis-like death in Leishmania donovani promastigotes. *Antimicrobial Agents and Chemotherapy, 48*(3), 852−859.

Pena, M. S., Cabral, G. C., Fotoran, W. L., Perez, K. R., & Stolf, B. S. (2017). Metacaspase-binding peptide inhibits heat shock-induced death in Leishmania (L.) amazonensis. *Cell Death & Disease, 8*(3), e2645.

Perrin, B. J., & Huttenlocher, A. (2002). Calpain. *The International Journal of Biochemistry & Cell Biology, 34*(7), 722−725.

Proto, W. R., Coombs, G. H., & Mottram, J. C. (2013). Cell death in parasitic protozoa: regulated or incidental? *Nature Reviews Microbiology, 11*(1), 58−66.

Rico, E., Alzate, J. F., Arias, A. A., Moreno, D., Clos, J., Gago, F., et al. (2009). Leishmania infantum expresses a mitochondrial nuclease homologous to EndoG that migrates to the nucleus in response to an apoptotic stimulus. *Molecular and Biochemical Parasitology, 163*(1), 28−38.

Rico, E., Oliva, C., Gutierrez, K. J., Alzate, J. F., Genes, C. M., Moreno, D., et al. (2014). Leishmania infantum EndoG is an endo/exo-nuclease essential for parasite survival. *PLoS One, 9*(2), e89526.

Rosenthal, E., & Marty, P. (2003). Recent understanding in the treatment of visceral leishmaniasis. *Journal of Postgraduate Medicine, 49*(1), 61−68.

Sen, N., Banerjee, B., Das, B. B., Ganguly, A., Sen, T., Pramanik, S., et al. (2007). Apoptosis is induced in leishmanial cells by a novel protein kinase inhibitor withaferin A and is facilitated by apoptotic topoisomerase I-DNA complex. *Cell Death and Differentiation, 14*(2), 358−367.

Sen, N., Das, B. B., Ganguly, A., Banerjee, B., Sen, T., & Majumder, H. K. (2006). Leishmania donovani: intracellular ATP level regulates apoptosis-like death in luteolin induced dyskinetoplastid cells. *Experimental Parasitology, 114*(3), 204−214.

Sen, N., Das, B. B., Ganguly, A., Mukherjee, T., Bandyopadhyay, S., & Majumder, H. K. (2004). Camptothecin-induced imbalance in intracellular cation homeostasis regulates programmed cell death in unicellular hemoflagellate Leishmania donovani. *The Journal of Biological Chemistry*, *279*(50), 52366−52375.

Samant, M., Sahu, U., Pandey, S. C., & Khare, P. (2021). Role of Cytokines in Experimental and Human Visceral Leishmaniasis. *Front Cell Infect Microbiol*, *11*, 624009. Available from https://doi.org/10.3389/fcimb.2021.624009.

Shaha, C. (2006). Apoptosis in Leishmania species & its relevance to disease pathogenesis. *The Indian Journal of Medical Research*, *123*(3), 233−244.

Singh, G., Jayanarayan, K. G., & Dey, C. S. (2005). Novobiocin induces apoptosis-like cell death in topoisomerase II over-expressing arsenite resistant Leishmania donovani. *Molecular and Biochemical Parasitology*, *141*(1), 57−69.

Smirlis, D., Duszenko, M., Ruiz, A. J., Scoulica, E., Bastien, P., Fasel, N., et al. (2010). Targeting essential pathways in trypanosomatids gives insights into protozoan mechanisms of cell death. *Parasites & Vectors*, *3*, 107.

Straarup, E. M., Schousboe, P., Hansen, H. Q., Kristiansen, K., Hoffmann, E. K., Rasmussen, L., et al. (1997). Effects of protein kinase C activators and staurosporine on protein kinase activity, cell survival, and proliferation in Tetrahymena thermophila. *Microbios*, *91*(368-369), 181−190.

Sudhandiran, G., & Shaha, C. (2003). Antimonial-induced increase in intracellular Ca2 + through non-selective cation channels in the host and the parasite is responsible for apoptosis of intracellular Leishmania donovani amastigotes. *The Journal of Biological Chemistry*, *278*(27), 25120−25132.

Tsiatsiani, L., Van Breusegem, F., Gallois, P., Zavialov, A., Lam, E., & Bozhkov, P. V. (2011). Metacaspases. *Cell Death and Differentiation*, *18*(8), 1279−1288.

Vardi, A., Berman-Frank, I., Rozenberg, T., Hadas, O., Kaplan, A., & Levine, A. (1999). Programmed cell death of the dinoflagellate Peridinium gatunense is mediated by CO(2) limitation and oxidative stress. *Current Biology*, *9*(18), 1061−1064.

Vercammen, D., Declercq, W., Vandenabeele, P., & Van Breusegem, F. (2007). Are metacaspases caspases? *The Journal of Cell Biology*, *179*(3), 375−380.

Verma, N. K., Singh, G., & Dey, C. S. (2007). Miltefosine induces apoptosis in arsenite-resistant Leishmania donovani promastigotes through mitochondrial dysfunction. *Experimental Parasitology*, *116*(1), 1−13.

Wanderley, J. L., Pinto da Silva, L. H., Deolindo, P., Soong, L., Borges, V. M., Prates, D. B., et al. (2009). Cooperation between apoptotic and viable metacyclics enhances the pathogenesis of Leishmaniasis. *PLoS One*, *4*(5), e5733.

Weingartner, A., Kemmer, G., Muller, F. D., Zampieri, R. A., Gonzaga dos Santos, M., Schiller, J., et al. (2012). Leishmania promastigotes lack phosphatidylserine but bind annexin V upon permeabilization or miltefosine treatment. *PLoS One*, *7*(8), e42070.

Welburn, S. C., Lillico, S., & Murphy, N. B. (1999). Programmed cell death in procyclic form Trypanosoma brucei rhodesiense—identification of differentially expressed genes during con A induced death. *Memorias do Instituto Oswaldo Cruz*, *94*(2), 229−234.

Zalila, H., Gonzalez, I. J., El-Fadili, A. K., Delgado, M. B., Desponds, C., Schaff, C., et al. (2011). Processing of metacaspase into a cytoplasmic catalytic domain mediating cell death in Leishmania major. *Molecular Microbiology*, *79*(1), 222−239.

Zangger, H., Mottram, J. C., & Fasel, N. (2002). Cell death in Leishmania induced by stress and differentiation: programmed cell death or necrosis? *Cell Death and Differentiation*, *9*(10), 1126−1139.

Chapter 13

Immunological determinants, host immune responses, and animal models of visceral leishmaniasis

Awanish Kumar
Department of Biotechnology, National Institute of Technology, Raipur, India

13.1 Introduction

Visceral leishmaniasis (VL) is a vector-borne disease caused by protozoan parasite Leishmania donovani (an obligate intracellular parasite). The parasite exists as flagellated procyclic promastigote form in vector sandflies (invertebrate host) and in vitro culture having $15-20$ μm in length, $1.5-3.5$ μm in breadth and metacyclic form (highly motile, long flagella, $5-8$ μm). The length of single and delicate flagellum is $15-28$ μm (Herwaldt, 1999). The form of *Leishmania* that occurs in mammalian hosts (vertebrate) is amastigote, which is a nonflagellated ($2-4$ μm diameter) form and resides/replicates in host macrophages. After an infected blood meal, the vector takes about $4-18$ days (according to the *Leishmania* species) and is able to transmit the infection to the victim. This disease is endemic in 88 countries of the world (American continent, Asia, the Middle East, southern Europe, and Africa). About 350 million people are at risk of *Leishmania* infection and annually about 500,000 new cases of visceral form of leishmaniasis occur every year. Ninety percent of VL cases are reported in Bangladesh, Nepal, northeastern India, northeastern Brazil, and Sudan. This disease is mainly restricted to Bihar, West Bengal, and northeastern areas of Uttar Pradesh province of India, but cases of VL have been also reported from Assam, Tamil Nadu, and Orissa state of India now (Torres-Guerrero, Quintanilla-Cedillo, Ruiz-Esmenjaud, & Arenas, 2017).

VL is also known as kala-azar and it includes a broad range of clinical manifestations (Pandey, Kumar, & Samant, 2020). VL remains subclinical or asymptomatic in many cases and the major cause of mortality and morbidity.

Pathogenesis, Treatment and Prevention of Leishmaniasis. DOI: https://doi.org/10.1016/B978-0-12-822800-5.00012-3

It may follow an acute, subacute, or chronic cased. VL is caused by species complex *Leishmania donovani* (i.e., *L. donovani* and *Leishmania infantum* in old world and *Leishmania chagasi* in new world) (Deak, Jayakumar, & Cho, 2010; Kumar, Pandey, & Samant, 2018). The etiological agents, vectors, host range, geographical distribution, and clinical manifestations of VL causing parasite are discussed in Table 13.1. VL is characterized by fever, hepatosplenomegaly, severe cachexia, hypergammaglobulinemia [mainly immunoglobulin G (IgG) from polyclonal B-cell activation] with hypoalbuminemia, and pancytopenia. The extreme scragginess develops, skin becomes dark, and hair becomes dry and certain complications may occur like dysentery, epistaxis, herpes zoster, and pulmonary tuberculosis. At many places, VL also primes to post-kala-azar dermal leishmaniasis (PKDL). PKDL is considered as a syndrome that develops at variable times after resolution of VL in a person. It is associated with the relapse of visceral disease and is manifested by the lesions of skin. Initially PKDL is most prominent on the face. People with chronic PKDL are served as reservoir hosts of infection (Zijlstra, Musa, Khalil, el-Hassan, & el-Hassan, 2003). A number of immunological determinants take part in the establishment of *L. donovani* infection in the host.

13.2 Immunological determinants of *Leishmania* infection

Various immunological determinants are involved at different levels of *Leishmania* infection and they are described below.

13.2.1 Host−parasite interaction

VL is an exceptional example of a complex parasite−host interaction and a number of molecular determinants are involved during this interaction. Promastigotes of *Leishmania* bind to macrophage surface molecules [complement receptor 1 and 3 (CR1 and CR3) and C3b] before they get internalized. CR1 is the major ligand of macrophage for mature promastigotes. *Leishmania* surface glycoprotein (e.g., gp63 membrane protease) and other macrophage receptors (e.g., CR3, mannose−fucose receptor) have been also reported in the interaction. Once promastigotes internalized, they transform into intracellular form known as amastigotes. Amastigotes multiplies by binary fission and ultimately macrophage ruptures and spreading takes place to the uninfected cells. The identification of natural antibodies coating amastigotes in vivo suggested that macrophage FcIg and CR3 receptors might contribute to the phagocytosis. As we know, *Leishmania* promastigotes are covered with a dense surface glycocalyx molecule which is anchored by the glycosylphosphatidylinositol (GPI). These GPI-anchored molecules include proteins such as gp63 (parasite surface protease) and proteophosphoglycan (PPG). The most profuse component is LPG (a large GPI-anchored

TABLE 13.1 The etiological agents, vectors, host range, geographical distribution, and clinical manifestations of visceral leishmaniasis.

Species	Regions of the world involved	Infection in	Vector	Reservoir	Clinical manifestations
Leishmania donovani	Eastern Asia, India, Africa	Humans	Phlebotomus argentipes, Lutzomyia longipalpis	Dogs, savannah rodents, humans	VL, PKDL
Leishmania infantum	Mediterranean basin, Middle East, and Asian countries	Wild canines and domestic dogs	Phlebotomus alexandri, Lutzomyia migonei	Dogs, cats, foxes, jackals	Zoonotic VL
Leishmania chagasi	South American countries	Human	L. longipalpis	Dogs, humans	Zoonotic VL

phosphoglycan called lipophosphoglycan) (Späth, Epstein, & Leader, 2000). LPG and gp63 is responsible for the virulence of the parasite (Fig. 13.1). LPG has been concerned with many steps required for the establishment infection inside macrophage and the survival. LPG has no role in the amastigotes stage, but amastigotes continue to make a glycoconjugates which is structurally related to LPG. On the other hand, gp63 helps *Leishmania* parasite to enter into the host cells and in survival. gp63 has the potential to degrade immunoglobulins, complement factors, and lysosomal proteins because it is a broad substrate spectrum endoproteinase. *Leishmania* amastigotes survive in the acidic environment of macrophage (phagolysosomes) because its proteolytic activity at pH 4 bears apparent relevance (Kumar, 2013). Toll-like receptor (TLR) was firstly reported in *Drosophila* but later they have been also reported on mammalian cells including macrophages and dendritic cells (DCs). TLRs are the components of the innate immunity and induce nonspecific immune response. *Leishmania* may also bind to TLRs of host macrophages surface and can switch on the early genes of the host to regulate the parasite and host interactions but the indepth mechanism is still unknown. After internalization of *Leishmania* parasite into phagosomes, secondary lysosomes of macrophage are fused to form the complete PV (Mogensen, 2009). At this stage promastigote rapidly transformed into intracellular amastigotes. Due to the transformation, promastigote LPG

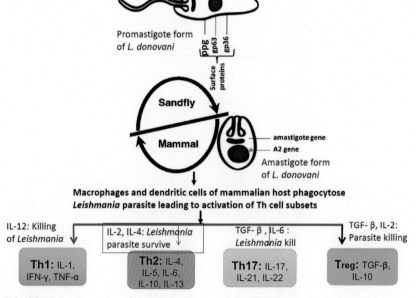

FIGURE 13.1   Generation of various responses and functioning of helper T-cell once macrophages and dendritic cells of host phagocytose *Leishmania* parasite.

shedding takes place and it is migrated to the surface of the infected macrophages. LPG inhibits the hydrolytic activity of the lysosomal enzymes and respiratory burst (a natural process of cell rupture that occurs after phagocytosis and) of macrophage possibly due to the inhibition of protein kinase C and chelation of calcium (Späth et al., 2000). Various markers (like proton ATPase34 and LAMP-1) are considered for intracellular compartmentalization due to which amastigotes replicate in macrophages. Major histocompatibility complex (MHC) class II molecules association to PV suggests a mechanism by which the immune response to this intracellular organism becomes class II and CD4 dependent.

13.2.2 Antigen presentation and immune components involved in *Leishmania* infection

Neutrophils or polymorphonuclear neutrophils are the first cells that migrate to the site of VL infection. It acts as a primary effector or phagocytic cells that phogocytoses *Leishmania* parasite. *Leishmania* phagocytosed neutrophils start secreting the chemokines like interleukin (IL)-842 which is very essential to bring more neutrophils to the site of infection. The second wave of cells (monocytes/macrophages) enters the site of infection 2−3 days later (Liu & Uzonna, 2012). DCs are also potent antigen-presenting cells and can induce T-cell activation very efficiently. It has also been shown that DCs are the source of different interleukins. Incubation of *Leishmania* promastigotes with DCs induced early production of IL-12 (shown in vitro) which might be contributed from the preexisting pool of IL-12 which was secreted soon after ligation of any microbial product. It is also reported that uptake of *Leishmania* amastigotes by skin-derived DCs induces IL-12. DCs are potent candidate for VL immunotherapy. DCs can induce immunity to infections upon loading with microbial antigens (McDowell, Marovich, Lira, Braun, & Sacks, 2002).

13.2.3 Survival and evasion strategies of *Leishmania* in host macrophages

Before entry into macrophages, most of the extracellular promastigotes are killed by complement system of host. However, some *Leishmania* parasite survives due to resistance to complement-mediated lysis. Resistance is achieved by LPG-associated spontaneous shedding of C5b-C9 complexes from the surface of *Leishmania* parasite. Serine/threonine protein kinase of metacyclic *Leishmania* inactivates C3, CS, and C9 of complement system by the process of phosphorylation (Gurung & Kanneganti, 2015). At the same time *Leishmania* also expresses gp63 (an mctzincin zinc proteinase also called as leishmanolysin), which converts C3b to iC3b (opsonic complement factor) and promotes the uptake of the parasites by host cells having iCR3

(CD11b/CDI8). The surviving *Leishmania* adheres to the host cells of the monocyte/macrophage including DCs, Langerhans cells, and human granulocytes. This adherence is mediated by several receptors like fibronectin receptor, mannose—fucose receptor, and the receptor for C-reactive protein. Type-I (CR1, CD3S) and Type-III (CR111, CD11b/CD18) Complement receptors bind to complement components attached to the parasite plasma membrane. This process is followed by the internalization of *Leishmania* parasite inside host cell either by "zipper like interactions or by "coiling phagocytosis" and creation of phagosome. The phagosomes fuse with endocytic organelle and form a vacuole structure known as PV (Walker et al., 2014). It contains β-glucuronidase, cathepsins, and hydrolases enzymes. Motile promastigote form of *Leishmania* transforms into nonmotile amastigote within 2 days in the PV. The numerous small PVs of *L. donovani* contain only one to few amastigotes in each. In place of LPG, amastigote synthesizes related compound PPG, acid phosphatase, and glycoinositolphospholipids that further establish disease in host. The environment of PV is acidic, and the acidic pH is maintained by an H^+-ATPase of the host cell origin and by a P-type H^+-ATPase of parasite cell membrane also. Even though *Leishmania* infection does not lead to full-fledged diseases, the outcome depends upon a complex network of interrelated host—parasite mechanisms. Once amastigote survived in macrophages, how the host responds against it is described in the following section.

13.3 Immune responses shown by host during infection

The initial human immune response to parasite infection is felicitated by innate immunity of host that plays a major role in local inflammatory response and regulation to stop the propagation of *Leishmania* parasite. Rapid dissemination of *Leishmania* amastigote is characteristic of infection in susceptible host and depends on the dose/content of infection and species of the parasite. In C57BL/6 mice it was shown that local natural killer (NK) cells rapidly produced interferon gamma (IFN-γ) after activation by parasite antigens and led to IL-12. Macrophage activation by T-cell-derived cytokines is required to destabilize the cellular infection of *Leishmania* (inside PV) and progression of disease. Inside the infected macrophage, killing of *Leishmania* amastigote or inhibition of parasite growth is mediated by production of nitric oxide (NO) from inducible nitric oxide synthase (iNOS). Transcription of iNOS is induced and enhanced by IFN-γ. It is a key cytokine in the control of *Leishmania* with the help of other synergic cytokines such as tumor necrosis factor (TNF) or IL-2. Such activation of macrophage resulted from a network of up- or downregulating chemokine signals which modulated immune cell activation, proliferation, and expansion (Kima & Soong, 2013).

Host also shows an adaptive immune response for antileishmanial effect and this protection is acquired via presentation of appropriate *Leishmania* antigens by antigen-presenting cells with MHC-II presentation. It triggers induction and expansion of Th1 lymphocytes and the activation of macrophages. Both in vivo and in vitro studies showed a significant difference in antigen presentation capacity of macrophages infected with promastigotes or amastigotes, the latter being inhibitorier to parasite antigen presentation including a protein LACK (*Leishmania* homolog of receptors for activated C kinase). A specific interaction between MHC-II molecule and parasites in the PV including internalization of MHC-II molecules by amastigote has been reported. There is a decrease in Cd80 expression on macrophages in susceptible mice after infection resulting in decreased protective T-cell response. Most studies suggest a critical role of initial cytokine scenes and corresponding Th-cell, B-cell, and antibody subset development. Induction of Th1 response is protective while Th2 response facilities *Leishmania* infection (Rodriguez-Pinto, Saravia, & McMahon-Pratt, 2014). Antigen-presenting cells (macrophages and DCs) phagocytose *Leishmania* lead to various response of helper T cell and different functional outcomes (Fig. 13.1). Infected DCs produce IL-12, which is critical for the induction of CD4 + Th1 cells and release of IFN-γ. IFN-γ acts on infected macrophages leading to their classical activation pathway that upregulates iNOS for the production of NO and other free radicals that are important for intracellular killing of parasite like *Leishmania*. In contrast, the production of IL-4 by other types of cell (keratinocytes) supports development of CD4 + Th2 response. Th2 cells release IL-4, IL-5, IL-6, IL-10, and IL-13 which leads to upregulation of arginase activity (alternative activation of macrophage) and the production of polyamines that favor proliferation of *Leishmania* (intracellular) parasite. On induction of TGF-β and IL-6, Th17 subsets of helper T cell release IL-17, IL-21, IL-22 which is associated with protection of VL. In addition, naturally occurring regulatory T cells (Treg) and infected macrophages also produce some immunoregulatory cytokines (IL-10, TGF-β), which further deactivate infected cells leading to the killing of *Leishmania* parasite.

The responsiveness of IL-12 in the early phase of infection promotes Th1-type development. Various studies revealed role of TGF-β for suppressing IFN-γ and subsequent development of Th2 response including IL-12 unresponsiveness. IL-12 expression is influenced by *Leishmania* parasites in a stage dependent and species independent. Peripheral blood mononuclear cells (PBMCs) from VL patients did not secret IL-12 after stimulated with leishmanial antigens in vitro. Amastigotes also inhibited secretion of IL-12 along with CD40 cross-linking. IL-12 is essential for protective immunity through IFN-γ production, NK cell activity, and IL-4 suppression. The role of antigen-induced production of IL-10 is elicited due to its antagonistic effects on IFN-γ. Some immunosuppressive proteins like papLe22 from *L. infantum* were found to produce IL-1 and exacerbate the disease (Szabo, Dighe, Gubler, & Murphy, 1997).

The production of superoxide (O^{2-}) and NO is the two major antileishmanial effector molecules/determinants. Parasite-infected macrophages have a decreased capacity to produce oxygen radicals and several proteins like LPG, gp63, and tryparedoxin peroxidase have been shown to inhibit production of O^{2-}. Parasite destruction in macrophages is carried out by NO most efficiently, after being activated by T-cell-derived cytokines. The data suggested that *Leishmania* inhibits nitric oxide synthase 2 (NOS2) activity in the early stages of infection, while in later stages it increased NOS2 production and became susceptible to Th1 cell—induced apoptotic death limiting the number of host cells. Prevention of parasite replication above a certain threshold and thereby preventing the disease progression is an active process and performed by Th-cell-mediated activation of NOS2. The role of T lymphocyte, cytokines, B cell, and immunoglobulin is discussed below (Horta, Mendes, & Roma, 2012).

13.3.1 Role of T lymphocytes

Immunity is predominantly mediated by T lymphocytes in human and experimental VL. Initial studies on mice using T-cell-depleted mice and nude BALB/c mice have shown the prominent role of T lymphocytes in *Leishmania* infection. Adoptive transfer and activation of T cells in presence of *Leishmania* antigen conferred resistance against this infection. Reconstitution experiments using nude BALB/c mice showed the necessity of CD4 + and CD8 + T cells both in the protection against infection of *L. donovani*. There was a time course-related participation of different T-cell populations to control *Leishmania* infection. When (CD4 +) cells and (CD8 +) cells progress during the infection it could interfere with parasite replication (Bogdan, 2012).

13.3.2 Role of cytokines

T lymphocytes participate in the immune response to *Leishmania* infection by producing different cytokines (Samant, Sahu, Pandey, & Khare, 2021). BALB/c mice infected with *L. donovani* have shown no production of IFN-γ/IL-2 and formation of granuloma while neither nude BALB/c mice neither shown granuloma formation or IFN-γ production. Furthermore, anti-IFN-γ antibody abolished granuloma formation, confirming the importance of this cytokine in the protection of host from *Leishmania* infection. Moreover, depletion experiments using anti-IL-2 monoclonal antibodies and reconstitution using recombinant IL-2 had shown a role of IL-2 in leishmanicidal activity apparently through the induction of IFN-γ. IL-12 is also linked to show protection against the *Leishmania* infection (Goto & Lindoso, 2004). *L. donovani*-infected BALB/c mice when treated with IL-12, a significantly reduction of the parasite burden was observed with the participation of

CD4 + , CD8 + T cells, NK cells, IFN-γ, IL-2, and TNF-α. But a distinct antileishmanial effect of IL-12 (independent of IFN-γ) was also shown in gene-disrupted mice. These mice also showed an induced capacity to reduce the parasite burden with the participation of TNF-α (Murray, 1997). Furthermore, increased levels of TGF-β were observed in IL-12-/- mice and were further increased in IL-12/IFN-γ double knockout mice, without expansion of the Th2 response (Wilson, Jeronimo, & Pearson, 2005).

The role of IL-4 cytokine is related to susceptibility of disease. IL-4 production was detected in the intermediary phase coinciding with the peak of parasite burden in the susceptible mouse strain and no production of IL-4 was observed in the resistant mouse strain (Saha et al., 2006). Furthermore, mice treated with anti-IL-4 monoclonal antibodies and mice with IL-4 gene disruption (Satoskar, Bluethmann, & Alexander, 1995) did not show better control of *Leishmania* infection. IL-10 (another Th2 cytokin) was related to progression of disease and was shown to have a role in susceptibility in experimental VL (Karp et al., 1993). IL-10 receptor blockade increased serum IFN-γ initially attributed to the nonsuppressed leishmanicidal effect of IFN-γ. However, suppression of parasite growth with IL-10 receptor blockade even in gene-disrupted mice suggested a broader effect of IL-10 on the IFN-γ suppression of multiple leishmanicidal mechanisms (Murray et al., 2002). IL-10 was shown to be important for the persistence of the parasite in the lesion, preventing its complete clearance from the lesion despite the presence of a protective immune response (Belkaid, Piccirillo, Mendez, Shevach, & Sacks, 2002). Furthermore, persistence of the parasite was shown to be of the utmost importance for the maintenance of protective immunity against reinfection, with CD4 + CD25 + Treg cells with IL-10-dependent and IL-10-independent mechanisms probably involving transforming growth factor TGF-β being involved in the suppression of IFN-γ production (Belkaid et al., 2002). IL-10 is secreted by the DCs, macrophages, and T lymphocytes chiefly, whereas IL-4 is mainly produced by lymphocytes but not by the macrophages.

13.3.3   Role of B cells and immunoglobulin

Active VL cases are characterized by the detection of elevated level of specific as well as nonspecific antibodies (humoral immune response). Primarily titers of IgG rise piercingly during VL condition, but these antibodies are not apparently protective. The enormous increase in the serum antibodies levels (hypergammaglobulinemia) in active VL is due to the polyclonal activation of immunoglobulin-producing cells. It leads to biosynthesis of IgG in higher extent and IgM to lesser extent (Klimpel & Baron, 1996). Most of the antibodies produced during *Leishmania* infection are not parasite specific, but the hypergammaglobulinemia is found during infection which have strong diagnostic value because at this stage gamma globulin comprise 50% of the total serum proteins (Stauber, 1963). Positive skin reactions were immediately reported during active infection, but delayed type of hypersensitivity was not reported. B-cell activation (polyclonal) was reported both in experimental VL and human but the actual role of B cells or immunoglobulins in case of VL immunity have been obtained with the mode of cutaneous leishmaniasis (CL), where resistance was observed with B-cell depletion. Circulating antibody is crucial for susceptibility to the development of VL. Internalization of IgG-coated amastigote by macrophages was shown to lead to IL-10 production and resulting into enhancement of intracellular parasite growth.

13.4 Animal models used for the study of VL

Various animals were developed as model and used to study VL. Different *Leishmania* species cause clinically distinct diseases and the severity of the disease caused by any given parasite can vary markedly between individual hosts. This chapter concisely illustrates the most common animal experimental models which have been employed to study the immune response in VL.

13.4.1 Murine models

Murine models are mice and other rodents and they are well established in case of VL.

13.4.1.1 Mice

L. donovani parasites are injected underneath the skin of the mice footpad. Mice strains used in VL are BALB/c, C57BL/6, CBA/J, C3H or BIOD2 and they show clinical symptoms like human VL. T-cell-immunodeficient BALB/c strains manifest a systemic VL leading to death (Howard, Hale, & Chan-Liew, 1980). Resistance and susceptibility of VL are closely related with the development of T-cell responses of Th1 or Th2 type, respectively. Studies have shown that *L. donovani* mice model does not reproduce the features of active human VL like chronic fever, profound cachexia hepatosplenomegaly, pancytopenia and have an ineffective antileishmanial cellular response (Melby, Chandrasekar, Zhao, & Coe, 2001). In susceptible BALB/c mice, *Leishmania major* infection incites a progressive disease with visceral dissemination which is associated with the parasite-specific appearance in the draining lymph nodes of Th2-type cells. Most inbred strains of mice (e.g., CBA, C3H, or C57BL/6) readily control infection and develop a robust response coupled with the Th1-type cells appearance. CD4 + effector T cells activate and release IFN-γ (no IL-4), and are required for activation of phagocyte-dependent immunity. The capacity of *Leishmania*-specific CD4 + T cells to transfer the disease passively or resistance of disease is directly correlated with the production of Th2 or Th1 cytokines. Some *Leishmania* antigens drive Th1- or Th2-type responses in susceptible mice (Scott, 2003). Most naive T cells can mature into either subset of effector cells. Early IL-12 production by macrophage suppresses IL-4 transcription, while activating IFN-γ and persistence of endogenous IL-12 is required to sustain Th1-type responses and long-term infection control (Stobie et al., 2000). Till date, two host systems have been classified for studying *Leishmania* infection on the basis of susceptibility and resistance of the host. It is well documented that Th1 immune response is the key factor to suppress infection of *Leishmania*. Activated Th1 cells induce IFN-γ that activates the macrophages and kill the parasites of VL. C57BL/6 mice increase early Th1 immune response and prevent the further growth of the parasite causes self-healing phenotype whereas susceptible BALB/c strain raises early Th2 response and results in nonhealing lesion and exaggeration of disease (Dey, Majumder, & Majumdar, 2007). Respective resistance and susceptibility of C57BL/6 and BALB/c strains depend not on the Th1 and Th2 type of immune response of CD4 + T cells only but also on the genetic background of the host. In general, the immune responses following infection of inbred mouse strains with viscerotropic *Leishmania* species (*L. donovani* or *L. infantum*) are similar to those observed in the mouse model generated with *L. major* infection (Watanabe, Numata, Ito, Takagi, & Matsukawa, 2004).

13.4.1.2   Hamster

Mice are either resistant intrinsically or susceptible to *Leishmania* infection and offer a well-characterized genetic makeup due to inbred, recombinant, and naturally/experimentally mutated strains but Syrian golden hamster (*Mesocricetus auratus*: an overtly susceptible host) is considered as the best and excellent model for VL. Therefore hamsters are used for histopathological studies, drug efficiency studies, and vaccine studies for the mechanistic exploration of immune responses to *L. donovani* infection (Garg & Dube, 2006). On the contrary, Syrian golden hamster model (closely relate the human counterpart) shown relatedness of parasite burden in visceral organ, progressive cachexia, hepatosplenomegaly, hypergammaglobulinemia, pancytopenia, and ultimately death just like human. Unfortunately, studies in hamster model are limited by the lack of immunological reagents (e.g., antibodies, cell markers, cytokines) of defined specificity (Kumar, 2013). Syrian golden hamster is easily visceralizing *Leishmania* species (*L. donovani*, *L. infantum*) and highly susceptible to infection with VL. *L. donovani* amastigotes and hamster macrophages invasion was studied and supported by occurrence of lysosome-phagosome fusion. To understand the immune response to *L. donovani* infection in this hamster model, there was a pronounced expression of the Th1 cytokine mRNAs (IFN-γ, IL-2) was detected as early as 1 week postinfection. IL-12 transcript expression was detected at low levels starting 7 days postinfection with parallel expression of IFN-γ.

Surprisingly, the IL-4 basal expression was detected in uninfected hamsters (Loría-Cervera & Andrade-Narváez, 2014). Additionally, TNF-α mRNA was increased within 1 week of infection but its levels did not increase further during the first month of infection. Expression of IL-10 (a potent macrophage deactivator) in spleen tissue increased over the first 4 weeks after infection of *L. donovani* in hamster, suggesting that this cytokine could contribute to progression of VL in hamsters and due to similarity, hamster offers important insights into human disease VL. Uncontrolled parasite replication in the bone marrow, liver, and spleen occurred during progressive disease in the hamster model of VL, despite the high activation of the strong Th1-like cytokine response (Melby, Tryon, Chandrasekar, & Freeman, 1998). In the latter stage dysfunction and inability of the infected antigen-presenting cells (to stimulate specific T cells) was observed. Later on, the lack of NO production was shown due to a defect in the transcriptional activation of NOS2. Luciferase reporter assays demonstrated that the NOS2 promoter of hamster is just like the NOS2 promoter of human and they reduced basal and IFN-γ/Lipopolysaccharide (LPS)-induced activity. Certainly, the hamster model is very useful model for VL it is widely used for the generation of therapeutic and vaccine against VL (Melby et al., 2001; Pandey, Kumar, et al., 2020; Pandey, Pande, & Samant, 2020).

13.4.2 Mammalian models

They are valuable VL models for *Leishmania* research because they are similar to humans in anatomy, immunology, and physiology. However, they are expensive animals, difficult to obtain, handle, and associated with strong ethical issues.

13.4.2.1 Dog

Experimental data for VL in bulk is generated in murine models but very less work on human leishmaniasis with dog model was done. Knowledge on the mechanisms involved in the immune response to *Leishmania* in dogs is still limited in comparison to mouse and hamster. This is mainly due to the lack of standardized immunological reagents and commercial products for the characterization of canine immunology and chemokines. DNA sequences of some dog cytokines have become available in data banks of dog genome (Loría-Cervera & Andrade-Narváez, 2014). Clinical resistance (natural and experimental) against *L. infantum* infection in dogs has long been reported. Clinically, three categories of VL infected asymptomatic dogs has been identified (1) those progressing towards explicit disease (prepatent cases), (2) those are asymptomatic for prolonged periods (even for life), and (3) those curing spontaneously. Dogs of the last two groups (2 and 3) are usually regarded as resistant and first group animals are prone to clinical disease and known as susceptible. Cross-sectional studies in endemic areas have shown that the ratio of above mentioned three categories of dogs is approximately 1:1:1 (Laurenti, Rossi, & da Matta, 2013). Immunologically, this broad category was confirmed by serological analysis of a large population of asymptomatic dogs living in an endemic area of Portugal. Dog genetics appears to have some influence in determining resistance to clinical VL. An attempt was taken by Pinelli et al. (1994) to characterize the cellular immune response in symptomatic dogs compared with asymptomatic dogs with leishmaniasis. Naturally infected dogs with *Leishmania* have shown different degrees of lymphoproliferative response and production of some cytokines. Lymphocytes from resistant dogs responded more vigorously to *Leishmania* antigen and shown higher levels of cytokines IL-2 and TNF-γ. Analysis of infected dog PBMC subsets has revealed that such immune cell restoration was associated with a significant increase in CD4 + T-cell percentage (Semião-Santos et al., 1996).

13.4.2.2 Nonhuman primates

Availability of a nonhuman primate (monkey, chimpanzee) model of VL would facilitate the study of different aspects of this disease. Monkeys are generally considered as final experimental animals to be used in studies of the safety and efficacy of drug/vaccine development. It would accelerate the development of vaccines and testing of new drug candidates against VL because nonhuman primate show VL symptom and disease as like human disease (Loría-Cervera & Andrade-Narváez, 2014). The Asian rhesus macaques (*Macaca mulatta*) are quite susceptible to *Leishmania* infection and also displayed *Leishmania* antibodies and parasite-specific T-cell-mediated immune responses both in vivo and in vitro, and can be protected from the disease VL by vaccination effectively. In the biopsy of *M. mulatta*, distinct histopathological patterns were observed, but healing lesions contained more organized epithelioid granulomas and activated macrophages during *Leishmania* infection. Interestingly immunological effectiveness in macaques had shown the presence of antigen-specific IFN-γ or TNF-α-producing CD4 + and CD8 + cells likely human (Grimaldi, 2008). The progression and resolution of skin lesions caused by *Leishmania* species observed to be very similar to humans. Additionally, macaques develop varying levels of resistance against homologous *Leishmania* reinfection as it happens in humans. New world primates, such as marmosets (*Callithrix jacchus*), owl monkeys (*Aotus trivirgatus*), and squirrel monkeys (*Saimiri sciureus*) have been believed potential hosts for the study of VL. Owl monkeys develop VL which is characterized by anemia, hepatosplenomegaly, and weight loss. Its high susceptibility to *L. donovani* infection further suggested that it could be a useful model for VL study. Squirrel monkey develops VL when infected with *L. donovani* but are able to recover from disease and became resistant to reinfection (Amaral et al., 2001). A little is known about immune response to *Leishmania* infection in monkeys but they are frequently used as models of *Leishmania* candidate vaccines for preclinical testing. Successful vaccination has been accomplished against VL by intradermal inoculation of autoclaved alum-precipitated *L. major* with Bacillus Calmette−Guérin (BCG) and autoclaved *L. donovani* with BCG in Indian langurs. Vaccinated langurs showed a delayed protection and significant lymphoproliferative response with high levels of IFN-γ and IL-2. Research attempts were made to reproduce the spectrum of human VL due to *L. donovani* in Vervet monkeys (*Chlorocebus pygerythrus*). Both symptomatic and asymptomatic/cryptic infections were observed in VL generated Vervet monkeys. The development of a nonhuman primate model for VL largely mimics the human situation (Mutiso et al., 2013). It described the different aspects of the disease that would not be possible in humans for ethical reasons. However, the use of primates in biomedical research is very limited for ethical reasons.

13.5 Immunosuppression in experimental visceral leishmaniasis

One of the immunopathological main outcomes of active VL in humans is T-cell responses suppression due to antigens of *Leishmania*. Although the *L. donovani*-infected mouse is not a good model for VL to study the immune suppression because negative *Leishmania* antigen−induced delayed-type hypersensitivity. It can be observed coinciding with the peak of parasite burden in the susceptible mouse strain (Mukhopadhyay, Bhattacharyya, & Majhi, 2000). However, the better VL model to study this aspect is a hamster. *L. donovani* and *L. chagasi* infected hamster develop progressive VL. Immunosuppression in hamsters infected with *L. chagasi* was observed and a concanavalin A−induced lymphoproliferative response in all experimental VL was observed along with absence of a *Leishmania* antigen−induced response. *Leishmania* antigen−induced response was found to be suppressed in previous studies (Fazzani et al., 2011; Mukhopadhyay et al., 2000). Antigen-specific T cell present during active VL recovers after treatment and cure. Various factors have been reported to cause immunosuppression in experimental models of VL (mouse and hamster). *Leishmania* parasite growth increased due to macrophage mediated suppression and it is related to defective antigen presentation (suppression of class I/class II MHC molecule). Adherent splenic cells have been shown to be important in *L. donovani*-infected hamsters, due to defective antigen presentation and the suppression of lymphoproliferation. TGF-β produced by adherent antigen-presenting cells was implicated in immunosuppression. In vitro data suggested the suppressor factor of macrophages leading to the decreased production of NO in *Leishmania*-infected macrophages (Rodrigues, Cordeiro-da-Silva, Laforge, Silvestre, & Estaquier, 2016). Using the RT-PCR primers for some cytokines change in the expression of different cytokine RNA was studied in VL-induced hamsters but more sensitive methods are needed.

T cells, TGF-β, possibly IL-10 and CD4 + CD25 + regulatory cells likely to participate in immunosuppression all through VL. Another aspect addressed in a number of studies of immunosuppression is decreased expression of costimulatory molecules B7-1 and Th1-specific M150 protein in antigen-presenting cells (Nakamura, Kitani, & Strober, 2001). However, apparent blockade of B7-1 or B7-2 molecules observed with the led to restoration of T-cell response and increased IFN-γ and IL-4 production in *L. chagasi* and *L. donovani*-infected mice respectively. TGF-β is one of the most important factors in susceptibility and immunosuppression leading to development of Th2 response through inhibition of T-bet in leishmaniasis. Apoptosis of T cells have been reported in experimental VL. More than 40% of CD4 + T cells undergo apoptosis, accompanied by a secretion (from susceptible but not from resistant mice) and in immunosuppression there is a significant decrease in IL-2 and IFN-γ during *L. donovani* infection (Fazzani et al., 2011; Mukhopadhyay et al., 2000; Rodrigues et al., 2016). During *L. donovani* infection, apoptosis was also detected in inflammatory cells of the spleen and liver. Since apoptosis of host lymphocytes of mice may have a role in immunosuppression leading to *Leishmania* growth, this question could be addressed in the hamster model also. A direct time-related correlation was not seen so far with the *Leishmania* antigen−induced suppression of the lymphoproliferative response. Apoptosis was present in the initial phase of the *Leishmania* infection and the suppression of the lymphoproliferative response throughout the experimental VL period (Potestio, D'Agostino, & Romano, 2004). This further indicated that the absence of a *Leishmania* antigen−specific lymphoproliferative response throughout the study period but the presence of apoptosis only in the initial phase of animal model. Survival of *Leishmania* depends on the proliferation and integrity of macrophages. In vivo studies suggested that apoptosis was induced in macrophages in the initial phase of infection in hamsters with VL (infected with *L. chagasi*) (Goto & Lindoso, 2004). However, as the infection progresses, apoptosis of macrophages disappears from both the liver and spleen, suggesting the protection of macrophages by *Leishmania* infection (Potestio et al., 2004). A clear-cut role of apoptosis in immunosuppression should be explored because that information is still indirect and incomplete.

13.6   Conclusions

Existing records in the field of immunoprophylaxis suggest that some of the vaccines developed for CL are now being explored in clinical trials. Major efforts to develop vaccines have been made against CL in comparison to VL. Though effects up to some extent have been made for the development of VL vaccines (Pandey, Kumar, et al., 2020; Pandey, Pande, et al., 2020) no promising results are reported. The immunological responses induced during experimental VL are markedly different from those induced in CL. A number of things are needed to understand how different species of *Leishmania* (determine different forms of leishmaniasis CL, mucocutaneous leishmaniasis, and VL) can generate such different immunological responses. Detailed analysis among the differences is very important in view of the fact that the ultimate goal in the fight against any forms of leishmaniasis, is the development of a vaccine that is effective in leishmaniasis caused by different species of *Leishmania*. Extensive studies are needed to identify parasite or host-related issues leading to these differences. In this context, studies of immunosuppression mechanism can contribute to a better understanding of this undesirable consequence of *Leishmania* infection. It indicated a type of immune response that should be avoided when induced by a candidate vaccine, that is, activation of Th1 cells and avoiding responses leading to IL-10 and TGF-β production.

The specific problem in VL is profound impairment of Th1 cell function. CD4 + T-cell populations were found to be a crucial factor either in progression of VL through IL-4 or in prevention through IFN-γ. IFN-γ is critical in the activation of macrophages to kill *Leishmania*. The successful protection from infection requires induction of cytotoxic T lymphocyte responses as well as Th-cell (IFN-γ, IL-12 secretion, and subsequent NO-mediated killing of parasite by infected macrophage) and humoral (antibody) type of responses. Macrophages are the proposed primary host cells for *Leishmania* but the role of these cells has not been well characterized. The fate of infected macrophages in pre-T-cell phase is not well known. Since T cells come later during infection, it is possible that *L. donovani* was adopted in the host in terms of signaling or antigen presentation for its own benefit and induced factors that provide an environment of disease progression and trigger T cells for Th2 differentiation. At the same time parasites starts modulating the macrophages and may induce IL-4 (disease inducing factors from T cells) for parasite survival in susceptible host. It is also known that *Leishmania* parasitized macrophages produce IL-10 but prior to IL-4 in susceptibility of the host and in disease progression. This suggests the crucial role of IL-10 in disease initiation and progression in combination with IL-4. From the study, it is obvious that parasites modulate the macrophages in terms of their antigen-presenting capacity and signaling capability. CD40 ligand (expressed by activated T cells) signaling pathway is skewed by the parasite towards the proparasitic pathway in macrophages. Interaction between CD40 ligand on activated T cells and CD40 on these macrophages may not be able to revert the signaling towards the antiparasitic pathway and thus, such macrophage—T cell interaction may not be host protective due to an imbalance in kinase or phosphatase activities.

The main scientific issues in the design of a VL vaccine are the same to any other infectious disease vaccines. It includes specificity and the induction of long-term immunological memory. As is the case for many other vaccines for achieving these goals, there is still much left unknown. However, there is progress in our understanding of the molecular nature of potential vaccine candidates but it is not indepth or clear-cut. To design a successful vaccine, the mechanisms that determine disease-preventing immune responses should be clear. However, our ability to control these responses in a reliable way is still at an early stage. Despite these caveats, there is a feeling of renewed optimism for VL vaccine in the scientific community.

Acknowledgment

The author is thankful to the National Institute of Technology Raipur, India for providing the facility, space, and an opportunity for this work.

References

Amaral, V. F., Teva, A., Porrozzi, R., Silva, A. J., Pereira, M. S., Oliveira-Neto, M. P., et al. (2001). Leishmania (Leishmania) major-infected rhesus macaques (Macaca mulatta) develop varying levels of resistance against homologous re-infections. *Memórias do Instituto Oswaldo Cruz, 96*(6), 795−804.

Belkaid, Y., Piccirillo, C. A., Mendez, S., Shevach, E. M., & Sacks, D. L. (2002). $CD4^+CD25^+$ regulatory T cells control Leishmania major persistence and immunity. *Nature, 420*, 502−507.

Bogdan, C. (2012). Natural killer cells in experimental and human leishmaniasis. *Frontiers in Cellular and Infection Microbiology, 2*, 69.

Deak, E., Jayakumar, A., Cho, K. W., et al. (2010). Murine visceral leishmaniasis: IgM and polyclonal B-cell activation lead to disease exacerbation. *European Journal of Immunology, 40*(5), 1355−1368.

Dey, R., Majumder, N., Majumdar, S., et al. (2007). Induction of host protective Th1 immune response by chemokines in Leishmania donovani-infected BALB/c mice. *Scandinavian Journal of Immunology, 66*(6), 671−683.

Fazzani, C., Guedes, P. A., Senna, A., Souza, E. B., Goto, H., & Lindoso, J. A. L. (2011). Dynamics of immunosuppression in hamsters with experimental visceral leishmaniasis. *Brazilian Journal of Medical and Biological Research, 44*(7), 666−670.

Garg, R., & Dube, A. (2006). Animal models for vaccine studies for visceral leishmaniasis. *Indian Journal of Medical Research, 123*, 439−454.

Goto, H., & Lindoso, J. A. L. (2004). Immunity and immunosuppression in experimental visceral leishmaniasis. *Brazilian Journal of Medical and Biological Research, 37*(4), 615−623.

Grimaldi, G., Jr. (2008). The utility of rhesus monkey (Macaca mulatta) and other non-human primate models for preclinical testing of Leishmania candidate vaccines. *Memórias do Instituto Oswaldo Cruz, 103*(7), 629−644.

Gurung, P., & Kanneganti, T. D. (2015). Innate immunity against Leishmania infections. *Cell Microbiology, 17*(9), 1286−1294.

Herwaldt, B. L. (1999). Leishmaniasis. *Lancet, 354*(9185), 1191−1199.

Horta, M. F., Mendes, B. P., Roma, E. H., et al. (2012). Reactive oxygen species and nitric oxide in cutaneous leishmaniasis. *Journal of Parasitology Research, 2012*, Article ID 203818.

Howard, J. G., Hale, C., & Chan-Liew, W. L. (1980). Immunological regulation of experimental cutaneous leishmaniasis. 1. Immunogenetic aspects of susceptibility to Leishmania tropica in mice. *Parasite Immunology, 2,* 303–314.

Karp, C. L., El-Safi, S. H., Wynn, T. A., Satti, M. M., Kordofani, A. M., Hashim, F. A., et al. (1993). In vivo cytokine profiles in patients with kala-azar. Marked elevation of both interleukin-10 and interferon-gamma. *Journal of Clinical Investigation, 91,* 1644–1648.

Kima, P. E., & Soong, L. (2013). Interferon gamma in leishmaniasis. *Frontiers in Immunology, 4,* 156.

Klimpel, G. R., & Baron, S. (1996). *Immune defenses. Medical Microbiology* (4th ed.). Texas, USA: University of Texas Medical Branch at Galveston.

Kumar, A. (2013). *Leishmania and leishmaniasis.* Springer USA. Available from http://doi.org/ 10.1007/978-1-4614-8869-9.

Kumar, A., Pandey, S. C., & Samant, M. (2018). Slow pace of antileishmanial drug development. *Parasitology Open, 4*(4), 1–11.

Laurenti, M. D., Rossi, C. N., da Matta, V. L., et al. (2013). Asymptomatic dogs are highly competent to transmit Leishmania (Leishmania) infantum chagasi to the natural vector. *Veterinary Parasitology, 196*(3-4), 296–300.

Liu, D., & Uzonna, J. E. (2012). The early interaction of Leishmania with macrophages and dendritic cells and its influence on the host immune response. *Frontiers in Cellular and Infection Microbiology, 2,* 83.

Loría-Cervera, E. N., & Andrade-Narváez, F. J. (2014). Animal models for the study of leishmaniasis immunology. *Revista do Instituto de Medicina Tropical de São Paulo, 56*(1), 1–11.

McDowell, M. A., Marovich, M., Lira, R., Braun, M., & Sacks, D. (2002). Leishmania priming of human dendritic cells for CD40 ligand-induced interleukin-12p70 secretion is strain and species dependent. *Infection and Immunity, 70*(8), 3994–4001.

Melby, P. C., Chandrasekar, B., Zhao, W., & Coe, J. E. (2001). The hamster as a model of human visceral leishmaniasis: progressive disease and impaired generation of nitric oxide in the face of a prominent Th1-like cytokine response. *Journal of Immunology, 166,* 1912–1920.

Melby, P. C., Tryon, V. V., Chandrasekar, B., & Freeman, G. L. (1998). Cloning of Syrian hamster (Mesocricetus auratus) cytokine cDNAs and analysis of cytokine mRNA expression in experimental visceral leishmaniasis. *Infection and Immunology, 66*(5), 2135–2142.

Mogensen, T. H. (2009). Pathogen recognition and inflammatory signaling in innate immune defenses. *Clinical Microbiology Reviews, 22*(2), 240–273.

Mukhopadhyay, S., Bhattacharyya, S., Majhi, R., et al. (2000). Use of an attenuated leishmanial parasite as an immunoprophylactic and immunotherapeutic agent against murine visceral leishmaniasis. *Clinical and Diagnostic Laboratory Immunology, 7*(2), 233–240.

Murray, H. W. (1997). Endogenous interleukin-12 regulates acquired resistance in experimental visceral leishmaniasis. *Journal of Infectious Diseases, 175*(6), 1477–1479.

Murray, H. W., Lu, C. M., Mauze, S., Freeman, S., Moreira, A. L., Kaplan, G., et al. (2002). Interleukin-10 (IL-10) in experimental visceral leishmaniasis and IL-10 receptor blockade as immunotherapy. *Infection and Immunity, 70,* 6284–6293.

Mutiso, J. M., Macharia, J. C., Kiio, M. N., Ichagichu, J. M., Rikoi, H., & Gicheru, M. M. (2013). Development of Leishmania vaccines: predicting the future from past and present experience. *Journal of Biomedical Research, 27*(2), 85–102.

Nakamura, K., Kitani, A., & Strober, W. (2001). Cell contact-dependent immunosuppression by CD4(+)CD25(+) regulatory T cells is mediated by cell surface-bound transforming growth factor beta. *Journal of Experimental Medicine, 194*(5), 629–644.

Pandey, S. C., Kumar, A., & Samant, M. (2020). Genetically modified live attenuated vaccine: a potential strategy to combat visceral leishmaniasis. *Parasite Immunology*, *42*(9), e12732.

Pandey, S. C., Pande, V., & Samant, M. (2020). DDX3 DEAD-box RNA helicase (Hel67) gene disruption impairs infectivity of *Leishmania donovani* and induces protective immunity against visceral leishmaniasis. *Scientific Reports*, *10*(1), 1−10.

Pinelli, E., Killick-Kendrick, R., Wagenaar, J., Bernadina, W., del Real, G., & Ruitenberg, J. (1994). Cellular and humoral immune responses in dogs experimentally and naturally infected with *Leishmania infantum*. *Infection and Immunity*, *62*, 229−235.

Potestio, M., D'Agostino, P., Romano, G. C., et al. (2004). CD4 + CCR5 + and CD4 + CCR3 + lymphocyte subset and monocyte apoptosis in patients with acute visceral leishmaniasis. *Immunology*, *13*(2), 260−268.

Rodrigues, V., Cordeiro-da-Silva, A., Laforge, M., Silvestre, R., & Estaquier, J. (2016). Regulation of immunity during visceral Leishmania infection. *Parasites & Vectors*, *9*, 118.

Rodriguez-Pinto, D., Saravia, N. G., & McMahon-Pratt, D. (2014). CD4 T cell activation by B cells in human Leishmania (Viannia) infection. *BMC Infectious Diseases*, *14*, 108.

Saha, S., Mondal, S., Banerjee, A., Ghose, J., Bhowmick, S., & Ali, N. (2006). Immune responses in kala-azar. *Indian Journal of Medical Research*, *123*, 245−266.

Samant, M., Sahu, U., Pandey, S. C., & Khare, P. (2021). Role of Cytokines in Experimental and Human Visceral Leishmaniasis. *Front Cell Infect Microbiol*, *11*, 624009. Available from http://doi.org/10.3389/fcimb.2021.624009.33680991.

Satoskar, A., Bluethmann, H., & Alexander, J. (1995). Disruption of the murine interleukin-4 gene inhibits disease progression during *Leishmania mexicana* infection but does not increase control of *Leishmania donovani* infection. *Infection and Immunity*, *63*(12), 4894−4899.

Scott, P. (2003). Development and regulation of cell-mediated immunity in experimental leishmaniasis. *Journal of Immunology Research*, *27*, 489−498.

Semião-Santos, S. J., Abranches, P., Silva-Pereira, M. C. D., Santos-Gomes, G. M., Fernandes, J. P., & Vetter, J. C. M. (1996). Reliability of serological methods for detection of leishmaniasis in portuguese domestic and wild reservoirs. *Memórias do Instituto Oswaldo Cruz*, *91*(6), 747−750.

Späth, G. F., Epstein, L., Leader, B., et al. (2000). Lipophosphoglycan is a virulence factor distinct from related glycoconjugates in the protozoan parasite Leishmania major. *Proceedings of the National Academy of Sciences of the United States of America*, *97*(16), 9258−9263.

Stauber, L. A. (1963). Immunity to leishmania. *Annals of the New York Academy of Sciences*, *113*, 409−417.

Stobie, L., Gurunathan, S., Prussin, C., Sacks, D. L., Glaichenhaus, N., Wu, C. Y., & Seder, R. A. (2000). The role of antigen and IL-12 in sustaining Th1 memory cells in vivo: IL-12 is required to maintain memory/effector Th1 cells sufficient to mediate protection to an infectious parasite challenge. *Proceedings of the National Academy of Sciences of the United States of America*, *97*, 8427−8432.

Szabo, S. J., Dighe, A. S., Gubler, U., & Murphy, K. M. (1997). Regulation of the interleukin (IL)-12R beta 2 subunit expression in developing T helper 1 (Th1) and Th2 cells. *Journal of Experimental Medicine*, *185*(5), 817−824.

Torres-Guerrero, E., Quintanilla-Cedillo, M. R., Ruiz-Esmenjaud, J., & Arenas, R. (2017). Leishmaniasis: a review. *F1000Research*, *6*, 750.

Walker, D. M., Oghumu, S., Gupta, G., McGwire, B. S., Drew, M. E., & Satoskar, A. R. (2014). Mechanisms of cellular invasion by intracellular parasites. *Cellular and Molecular Life Sciences*, *71*(7), 1245−1263.

Watanabe, H., Numata, K., Ito, T., Takagi, K., & Matsukawa, A. (2004). Innate immune response in Th1- and Th2-dominant mouse strains. *Shock, 22*(5), 460–466.

Wilson, M. E., Jeronimo, S. M., & Pearson, R. D. (2005). Immunopathogenesis of infection with the visceralizing Leishmania species. *Microbial Pathogenesis, 38*, 147–160.

Zijlstra, E. E., Musa, A. M., Khalil, E. A., el-Hassan, I. M., & el-Hassan, A. M. (2003). Post-kala-azar dermal leishmaniasis. *The Lancet Infectious Disease, 3*(2), 87–98.

Index

Note: Page numbers followed by "*f*" and "*t*" refer to figures and tables, respectively.